MULTIPLE RISK FACTORS IN CARDIOVASCULAR DISEASE

VASCULAR AND ORGAN PROTECTION

Medical Science Symposia Series

Volume 8

The titles published in this series are listed at the end of this volume.

Multiple Risk Factors in Cardiovascular Disease

Vascular and Organ Protection

Edited by

A. M. Gotto, Jr.
Baylor College of Medicine, The Methodist Hospital,
Houston, U.S.A.

C. Lenfant
National Heart, Lung, and Blood Institute, NIH,
Bethesda, Maryland, U.S.A.

A. L. Catapano
Institute of Pharmacological Sciences, University of Milan,
Milan, Italy

and

R. Paoletti
Institute of Pharmacological Sciences, University of Milan,
Milan, Italy

SPRINGER-SCIENCE+BUSINESS, MEDIA, B.V.

Library of Congress Cataloging-in-Publication Data

Multiple risk factors in cardiovascular disease : vascular and organ
  protection / edited by A.M. Gotto, Jr. ... [et al.].
      p.   cm. -- (Medical science symposia series ; v. 8)
    Based on the 3rd International Symposium on Multiple Risk Factors
  in Cardiovascular Disease held in Florence, Italy, July 6-9, 1994.
    Includes index.
    ISBN 978-94-010-4022-8   ISBN 978-94-011-0039-7 (eBook)
    DOI 10.1007/978-94-011-0039-7
    1. Cardiovascular system--Diseases--Risk factors--Congresses.
  I. Gotto, Antonio M. II. International Symposium on Multiple Risk
  Factors in Cardiovascular Disease (3rd : 1994 : Florence, Italy)
  III. Series.
    [DNLM: 1. Cardiovascular Diseases--epidemiology--congresses.
  2. Risk Factors--congresses. 3. Cardiovascular Diseases--prevention
  & control--congresses.   W1 ME46RD v.8 1995 / WG 100 M962 1995]
  RC669.M84   1995
  616.1'071--dc20
  DNLM/DLC
  for Library of Congress   95-2833

ISBN 978-94-010-4022-8

Printed on acid-free paper

CONTENTS

VI. DIABETIC DYSLIPIDEMIA AND ATHEROSCLEROSIS: CURRENT CLINICAL FINDINGS AND TREATMENT STRATEGIES

VII. HYPERTENSION

PREFACE

This book includes the most significant contributions of the 3rd International Symposium on MULTIPLE RISK FACTORS IN CARDIOVASCULAR DISEASE held in Florence, Italy, July 6-9, 1994. The meeting focused on the risk factors for cardiovascular disease and their interactions. The need for this symposium is based on the epidemiological evidence that individuals from industrialized countries often possess two or more risk factors which synergistically increase the global risk profile. This has become more evident in recent years with the increase in life expectancy of the general population. The evidence that in high risk patients, a combination of risk factors often is detected, is highlighted in these *Proceedings*. Many recent epidemiological data identifying the intrinsic and environmental factors contributing to the development of atherosclerosis are discussed. These results, in parallel with basic and clinical research, underline how atherosclerosis is a complex and multifactorial process involving the influences of lipids, including lipoprotein subfractions, blood pressure, rheologic forces, carbohydrate tolerance, and thrombogenic factors. Furthermore, the risk associated with any one of these risk factors varies widely depending on level of the associated atherogenic risk factors.

It is emphasized that, at the present time, the knowledge of the role of lipids in atherosclerosis still greatly exceeds that of any other factor involved. Thus, it is not surprising that most data on regression of atherosclerotic lesions in humans come from studies on the efficacy of lipid lowering therapy. Hypercholesterolemia and hypertriglyceridemia are more common than would be expected by chance among hypertensive patients. Hypertension also is more prevalent in those with abnormal lipid levels than in those with normal lipid levels. The association of many of these risk factors (upper body obesity, glucose intolerance, hyperlipemia, and high blood pressure) has been defined as the plurimetabolic syndrome or syndrome X, and is discussed in depth in this volume.

It is essential to consider a reduction in all risk factors involved in the development of atherosclerosis as the real end-point in any treatment. Special care should be used in selecting the pharmacological or nonpharmacological therapy without affecting adversely the cardiovascular profile. Hence, preventive management as well as risk estimation in individuals should be multifactorial with the goal of improving the cardiovascular risk profile, thus retarding or preventing the onset of heart or vascular disease. This is accomplished ultimately by causing existing lesions to regress, become stabile, or progress more slowly, and also by preventing the formation of new lesions.

The symposium concluded with strategies which include: population screening, so as to shift the whole distribution of risk factors closer to more favorable levels; health education to enable people to take care of their health; and preventive medicine for higher risk coronary candidates. These strategies should be useful not only to specialists but to practicing physicians.

The Editors

LIPID RISK FACTORS AND THE REGRESSION OF ATHEROSCLEROSIS

Antonio M. Gotto, Jr.
Department of Medicine
Baylor College of Medicine
The Methodist Hospital
6550 Fannin, M.S. SM-1423
Houston, Texas 77030
USA

Introduction

Although autopsy studies and experiments in animal models have long suggested that atherosclerosis may be reversible, convincing evidence in humans remained absent because sufficient means of altering the lipid profile or documenting changes in coronary vessels were not available. Over the past decade, however, advances in antilipidemic therapy and vascular imaging have made possible the accurate assessment of the impact of therapy on coronary arteries. Angiographically monitored trials have indeed shown a small but significant anatomic benefit of therapy over a broad range of interventions. Less lesion progression and more lesion regression have consistently been observed in the experimental groups versus controls. Unexpectedly, a large clinical benefit of therapy has also been observed in several of these trials, despite relatively short periods of interventions. The results of regression studies and possible mechanisms for the observed clinical benefit are summarized below.

Results of Regression Studies

The Familial Atherosclerosis Treatment Study [1] (FATS) did not enroll patients according to classic lipid parameters; entry criteria included an apolipoprotein B-100 level greater than 125 mg/dL, documented CAD, and a positive family history of CAD. Participants were all men 62 years of age or younger (mean age, 47). There were two intervention groups: in addition to dietary counseling, one group received 4 g/d of nicotinic acid and 30 g/d of the bile-acid resin colestipol and the other 40 mg/d of the HMG-CoA reductase inhibitor lovastatin and 30 g/d of colestipol. The conventional-therapy group received dietary therapy and placebo or, if low-density lipoprotein (LDL) cholesterol remained above the 90th percentile for age, colestipol. Nicotinic acid plus colestipol produced a 32% reduction

1

A.M. Gotto et al. (eds.), Multiple Risk Factors in Cardiovascular Disease, 1-5.

in LDL cholesterol and 43% increase in high-density lipoprotein (HDL) cholesterol, whereas lovastatin plus colestipol produced a 46% reduction in LDL cholesterol and a 15% increase in HDL cholesterol. Triglyceride levels were significantly decreased in the nicotinic acid–colestipol group.

Angiograms were obtained at baseline and at 30 months. Average change in percent stenosis of coronary artery segments was -0.9 with niacin–colestipol therapy and -0.7 with lovastatin–colestipol therapy, versus +2.1 in the conventional-therapy group. Definite regression, defined as a change in stenosis of 10 or more percentage points in one or more lesions, was more frequent with combination-therapy: 32% of those taking lovastatin and colestipol and 39% of those taking nicotinic acid and colestipol showed definite regression versus 11% of the conventional-therapy group. These statistically significant but nonetheless modest effects of therapy were accompanied by a marked reduction in coronary events (defined as cardiac death, myocardial infarction, or revascularization): 2 events in the nicotinic acid-plus-colestipol group and 3 in the lovastatin-plus-colestipol group were recorded, versus 10 in the conventional-therapy group.

The St. Thomas' Atherosclerosis Regression Study [2] (STARS) also assessed the impact of two distinct interventions: dietary therapy alone or with cholestyramine, both compared with controls who received usual care. STARS enrolled 90 men less than 66 years of age with coronary atherosclerosis and mild-to-moderate hypercholesterolemia; the mean interval between angiograms was 39 months. Dietary therapy restricted total fat intake to 27% of total calories, saturated fat to 8–10% of total calories, and dietary cholesterol to 100 mg/1000 calories. Omega-6 and omega-3 polyunsaturated fatty acids constituted 8% of calories and intake of plant-derived soluble fiber was the equivalent of 3.6 g/1000 calories. The second intervention group was prescribed the same diet as well as 8 g of cholestyramine twice a day. Dietary therapy resulted in a 16% decrease in LDL cholesterol and a 20% decrease in triglyceride. In the diet–cholestyramine group, LDL cholesterol fell 36% and triglyceride did not change. HDL cholesterol levels did not change significantly in either intervention group. There were essentially no changes in lipid levels in control patients.

The mean absolute width of coronary segments decreased 0.201 mm in controls, indicating progression, and increased 0.003 mm in the diet group and 0.103 mm in the diet-plus-cholestyramine group. Overall progression was seen in 11 of 28 usual-care patients versus 4 of 27 diet-only patients and 3 of 26 patients receiving both interventions. Both trends were significant. As in FATS, significant decreases in cardiovascular events accompanied these anatomic benefits: 10 events (defined as cardiac death, myocardial infarction, coronary surgery, angioplasty, or stroke) occurred in the usual-care group, compared with 3 in the diet-only group and 1 in the diet-plus-cholestyramine group.

The Program on the Surgical Control of the Hyperlipidemias [3] (POSCH) evaluated the benefits of partial ileal bypass in a randomized trial in 838 survivors (mean age, 51) of myocardial infarction, 90% of whom were men. All patients were instructed on the American Heart Association Step II Diet and 421 were randomized to the intervention group. Surgery entailed bypass of the distal one third of the ileum, to interrupt the enterohepatic circulation and increase the fecal loss of cholesterol-rich bile acids. At 5 years, LDL cholesterol was reduced by 38%, and HDL cholesterol and triglyceride were significantly increased by 4% and 20%, respectively.

POSCH differed from other regression studies in that overall mortality was the primary endpoint. While there was a 22% reduction in overall mortality in the intervention group at a mean follow-up of 9.7 years, the trend did not achieve significance. However, the combined endpoint of confirmed myocardial infarction and CAD death was a statistically significant 35% less frequent in the surgery group. Additionally, in the subgroup of the intervention cohort with an ejection fraction ≥ 50%, there was a significant decrease in overall mortality that was not observed in the subgroup with an ejection fraction < 50%.

In terms of the number of angiograms obtained and period of intervention, POSCH provides the most comprehensive angiographic data available. Angiograms were obtained at 3-, 5-, 7-, and 10-years and a global coronary score was used to describe the severity of atherosclerosis. Global change scores were consistently lower in the surgery group, indicating a slower rate of progression. Importantly, a graded correlation between global change score at 3 years and event rates over the next 7 years was observed irrespective of treatment [4]. Thus, POSCH demonstrated that angiographic endpoints are viable surrogates for clinical endpoints. A similar correlation was recently reported for the Cholesterol Lowering Atherosclerosis Study (CLAS) [5].

The Monitored Atherosclerosis Regression Study [6] (MARS) was the first trial with anatomic endpoints utilizing HMG-CoA reductase inhibitor monotherapy. Entry criteria required that patients be < 70 years of age and have angiographically demonstrable coronary disease; 91% were male and the mean age of participants was 58. In addition to dietary therapy, participants received either 80 mg/d lovastatin or placebo. LDL cholesterol, triglyceride, and apolipoprotein B levels were significantly decreased and HDL cholesterol significantly increased by lovastatin compared with placebo.

The overall patient average percent diameter stenosis increased by 1.6% in the lovastatin group versus 2.2% in the control group. This difference did not achieve statistical significance, nor did a trend for decreased coronary events in the intervention group. In subgroup analysis of lesions ≥ 50%, however, a 4.1% reduction in percent stenosis with lovastatin therapy was noted, compared with an increase of 0.9% in controls; this difference was statistically significant. A greater benefit of treatment on more severe lesions has been noted in other trials as well. In contrast, the Canadian Coronary Atherosclerosis Intervention Trial [7] (CCAIT) showed a greater impact of therapy on lesions < 50% stenosed than on those > 50% stenosed.

Studies have shown that lesions associated with rapid occlusion and acute events are most often < 50% stenosed [8]. These culprit lesions have several characteristic pathologic features, including hemorrhage into the lipid-rich core, formation of a mural thrombus, and fissuring of the fibrous cap, which is associated with vascular obstruction due to the composite mass of an expanding clot and the lipid-rich plaque. The most common fissuring site seems to be an area of high foam-cell density in a lipid-rich plaque that is exposed to strong circumferential shearing.

In each of the 15 coronary events documented in FATS, a lesion of this type was identified in the area of increased ischemia that had progressed substantially from baseline [8]. Only 5 of these events occurred in the intervention groups, suggesting that the benefit of intensive lipid-lowering therapy is attributable in part to the stabilization of culprit lesions.

Possible Mechanisms for the Observed Clinical Benefit

Several mechanisms have been proposed for this stabilizing effect. One possibility is that the lipid core of culprit lesions is depleted as a result of cholesterol-lowering, which is compatible with the concept of reverse cholesterol transport. A reduction in circulating LDL levels would presumably decrease foam-cell formation and allow HDL-mediated removal of lipid to predominate, particularly if HDL levels are increased by therapy. Because large, eccentric lipid pools are associated with increased shear stress and a thin fibrous cap, a reduction in lipid content would lessen the probability of rupture.

This possibility is supported by FATS and STARS. In FATS, changes in apolipoprotein B level and HDL cholesterol level were the strongest multivariate predictors of anatomic change [1]. In STARS, changes in mean absolute width of coronary segments correlated with changes in LDL cholesterol level and the ratio of LDL cholesterol to HDL cholesterol [2]. Interestingly, CLAS data suggest that triglyceride-rich lipoproteins may also be important risk factors for progression [9]. On multivariate analysis, non-HDL cholesterol predicted progression in the placebo group, likely reflecting the combined contributions of LDL cholesterol and very-low-density lipoprotein (VLDL) cholesterol (a marker of VLDL), which were both univariate predictors. In the drug-treated group, nonprogressors had significantly higher levels of apolipoprotein C-III in HDL than did progressors. Because apolipoprotein C-III inhibits lipoprotein lipase activity, its sequestration in HDL presumably indicates increased lipolysis and clearance of VLDL.

Cholesterol lowering may also improve endothelial function. Paradoxical vasoconstriction in response to endothelium-dependent vasodilators such as acetylcholine is associated with both hypercholesterolemia and coronary atherosclerosis, and likely contributes to vasospasm and plaque rupture. Egashira et al. [10] recently reported that the HMG-CoA reductase inhibitor pravastatin improved endothelium-dependent vasoregulation in 9 patients with hypercholesterolemia. The initial dose of 10 mg/d was increased to 20 mg/d if serum cholesterol remained $\geq$ 200 mg/dL. Mean serum cholesterol levels were reduced from 272 to 187 mg/dL. Changes in the diameter of the epicardial coronary artery and in coronary artery blood flow in response to the infusion of acetylcholine were assessed by angiography and an intracoronary Doppler catheter. The investigators demonstrated that acetylcholine-induced vasoconstriction of the epicardial artery was reduced ($P < 0.05$) and acetylcholine-induced increases in coronary blood flow were greater ($P < 0.001$) after pravastatin therapy.

Other possible mechanisms whereby cholesterol-lowering stabilizes plaques include reduced thrombotic potential, reduced cytotoxicity, and a reduced inflammatory response. For example, because minimally oxidized LDL are chemotactic for monocyte-macrophages and highly oxidized LDL are directly cytotoxic, antilipidemic therapy may slow progression by reducing the concentration of these particles. Oxidized LDL has also been reported to be chemotactic for T cells *in vitro* [11], although whether this inflammatory response is proatherogenic is unclear.

Summary

Angiographically monitored clinical trials of antilipidemic therapy have demonstrated that the progression of atherosclerosis may be slowed or even reversed. The clinical benefit observed in these trials strengthens the rationale for aggressive therapy in patients with known atherosclerotic disease. Additionally, these trials have provided further insight on the basis of clinical events and the risk factors associated with progression.

References

1. Brown G, Albers JJ, Fisher LD, et al. Regression of coronary artery disease as a result of intensive lipid-lowering therapy in men with high levels of apolipoprotein B. N Engl J Med 1990;323:1289–1298.
2. Watts GF, Lewis B, Brunt JNH, et al. Effects on coronary artery disease of lipid-lowering diet, or diet plus cholestyramine, in the St. Thomas' Atherosclerosis Regression Study (STARS). Lancet 1992;339:563–569.
3. Buchwald H, Varco RL, Matts JP, et al. Effect of partial ileal bypass surgery on mortality and morbidity from coronary heart disease in patients with hypercholesterolemia. Report of the Program on the Surgical Control of the Hyperlipidemias (POSCH). N Engl J Med 1990; 323:946–955.
4. Buchwald H, Matts JP, Fitch LL, et al. Changes in sequential coronary arteriograms and subsequent coronary events. JAMA 1992;268:1429–1433.
5. Cashin-Hemphill L, Mack W, LaBree L, et al. Coronary progression predicts future cardiac events. Circulation 1993;88:I363. Abstract.
6. Blankenhorn DH, Azen SP, Kramsch DM, et al. Coronary angiographic changes with lovastatin therapy. The Monitored Atherosclerosis Regression Study (MARS). Ann Intern Med 1993;119:969–976.
7. Waters D, Higginson L, Gladstone P, et al. Effects of monotherapy with an HMG-CoA reductase inhibitor on the progression of coronary atherosclerosis as assessed by serial quantitative arteriography. The Canadian Coronary Atherosclerosis Intervention Trial. Circulation 1994;89:959–968.
8. Brown BG, Zhao X-Q, Sacco DE, Albers JJ. Lipid lowering and plaque regression. New insights into prevention of plaque disruption and clinical events in coronary disease. Circulation 1993;87:1781–1791.
9. Blankenhorn DH, Alaupovic P, Wickham E, Chin HP, Azen SP. Prediction of angiographic change in native human coronary arteries and aortocoronary bypass grafts. Lipid and nonlipid risk factors. Circulation 1990;81:470–476.
10. Egashira K, Hirooka Y, Kai H, et al. Reduction in serum cholesterol with pravastatin improves endothelium-dependent coronary vasomotion in patients with hypercholesterolemia. Circulation 1994;89:2519–2524.
11. McMurray HF, Parthasarathy S, Steinberg D. Oxidatively modified low density lipoprotein is a chemoattractant for human T lymphocytes. J Clin Invest 1993;92:1004–1008.

MULTIPLE RISK FACTORS: WHAT IS NEXT?

Millicent Higgins and Claude Lenfant
National Heart, Lung, and Blood Institute
National Institutes of Health
Bethesda, Maryland 20892-9090
USA

Introduction

The continuing decline in cardiovascular disease (CVD) mortality, and progressive reductions in prevalence of most major risk factors in the United States, suggest that further improvements can be made. Better understanding of risk factors and their role in the etiology and pathogenesis of CVD should lead to improvements in prediction, treatment, and prevention of CVD.

Investigations of risk and protective factors indicate that genetic susceptibility interacts with behavioral and environmental factors to determine risk of CVD. Noninvasive methods to detect preclinical disease enhance ability to differentiate risk factors for atherosclerosis from precipitants of acute clinical events, and make it possible to intervene at an earlier stage in the disease process. Opportunities to improve public health include wider application of what we know about ways to prevent or reduce risk factors, so that their excess prevalence in less well-educated and less affluent members of the population is reduced.

Multiple Risk Factors

Consideration of multiple risk factors as determinants of CVD risk began with the simple approach of categorizing each risk factor as present or absent and adding up the number present. The first estimates from Framingham, published in 1961, provided mortality ratios for middle-aged men and women according to the existence of major risk factors: hypercholesterolemia, hypertension, and cigarette smoking [1]. Any one risk factor increased risk of a heart attack, and there was an increment in risk for men having two or all three risk factors; it amounted to about a three-fold increase for any two risk factors and nearly an eight-fold increase in risk if all three risk factors were present. Absolute risks of heart attacks were lower in women, but relative risks increased with increasing numbers of risk factors, and the gradients were similar or steeper than those in men.

7

A.M. Gotto et al. (eds.), Multiple Risk Factors in Cardiovascular Disease, 7-15.
© 1995 *Kluwer Academic Publishers and Fondazione Giovanni Lorenzini.*

By 1981, Hopkins and Williams [2] were able to find published references to 246 risk factors, and five years later they had accumulated another 30 to 40 potential risk factors. They characterized risk factors as: initiators of atherogenesis, promoters of the build-up of cholesterol in the artery wall, potentiators of thrombus, and precipitators of heart attack via acute ischemia or arrhythmia. The number of putative risk factors has increased since then, and the media continue to bombard and confuse the public with reports of new, rediscovered, or discounted risk factors, as well as advice on how to reduce chances of having a heart attack.

Recent publications from Framingham treat risk factors as continuous variables in multivariable analyses and show that risk is graded and rises continuously with increasing levels and numbers of risk factors [3]. The current Framingham composite risk factor profile uses total cholesterol, HDL cholesterol, systolic blood pressure, cigarette smoking, glucose intolerance, and ECG evidence of left ventricular hypertrophy, as well as sex and age to estimate the probability of developing coronary heart disease (CHD) in the next 10 years. The stroke risk factor profile also incorporates information on antihypertensive drug treatment, atrial fibrillation, and prevalent heart disease to predict incident stroke [4].

Table 1. "New" Risk and Protective Factors for CHD.

Risk Factors	Protective Factors
Lipids/Lipoproteins/Apolipoproteins	Stopping Smoking
Body Size: Weight, Fat Distribution, Low Birth Weight	Physical Activity
	Moderate Alcohol Consumption
Multiple Metabolic Risk Factor Syndrome (Syndrome X)	Antioxidants
	Flavonoids
Hemostasis/Thrombosis/Platelet Activity	Other Dietary Constituents
	Weight Control
Infectious Agents	Social Support
Inflammation	Aspirin
Preclinical Atherosclerosis	High SES
Precipitants of Acute Events	Hormone Replacement Therapy
Genes/Environment Interaction	(Women)

In discussing what is next in multiple risk factors, we present examples of recent findings and ongoing research, including some recent evidence on protective factors. Potential "new" risk factors are listed in Table 1. They include Lp(a), apolipoproteins such as apo(a), and apoE, LDL particle size and density, oxidized LDL, and postprandial lipemia. Elements of body size receiving attention are height, weight, obesity, fat distribution, especially intra-abdominal fat, changes in weight resulting in weight gain or weight loss, as well as fluctuations in weight over repeated cycles of loss and gain. Long-term adverse consequences of low birth weight and weight at one year have been postulated to include increased rates of CVD. Hemostatic factors, including measures of coagulation, fibrinolysis, platelet activity, and balance between pro-coagulant and fibrinolytic states are being investigated to assess their role in the onset and progression of atherosclerosis, as well as their contribution to precipitating acute clinical events. Recent evidence suggests that infectious agents and inflammation may increase risk of CVD, for example chronic Chlamydia Pneumonia infection was a risk factor for CHD in the Helsinki Heart Study. Elevated IgG and IgA titers were present in higher proportions in cases than controls at baseline and six months before a coronary event [5].

Clustering of Risk Factors

Dyslipidemia, hypertension, and diabetes mellitus are among the established risk factors, which are more prevalent among obese than lean people. High blood pressure and high cholesterol levels are more than twice as frequent in overweight men and women as in the rest of the US population, using BMI to define overweight [6]. Data from the CARDIA study of 18–30-year-old black and white men and women show that BMI is correlated positively with blood pressure, cholesterol, triglycerides, glucose, and uric acid and negatively with HDL cholesterol. Fasting insulin is also correlated with blood pressure, lipids and lipoproteins, and blood glucose [7]. Constellations of these risk factors have been named dyslipidemic hypertension, syndrome X, the Insulin Resistance Syndrome, and the multiple metabolic risk factor syndrome by various investigators. Its components are dyslipidemia, hypertension, obesity, glucose intolerance, and disturbances of insulin levels and utilization [8].

Fasting serum insulin levels were highest in young adults when systolic blood pressure, HDL cholesterol, and glucose were all in the least favorable quartiles of the distributions. Levels were lower in people with two or one of the three risk factors in the high range. Insulin levels declined further as the number of other risk factors in the optimum quartile increased. The pattern persisted after controlling for age, sex, race, and BMI, but the gradient was less steep [9]. The CARDIA study reexamined participants two years and five years after the initial examination, and found that individual CVD risk factors are highly correlated over these intervals ($r = .6$ and .7 for blood pressure and lipids, .9 for BMI). Risk factor clusters (SBP, total and HDL cholesterol and triglycerides) tracked over time. Clustering persisted at both high and low ends of the distribution and in people with BMIs above and below the median [10]. The composite risk factor score and BMI at the first exam predicted risk scores at subsequent exams; change in weight was also a predictor.

Familial and Genetic Factors

Although the importance of familial, constitutional, and genetic factors has been recognized for a long time, there are new opportunities to determine how nature and nurture interact, and to identify and measure genetic factors associated with increased susceptibility to CVD. Disease genes with large effects are rare, but the combination of several genes, each with a small effect, is likely to be more important in complex diseases like CVD, which are of multifactorial etiology and determined also by behavioral and environmental risk factors.

A positive family history of CHD, especially at an early age, is recognized as an independent risk factor, and major risk factors such as dyslipidemia, hypertension, diabetes mellitus, obesity, and cigarette smoking aggregate in families. The primary goal of the NHLBI-initiated Family Heart Study is to identify and evaluate genetic and nongenetic determinants of CHD, preclinical atherosclerosis, and CVD risk factors [11]. Family risk scores have been calculated for 45–69-year-old men and women (probands) participating in ongoing epidemiological studies at four sites (Minneapolis MN, Forsyth County NC, Framingham MA, and Salt Lake City UT). Scores are higher when reported events are more frequent than expected, based on family size and Framingham incidence rates by age and sex. Members of random samples of families, and of families with high rates of CHD are having extensive examinations to detect CHD and related conditions, and to measure established and putative risk factors, including genetic polymorphisms. Preliminary classification of probands by family risk scores shows higher mean levels and prevalence rates of established and newer risk factors among CHD negative probands from families with higher risk scores (Table 2). Mean levels of total cholesterol, HDL cholesterol, triglycerides, and Lp(a) were less favorable in non-CHD probands with higher family risk scores. There were no differences in mean blood pressure or BMI. However, family risk score was associated with prevalence of hypertension, when use of blood-pressure-lowering drugs was counted as evidence of hypertension. Overweight as well as hypertension, hypercholesterolemia, and cigarette smoking were more prevalent among CHD negative probands from families with CHD, even though they, themselves, were free of this condition.

Advances in molecular and population genetics, cardiovascular, and genetic epidemiology are increasing our understanding of multiple risk factors and opening up new research opportunities. Both myocardial infarction and cardiac hypertrophy have been related to a deletion polymorphism of the ACE gene [12,13]. Cambien and colleagues found an odds ratio of 3:1 for myocardial infarction among low risk homozygotes for the D allele [12].

An association between a mutation (M235T) in the angiotensinogen gene and severe familial hypertension was reported by Jeunemaitre and colleagues [14] and subsequently confirmed in a Japanese population and in women with pre-eclampsia. In the study involving US and French populations, the mutation was associated with higher levels of angiotensinogen, more frequent in hypertensives than normotensives, and there was an excess frequency of shared alleles in affected sib pairs [14]. A more recent publication reported linkage and association of the angiotensinogen-gene locus with essential hypertension in families, but neither M235T or T174M variants was associated with hypertension; however, several G-T repeat sequences flanking the angiotensinogen gene were more frequent in hypertensive patients than controls. The excess of shared alleles was greater among patients with diastolic pressures above 100 mm Hg and in female pairs than in male pairs [15].

Caution has been advised in accepting and interpreting as causal, associations based on small numbers of subjects, until they are replicated in other populations and their contribution to pathogenesis clarified [16].

Table 2. The Family Heart Study. Risk Factors In Non-CHD Probands by Family Risk Score.

Risk Factor	Family Risk Score		
	Low n=2,330	Medium n=4,596	High n=527
Means			
Cholesterol	211	213	220
HDL-C	54	54	53
Triglycerides	129	131	132
LDL-C	132	133	140
Lp(a)	78	85	92
Systolic BP	119	118	119
Diastolic BP	72	72	72
BMI	26.5	26.7	26.8
Waist/Hip Ratio	0.92	0.91	0.91
Prevalence %			
High Cholesterol	21	23	29
Hypertension	24	25	32
Cigarette Smoking	24	27	30
Overweight	34	35	37
High Waist/Hip Ratio	34	33	38

High Cholesterol = ≥ 240 mg/dl (6.21 mmol/L); Hypertension = SBP or DBP≥ 140/90 or on meds; Overweight = BMI > 27.8 for men, 27.3 for women; High WHR = ≥ for men; ≥.9 for women.

Associations between higher plasma homocysteine concentrations and occlusive vascular disease have been reported in several studies. In the Physicians Health Study, the risk of myocardial infarction was 3.4 times higher in men with elevated plasma homocysteine levels (above 15.8 umol/L) than in men with normal levels (below 14.1 umol/L) and the elevated risk persisted after controlling for age, hypertension, cholesterol, BMI, and diabetes [17]. Stampfer and, more recently, Selhub and colleagues [18] showed that high homocysteine levels were more frequent when plasma concentrations of B vitamins (folate, vitamin B_{12} and vitamin B_6) were low. Homocysteine levels increased with age, independent of vitamin status. These data suggest that, in addition to genetically determined cystathionine B-synthase deficiency, age and nutrition (specifically vitamin intake) influence homocysteine concentrations, and that genes, environment, behavior and their interaction, should be assessed as newer risk factors for CVD.

The Lewis blood group phenotype (a-b-) has been linked with increased risk of ischemic heart disease. An interaction involving the protective effect of alcohol against CHD has been suggested [19]. In Le (a-b-) men, alcohol consumption was associated with reduced incidence of CHD, possibly through an effect of alcohol on insulin resistance.

These examples illustrate some new directions which require collaboration of epidemiologists, clinicians, and molecular geneticists for advancing understanding of the complex multifactorial etiology of CVD and the interaction between genetic susceptibility and exposure to environmental insults and adverse lifestyles.

Preclinical Disease

Ability to detect preclinical atherosclerosis before disease is apparent through noninvasive techniques, such as ultrasound imaging of peripheral arteries, ultrafast computerized tomography, and measurement of the ratio of ankle to arm blood pressure, means that carotid artery wall thickness, calcification of coronary arteries, and reduced blood supply to the legs can be considered as risk factors for CHD, stroke, and peripheral arterial disease. In addition, risk factors can be related to preclinical evidence of disease and preclinical disease can also be used as an intermediate endpoint to evaluate preventive or therapeutic interventions. Risk factors for atherosclerosis can be differentiated from precipitants of clinical events [20]. Risk factors for atherosclerosis of coronary arteries and aortas have been identified in 15–34-year-old males who died of external causes: serum cholesterol, LDL cholesterol, and apolipoprotein E isoforms, as well as cigarette smoking, were related to the percent surface area involvement with lesions [21]. Other genotypic effects will be assessed, and similar investigations will be done in young women, when more autopsies accrue.

Precipitants of Clinical Events

Precipitants of heart attacks have been incriminated using innovative methods [22]. Unusual levels of physical exertion and outbursts of anger occurred shortly before the onset of myocardial infarction in recent studies. Physical activity protects against CHD in the long run, but extreme exertion may precipitate a myocardial infarction within the first hour or two [22]. Several investigators have drawn attention to circadian rhythms and the excess frequency of heart attacks in the early morning hours, especially in the first hours after waking.

Protective Factors

Vitamins, flavonoids, and antioxidants are examples of nutrients which have been linked to lower rates of coronary heart disease (Table 1) [23–25]. Physical activity, abstinence from smoking, and maintenance of a lean body weight are also beneficial. Relationships of alcohol to CVD are more complex. Moderate intake is associated with reduced incidence of CHD, but heavy consumption increased incidence of hypertension and cerebrovascular disease, especially hemorrhagic stroke [26].

Observational studies indicate that hormone replacement therapy (HRT) protects postmenopausal women [27]. Randomized controlled clinical trials are underway to provide more definitive evidence on the effect of estrogen and progestin on lipids, blood pressure, insulin, and fibrinogen in the PEPI trial and on incidence of CHD, certain cancers, and osteoporosis in the Womens' Health Initiative. Results from PEPI are due this year, but results of the HRT clinical trial component of the Womens' Health Initiative will not be available for at least 10 years. The use of low-dose aspirin was protective against heart attacks in a clinical trial of male physicians and in an observational study of female nurses [28,29].

What Is Next?

In answer to the question, what is next for multiple risk factors, we suggest that results of ongoing research and new opportunities arising from advances in molecular genetics, clinical and laboratory medicine, and new technologies, can be applied in population-based studies to improve assessment of risks for individuals, and prevention of CVD for individuals, families, and the population as a whole. Increased understanding of risk factors and their role in the etiology, pathogenesis, and course of CVD will lead to more focussed interventions for preclinical and overt disease, and contribute to further declines in morbidity and mortality.

At the same time, wider and more effective application of what we know now can reduce the burden of risk factors and disease in segments of society where they are still highly prevalent; these segments include less well-educated and less affluent people, and also patients with overt cardiovascular disease [6].

The goal is not only to reduce or postpone morbidity, disability, and mortality, but also to promote longer, healthier life spans.

References

1.   Kannel WB, Dawber TR, Kagan A, et al. Factors of risk in the development of coronary heart disease - six-year follow-up experience. Annals Int Med 1961;55: 33-50.

2.   Hopkins PN, Williams RR. A survey of 246 suggested coronary risk factors. Atherosclerosis 1981;40:1-52.

3.   Anderson KM, Wilson PWF, Odell PM, Kannel WB. An updated coronary risk profile. Circulation 1991;83:356-62.

4.   Wolf PA, D'Agostino RB, Belanger AJ, Kannel WB. Probability of stroke: A risk profile from the Framingham Study. Stroke 1991;22:312-8.

5.   Saikku P, Leinonen M, Tenkanew L, et al. Chronic Chlamydia pneumonia infection as a risk factor for coronary heart disease in the Helsinki Heart Study. Annals Int Med 1992;116:273-8.

6.   National Center for Health Statistics, Health, United States, 1992. DHHS Pub No (PHS)93-1232.

7.   Manolio TA, Savage PJ, Burke GL, et al. Association of Fasting insulin with blood pressure and lipids in young adults. The CARDIA Study. Arteriosclerosis 1990;10:

430-6.

8. Reaven GM. Role of insulin resistance in human disease. Diabetes 1988;37: 1495-507.

9. Savage PJ, Sholinsky P, Flack JM, Liu K. Tracking of CVD risk factor clusters in young adults: The CARDIA Study. Circulation 1992;86(Suppl.I):4:I-198.

10. Savage PJ, Manolio TA, Burke GL, et al. Insulin andclusters of CVD risk factors in young adults:The CARDIA Study. Circulation 1989;80(Suppl.II):4 II-205.

11. Higgins MW, Province M, Heiss G, et al. The Family Coronary Heart Disease Study: Objectives and design. In preparation.

12. Cambien F, Poirier O, Lecerf L, et al. Deletion polymorphism in the gene for angiotensin-converting enzyme is a potent risk factor for myocardial infarction. Nature 1992;359:641-4.

13. Schunkert H, Hense H-W, Holmer SR, et al. Association between a deletion polymorphism of the angiotensin-converting-enzyme gene and left ventricular hypertrophy. N Engl J Med 1994;330:1634-8.

14. Jeunemaitre X, Soubrier F, Kotelevtsev YV, et al. Molecular basis of human hypertension: Role of angiotensinogen. Cell 1992;71:169-80.

15. Caulfield M, Lavender P, Farrall M, et al. Linkage of angiotensinogen gene to essential hypertension. N Engl J Med 1994;330:1629-33.

16. Lindpaintner K. Genes, hypertension, and cardiac hypertrophy. N Engl J Med 1994;330:1678-9.

17. Stampfer MJ, Malinow MR, Willett WC, et al. A prospective study of plasma homocysteine and risk of myocardial infarction in U.S. physicians. JAMA 1992;268:877-81.

18. Selhub J, Jacques PF, Wilson PWF, Rush D, Rosenberg IH. Vitamin status and intake as primary determinants of homocysteinemia in an elderly population. JAMA 1993;270:2693-8.

19. Hein HO, Sørensen H, Suadicani Poul, Gyntelberg F. Alcohol consumption, Lewis phenotypes, and risk of ischaemic heart disease. Lancet 1993;341:392-6.

20. Heiss G., Sharrett AR, Barnes R, Chambless LE, Szklo M, Alzola C and the ARIC Investigators. Carotid atherosclerosis measured by B-made ultrasound in populations: associations with cardiovascular risk factors in the ARIC study. Am J Epidemiol 1991;134:250-6.

21. Hixson JE and the Pathobiological Determinants of Atherosclerosis in Youth (PDAY) Research Group. Arteriosclerosis and Thrombosis 1991;11:1237-44.

22. Mittleman MA, Maclure M, Tofler GH, Sherwood JB, Goldberg RJ, Muller JE for the Determinants of Myocardial Infarction Onset Study Investigators. Triggering of acute myocardial infarction by heavy physical exertion. Protection against triggering by regular exertion. N Engl J Med 1993;329:1677-83.

23. Hertog MGL, Feskens EJM, Hollmann PCH, Katan MB, Kromhout D. Dietary antioxidant flavonoids and risk of coronary heart disease: The Zutphen Elderly Study. Lancet 1993;342:1007-11.

24. Rimm EB, Stampfer MJ, Ascherio A, Giovannucci E, Colditz G, Willett W. Vitamin E consumption and the risk of coronary heart disease in men. N Engl J Med 1993;328:140-6.

25. Stampfer MJ, Hennekens CH, Manson JE, Golditz GA, Rosner B, Willett WC. Vitamin E Consumption and the risk of coronary heart disease in women. N Engl J Med 1993;328:1444-9.
26. Boffetta P, Garfinkel L. Alcohol Drinking and mortality among men enrolled in an American Cancer Society Prospective Study. Epidemiology 1990;1:342-8.
27. Stampfer MJ, Colditz GA. Estrogen replacement therapy and coronary heart disease: A quantitative assessment of the epidemiological evidence. Prev Med 1991; 20:47-63.
28. Final Report on the Aspirin Component of the Ongoing Physicians Health Study. N Engl J Med 1989;321:129-35.
29. Manson JE, Stampfer MJ, Colditz GA, et al. A prospective study of aspirin use and primary prevention of cardiovascular disease in women. JAMA 1991;266;(4):521-7.

MULTIPLE RISK FACTORS IN NORTHERN ITALY

Giorgio-Antonio Feruglio, Diego Vanuzzo, Giancarlo Cesana, Marco Ferrario, on behalf of the MONICA-Friuli and MONICA-Brianza Study Groups (*).

The World Health Organization (WHO) MONICA Project is a major international collaborative study with the objective of evaluating over ten years and in many different populations, the trends and determinants of cardiovascular disease [1]. Specifically the aim of the Project is to measure trends in mortality and morbidity from coronary heart disease and stroke and to assess the extent to which they are related to changes in known risk factors, daily living habits, and health care, in men and women aged 25-64 in defined communities [1]. In the early 1980s, 39 MONICA Collaborating Centers, using a standardized protocol [2], began the program in 27 countries, with a total study population (both sexes) of about 15 million. Risk factors in the WHO MONICA Project are monitored through three independent cross-sectional population surveys [3]. The first survey is mounted at the beginning, the second in the middle, and the third at the end of the ten-year study period. In northern Italy two MONICA Collaborating Centers have been running the Project in two geographical areas, Friuli and Brianza, since 1984. Friuli is an historical part of northeastern Italy, located along the Austrian and Slovenian borders, with a mixed economy, heavy and light industry, agriculture, trades and services; the population under surveillance is over 500,000 inhabitants. Brianza is located between Milan and the Swiss border; it is a highly industrialized and commercial area with urban characteristics, inhabited by about 450,000 people aged 25-64. In each of these areas two surveys of 1,800 subjects (200 in each five-year age and sex group) were completed, respectively in 1986 and 1989, while the third is ongoing (1994). This paper deals with the mean levels and prevalence of the principal risk factors in the two areas in 1986 and 1989; moreover it presents

---

(*)
MONICA FRIULI Study Group: GA Feruglio (principal investigator), D Vanuzzo, L Pilotto, GB Cignacco, M Rovere, M Ghersetti, F Marchesini, G Zanata, M Scarpa, Mario Spanghero, R Marini, Massimo Spanghero, M Palmieri, P Moratti, G Zilio.

MONICA BRIANZA Study Group: GC Cesana (principal investigator), M. Ferrario, F Achilli, O Agostoni, P Brambilla, C Bravi, A Busnelli, P Bertocchi, P Cannatelli, G De Vito, F Duzioni, I Ghezzi, MT Gussoni, P Mocarelli, G Monaco, L Merlino, E Pirola, R Sega, F Valagussa, A Villa, C Vimercati, R Zanettini.

A.M. Gotto et al. (eds.), Multiple Risk Factors in Cardiovascular Disease, 17-25.
© 1995 Kluwer Academic Publishers and Fondazione Giovanni Lorenzini.

other lipidic risk factors evaluated in 1989 in Friuli and the distribution of hyperlipidemias in this area according to the new classification of the European Atherosclerosis Society (EAS) [4].

Materials and Methods

The methodology of the WHO MONICA Project has been described elsewhere [1]; only a brief description of measurements and procedures used in population surveys is given here. Data on smoking were obtained through a standard questionnaire following accurate instructions; in the present analysis the prevalence of regular cigarette smokers will be illustrated. Height and body weight were measured with the subject in a standing position without shoes and heavy outer garments; body mass index (BMI) was calculated as weight divided by height squared (kg/m2). Waist and hip circumferences were measured in a standardized way, in centimeters and a decimal, rounded to the nearest 0 or 5; waist-to-hip ratio was then computed. Blood pressure was measured on the right arm, with the subject in a sitting position and after a minimum of 5 minutes of rest. Two consecutive observations of systolic blood pressure (SBP) and diastolic blood pressure (DBP) were recorded to the nearest 2 mmHg. DBP was read at the beginning of Korotkoff phase V. The mean value of two readings was used in this analysis. Participants were asked whether they had been taking antihypertensive drugs within two weeks prior to the examination. In this presentation a participant was considered hypertensive if: SBP > 159 mmHg and/or DBP > 94 mmHg, or on treatment for hypertension. A venous blood sample was drawn with the subject in a sitting position, with limited use of tourniquet. For total and HDL cholesterol determination, the recommended enzymatic method was chosen, and all the MONICA Collaborating Centers were standardized to the MONICA Quality Control Center for Lipid Measurements in Prague-Udine. In the second survey performed in 1989, a substudy on other lipids was carried out in the province of Udine, which covers about half of the Friuli area. Subjects were fasting and triglycerides were determined with the enzymatic method, while Lp(a) was assayed with radial immunodiffusion. In the substudy LDL cholesterol was calculated according to the Friedewald formula [5] when applicable and participants were classified in the three-group scheme of hyperlipidemias proposed by the European Atherosclerosis Society (EAS) [4], summarized in Table 1.

In this presentation the mean levels and the prevalence of the principal risk factors in the areas Friuli and Brianza will be compared with the MONICA Collaborating Centers with respectively the lowest and the highest level of the given variable for each survey (1st [6] and 2nd). It should be noted that the data of the second survey are only preliminary. Moreover the descriptive trends in the two northern Italian areas will be considered. All data are age-standardized according to the world standard population, thus including participants aged 35-64 years.

Table 1. Classification of hyperlipidemias according to the EAS [4].

	Total Cholesterol (mg/dl)	LDL Cholesterol (mg/dl)	Triglycerides (mg/dl)
Normolipidemia	< 200	< 135	< 200
Hypercholestrolemia			
mild	200-250	135-175	< 200
Moderate	250-300	175-215	< 200
Severe	> 300	> 215	< 200
Combined Hyperlipidemia			
Mild-Moderate	200-300	135-215	200-400
Severe*	> 300	not applicable	> 400
Hypertriglyceridemia			
Mild-Moderate	< 200	< 135	200-400
Severe	< 300	not applicable	> 400

* cases with total cholesterol > 300 mg/dl (or LDL cholesterol > 215 mg/dl) and triglycerides 200-400 mg/dl were considered in the severe form of combined hyperlipidemia

Results

The participation rate in the areas Friuli and Brianza was over 75% in both surveys (1986 and 1989). The precise number of participants aged 35-64 is reported in Table 2.

Table 2. Number of participants in the two surveys carried out in northern Italy.

	1986		1989	
	Men	Women	Men	Women
Friuli	719	724	694	704
Brianza	618	639	609	616

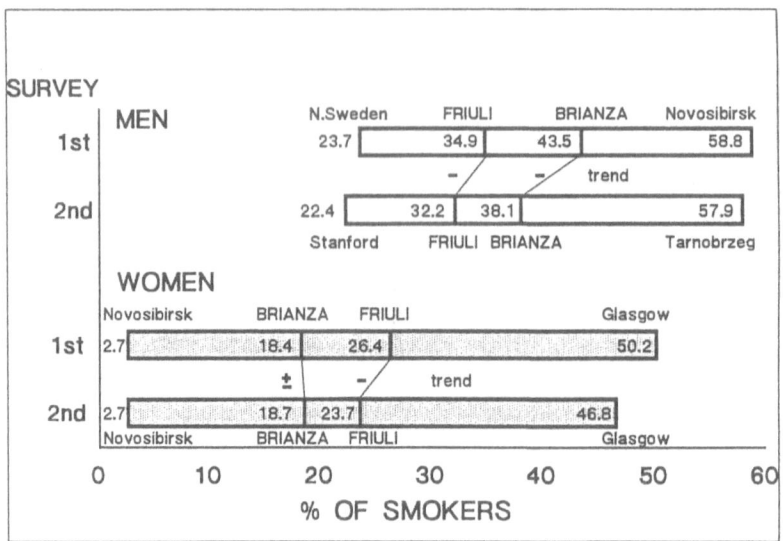

Figure 1. Age-standardized prevalence of current cigarette smokers. N.Sweden=Northern Sweden, Novosibirsk (Russia), Stanford (USA), Tarnobrzeg (Poland), Glasgow (UK).

In the province of Udine, the prevalence of men with a waist/hip ratio > 0.95 [7] is 26.4%, that of women with a waist/hip ratio > 0.85 [7], 24.2%.

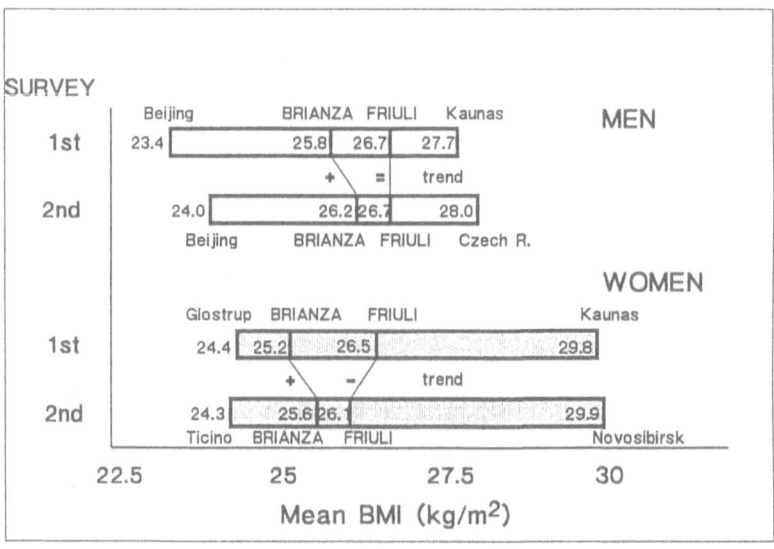

Figure 2. Age-standardized mean levels of body mass index. Beijing (China), Kaunas (Lithuania), Glostrup (DK), Ticino (CH), Novosibirsk (Russia).

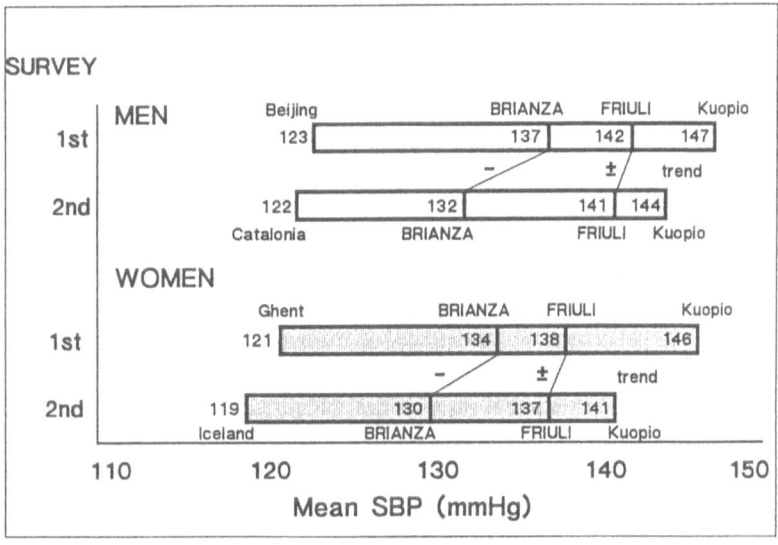

Figure 3. Age-standardized mean levels of systolic blood pressure. Beijing (China) Kuopio (Finland), Catalonia (Spain), Ghent (Belgium).

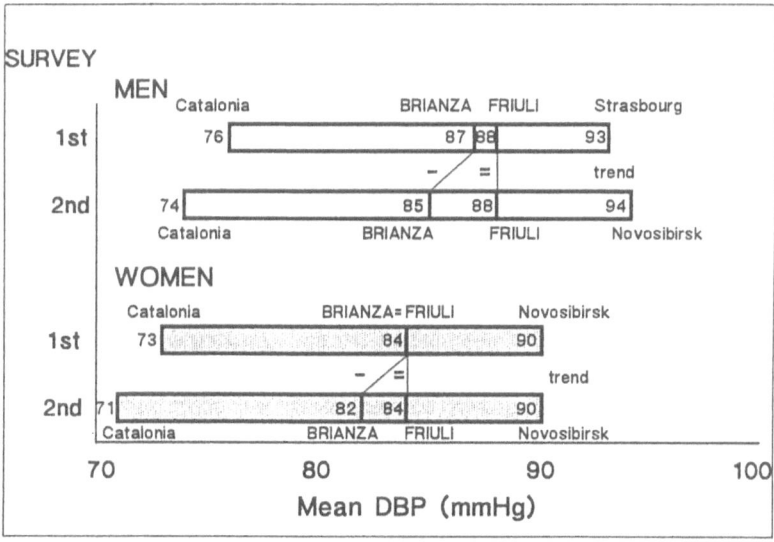

Figure 4. Age-standardized mean levels of diastolic blood pressure. Catalonia (Spain), Strasbourg (France), Novosibirsk (Russia).

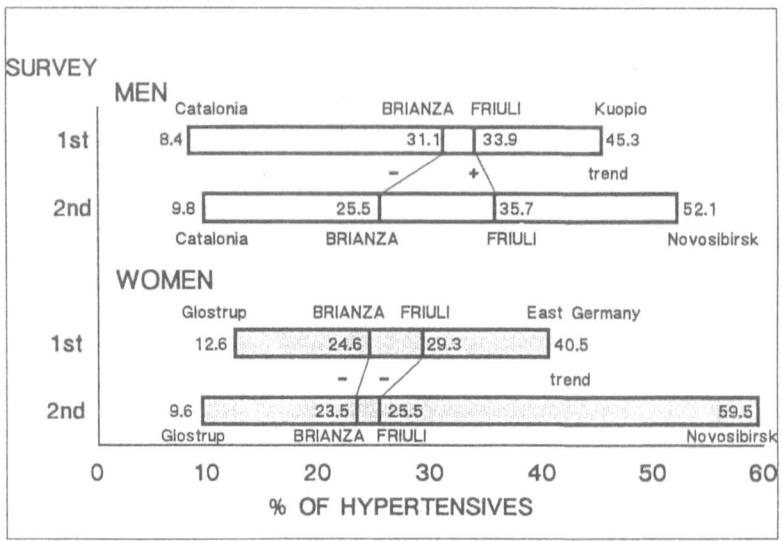

Figure 5. Age-standardized prevalence of hypertensives. Catalonia (Spain), Kuopio (Finland), Novosibirsk (Russia), Glostrup (DK).

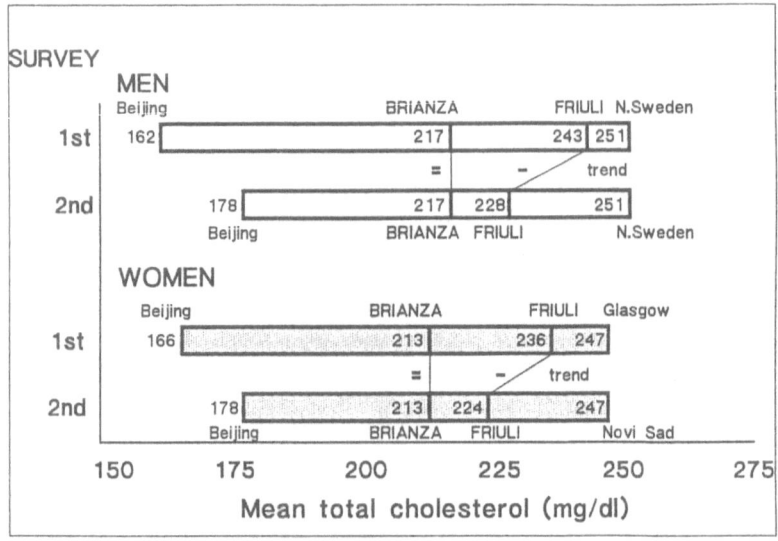

Figure 6. Age-standardized mean levels of total cholesterol. Beijing (China), N. Sweden=Northern Sweden, Glasgow (UK), Novi Sad (Yugoslavia).

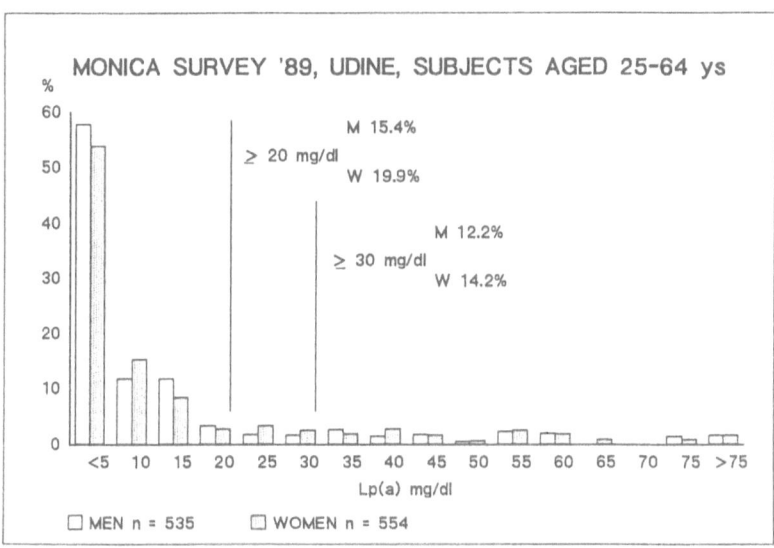

Figure 7. Distribution of Lp(a) in the province of Udine (northeastern Italy).

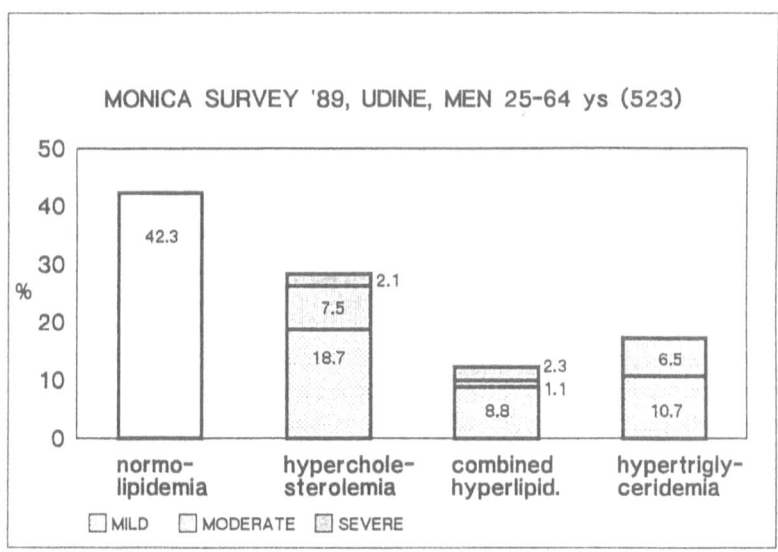

Figure 8. Prevalence of hyperlipidemias according to the EAS [4] in the province of Udine (northeastern Italy), men.

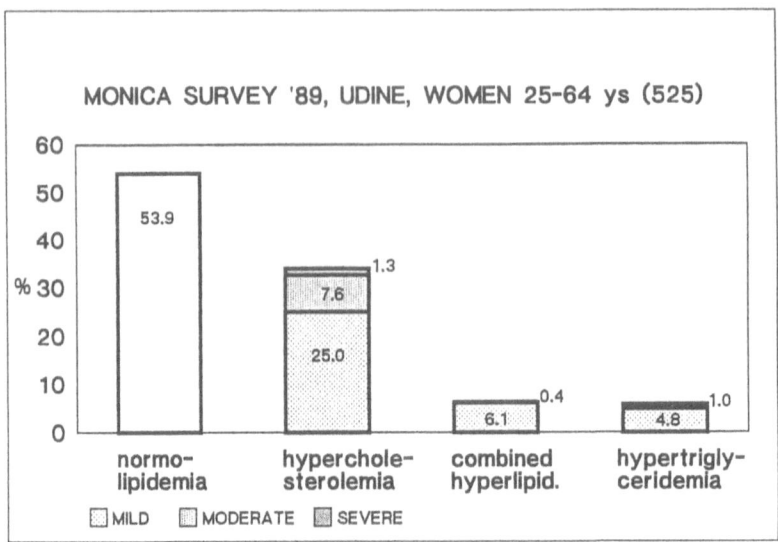

Figure 9. Prevalence of hyperlipidemias according to the EAS [4] in the province of Udine (northeastern Italy), women.

Discussion

Considering the distribution of the multiple risk factors described, the two areas of northern Italy, Friuli and Brianza, generally show a central position, even if Brianza is more often located in the middle-low part of the range and Friuli in the middle-high one. The only exception to these patterns is represented by the higher prevalence of male smokers in Brianza. As far as trends are concerned, they are slightly downward or stable in the two northern Italian areas, except for the mean levels of total cholesterol, which dropped markedly in Friuli. Analyzing other indicators of cardiovascular risk, it is noteworthy that in northeastern Italy a quarter of the people aged 25-64 have an abnormal waist-to-hip ratio [7] and that the prevalence of subjects with Lp(a) equal or greater than 30 mg/dl is, respectively, 12.2% in men and 14.2% in women. In Friuli, according to the new classification of hyperlipidemias proposed by the EAS [4], 60% of men and 45% of women are hyperlipidemic, even taking into account only one lipid measurement; moreover 10% of men and 3% of women have a severe hyperlipidemia. This overview shows that a hazardous risk factor pattern is present in northern Italy. This situation is roughly paralleled by cardiovascular mortality which is higher in northern Italy compared to the rest of the country. In the nineties a great potential for prevention is therefore evident also for Italy, traditionally considered more favorite from an ischemic-heart-disease point of view.

References

1.   WHO MONICA Project Principal Investigators. The World Health Organization MONICA Project (monitoring trends and determinants in cardiovascularv disease):

A major international collaboration. J Clin Epidemiol 1988;41:105-114.

2. WHO. Proposal for the multinational monitoring of trends and determinants in cardiovascular disease (MONICA Project). WHO/MNC/82. Geneva: WHO, 1983.

3. The WHO MONICA Project. MONICA Manual. Geneva: WHO, 1988.

4. European Atherosclerosis Society. Prevention of coronary heart disease: Scientific background and new clinical guidelines. Nutr Metab Cardiovasc Dis 1992;2:113-156.

5. Friedewald WT, Levy J, Fredrickson DS. Estimation of the concentration of low-density- lipoprotein cholesterol in plasma, without use of the preparative ultracentrifuge. Clin Chem 1972;18:499-509.

6. The WHO MONICA Project. Geographical variation in the major risk factors of coronary heart disease in men and women aged 35-64 years. Wld Health Statist Quart 1988;41:115-140.

7. Joint National Committee on Detection, Evaluation and Treatment of High Blood Pressure. The Fifth Report of the Joint National Committee on Detection, Evaluation and Treatment of High Blood Pressure. Arch Intern Med 1993;153: 154-183.

LONG-TERM ASSOCIATIONS BETWEEN HEMOSTATIC VARIABLES AND ISCHEMIC HEART DISEASE

T.W. Meade
MRC Epidemiology and Medical Care Unit
Wolfson Institute of Preventive Medicine
The Medical College of St. Bartholomew's Hospital
Charterhouse Square
London EC1M 6BQ
UNITED KINGDOM

Introduction

Recognition of a thrombotic component in ischemic heart disease (IHD) is now universal though comparatively recent [1,2] and the involvement of the coagulation system as well as of platelets is also accepted. Studies in survivors of myocardial infarction (MI) have suggested that measures of spontaneous platelet aggregation [3] and of platelet size [4] may predict recurrent IHD but it is the coagulation system that has proved more rewarding in studies of first episodes. Indeed, since thrombin is a potent platelet-aggregating agent and bearing in mind that fibrinogen is a cofactor for platelet aggregability [5], the coagulation system probably exerts a significant influence on platelet function as well as on the production of fibrin. Numerous clinical studies and a growing number of prospective population-based studies now leave little doubt that high levels of some pro-coagulant clotting factors, particularly fibrinogen and factor VII, are associated with the incidence of IHD over a period of a few years. More familiar indices of risk such as the blood pressure and blood cholesterol levels predict IHD over a matter of decades. Clotting factors tend to fluctuate more markedly than the blood cholesterol level, for example, in response to potential requirements for hemostasis with the consequence that long-term relations between clotting factor levels and IHD may be less easily demonstrable. It is now therefore useful to consider whether or not this is so. The main part of this review consists of long-term results from the Northwick Park Heart Study (NPHS) on first events of IHD but is preceded by a section on the contribution of the coagulation system to the arterial changes leading to clinically manifest IHD and is followed by a summary of studies relating measures of hemostatic function to recurrent IHD.

27

A.M. Gotto et al. (eds.), Multiple Risk Factors in Cardiovascular Disease, 27-33.
© *1995 Kluwer Academic Publishers and Fondazione Giovanni Lorenzini.*

Clotting Factors and IHD

VESSEL WALL CHANGES

Fibrinogen and fibrin are demonstrable at quite early stages of changes in the arterial wall and the contribution of the hemostatic system to the further development of the atheromatous lesion is clear. The presence of fibrin implies that the coagulation system has been activated. A number of angiographic studies have now shown an association between high fibrinogen levels and the extent of atheromatous changes in the coronary and carotid arteries. One of these studies has also shown that high factor VII activity levels may be involved [6]. Interpreting the fibrinogen results, in particular, has to take account of the possibility that high levels may be the result rather than the cause of vessel wall changes. However, the findings of one of the largest of the angiographic studies, the ECAT study in patients with angina pectoris, indicated that high fibrinogen levels were more closely associated with vascular occlusion than with mural changes [7], suggesting that raised levels are thrombogenic.

LONG-TERM ASSOCIATIONS

Three prospective studies have reported long-term findings on fibrinogen and IHD [8,9,10]. Their results are similar and will therefore be exemplified by findings from NPHS which, besides having been initiated specifically to focus on the thrombotic contribution to IHD, included a wider range of hemostatic variables than the other two studies. The main NPHS results come from 1,511 men aged between 40 and 64 years at the time of recruitment. Of these, 52 had previously experienced MI, leaving 1,459 men free of major, clinically manifest IHD at entry. By the end of 1991, they had been followed up for an average of 16.1 years and 192 of these men had developed major IHD. Of these, 92 had died of IHD and 100 had experienced nonfatal MI. The interval from entry to event was 9.5 years and 7.9 years for those experiencing fatal and nonfatal events, respectively. Fibrinogen was measured by the clot weight method, fibrinolytic activity by the dilute blood clot lysis time (results being expressed as 100/lysis time in hours), factor VII activity by an automated one-stage biological assay, and factor VIII activity by a semi-automated two-stage assay [8,11,12].
　　　　Figure 1 summarizes the findings for fibrinogen, fibrinolytic activity, and, for comparative purposes, total cholesterol. Besides the expected relation of high cholesterol levels with IHD, high entry fibrinogen levels were independently associated with IHD risk over the 16.1 year period. Low fibrinolytic activity was also independently associated with IHD incidence, particularly in the younger men though the finding for all men aged between 40 and 64 was significant as was the interaction between fibrinolytic activity and age.

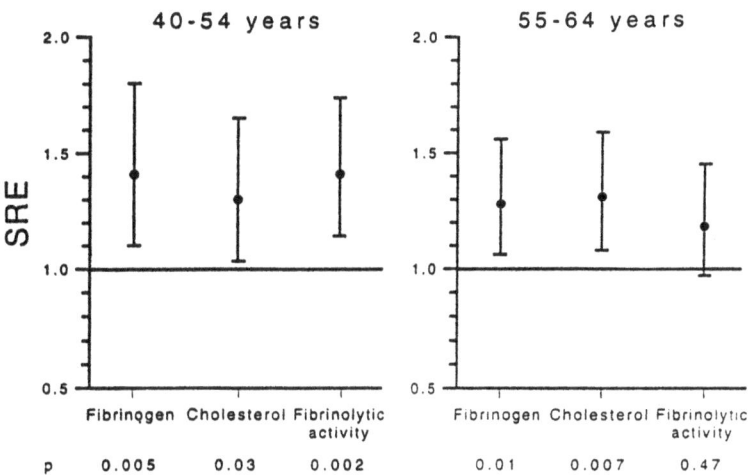

Figure 1. Standardized regression effects (SRE), 95% confidence intervals, and p values for relation of variables with IHD incidence. SRE indicates difference in risk of IHD associated with a difference of 1SD in variable, i.e. with high fibrinogen and cholesterol levels, and low fibrinolytic activity.

When NPHS began in 1972, measures of individual components of the fibrinolytic system were not available and the dilute blood clot lysis time was carried out as a "global" measure generally considered at that time to reflect activators rather than inhibitors. Further work has now demonstrated that the dilute clot lysis time is almost certainly a reflection of plasminogen activator inhibitor, PAI-1, as illustrated in Figure 2 [13].

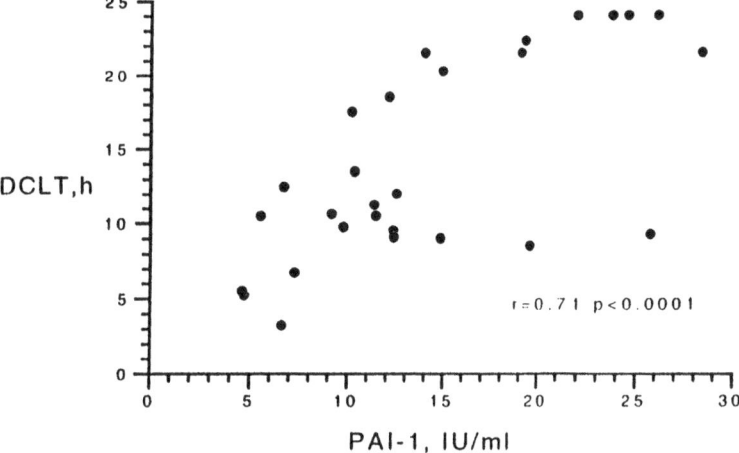

Figure 2. Dilute clot lysis time and plasminogen activator inhibitor [13].

The strong relation between VII_c and IHD previously reported in NPHS is confined to fatal events, as shown in Figure 3. This finding receives some support from the PROCAM study [14] in which the association of VII with fatal IHD was somewhat stronger than with nonfatal events. The NPHS factor VII activity assay is sensitive to the two-chain form, VII_a [15], which is many times more active than the single-chain zymogen, and more sensitive in this respect than the PROCAM factor VII assay. There is growing evidence that VII_a is the most appropriate measure for VII activity [15,16,17] and that VII_a is associated with the rate of thrombin generation [18]. One explanation for the particular association of VII_c with fatal events may lie in the degree of coagulability when tissue factor levels increase as a result of plaque fissuring or rupture. When this happens, a high VII_a level might, by leading to a high level of thrombin generation, increase the size and stability of occlusive thrombi through effects on both platelet aggregability and fibrin deposition.

NPHS has also recently shown a relation between factor VIII activity, VIII_c, and IHD again (as with VII_c) more noticeably for fatal than nonfatal events [12]. This finding is supported by several observations suggesting that patients with hemophilia experience less than the expected incidence of IHD. This apparent protection was most marked in a

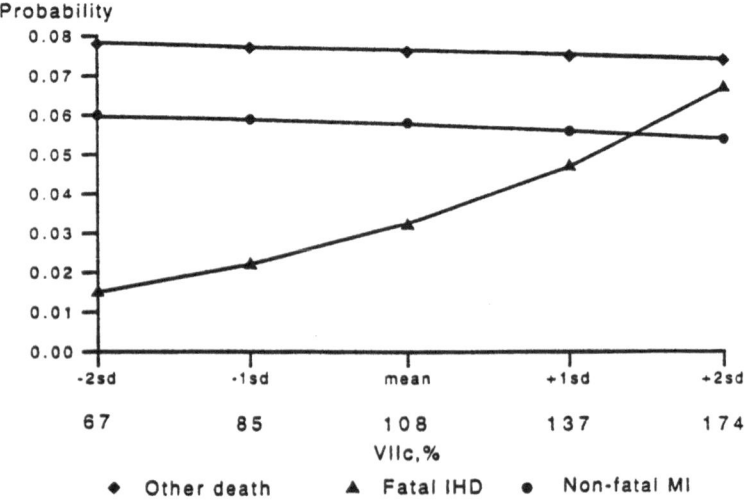

Figure 3. Estimated relationship between VIIc and probability of various outcomes during 16-year follow-up for a man aged 50.

Dutch study [19] which suggested that since these patients are probably not protected against atheroma, the involvement of factor VIII is through its effect on thrombogenic potential. In passing, it is important to allow for the strong effect of ABO blood group on factor VIII levels in assessing the relation between factor VIII itself and IHD, bearing in mind that ABO blood group is also probably associated with IHD incidence.

The NPHS findings on the coagulation system and IHD can be summarized as follows:

- Increased coagulability
  High VII_c
  High VIII_c $\}$ particularly for fatal events
  High thrombin
- Increased plasma fibrinogen
  As substrate for coagulation system : fibrin
  Other effects : viscosity, platelet aggregation, atheroma
- Decreased fibrinolytic activity
  Long lysis time = high PAI-1

RECURRENT EVENTS

Quite consistently, high fibrinogen levels are associated not only with the initial onset of clinical disease but also with recurrent MI [4,20], recurrent stroke [21,22], and with the progression of lower extremity arterial disease (LEAD) either in the form of an increased mortality from cardiovascular disease (mainly IHD and stroke) [23] or of increased incidence of graft occlusion following bypass surgery [24]. A relation of high factor VIII activity with recurrent MI has also been demonstrated [20]. The possibility that spontaneous platelet aggregation and large platelet volume may predict recurrent MI has already been referred to.

Conclusion

High levels of pro-coagulatory clotting factors and poor fibrinolytic activity are associated with the incidence of IHD in the long as well as in the short term. Because of the generally large within-person and laboratory components of variability in clotting factors compared with cholesterol, for example, the observed associations of these clotting factors with IHD probably underestimate the true strength of the relevant relationships to a somewhat greater extent than underestimation of the link between cholesterol and IHD. Clearly, both lipid and thrombogenic pathways contribute to IHD and there is nothing to be gained by emphasizing the importance of one at the expense of the other. At the same time, the role of the coagulation system in IHD is relatively unfamiliar so that considerations relevant to interpreting data on clotting factors and vascular disease should be borne in mind. There is increasing reason to believe that the associations of high fibrinogen and high factor VII activity levels with IHD are of causal significance, indicating the growing need for randomized controlled trials not only to evaluate the clinical value of the agents used but also to test the etiological hypotheses posed by the associations of clotting factors with IHD.

References

1.   DeWood MA, Spores J, Notske R, et al. Prevalence of total coronary occlusion during the early hours of transmural myocardial infarction. N Engl J Med 1980;303:897-902.

2.   Davies MJ, Thomas A. Thrombosis and acute coronary-artery lesions in sudden cardiac ischemic death. N Engl J Med 1984;310:1137-1140.

3.   Trip MD, Cats VM, van Capelle FJL, Vreeken J. Platelet hyperactivity and prognosis and survivors of myocardial infarction. N Engl J Med 1990;332: 1549-1554.

4.   Martin JF, Bath PM, Burr ML. Influence of platelet size on outcome after myocardial infarction. Lancet 1991;338:1409-1411.

5.   Meade TW, Vickers MV, Thompson SG, Seghatchian MJ. The effect of physiological levels of fibrinogen on platelet aggregation. Thromb Res 1985; 38:527-534.

6.   Broadhurst P, Kelleher C, Hughes L, Imeson JD, Raftery EB. Fibrinogen, factor VII clotting activity and coronary artery disease severity. Atherosclerosis 1990;85:169-173.

7.   ECAT Angina Pectoris Study Group. ECAT angina pectoris study: Baseline associations of Hemostatic factors with extent of coronary arteriosclerosis and other coronary risk factors in 3000 patients with angina pectoris undergoing coronary angiography. Euro Heart J 1993;14:8-17.

8.   Meade TW, Mellows S, Brozovic M, et al. Hemostatic function and ischemic heart disease; principal results of the Northwick Park Heart Study. Lancet 1986;2:533-537.

9.   Kannel WB, Wolf PA, Castelli WP, D'Agostino RB. Fibrinogen and risk of cardiovascular disease. JAMA 1987;258:1183-1186.

10.   Wilhelmsen L, Svardsudd K, Korsan-Bengtsen K, Welin L, Tibblin G. Fibrinogen as a risk factor for stroke and myocardial infarction. N Engl J Med 1984;311:501-505.

11.   Meade TW, Ruddock V, Stirling Y, Chakrabarti R, Miller GJ. Fibrinolytic activity, clotting factors, and long-term incidence of ischemic heart disease in the Northwick Park Heart Study. Lancet 1993;324:1076-1079.

12.   Meade TW, Cooper JC, Stirling Y, Howarth DJ, Ruddock V, Miller GJ. Factor VIII, ABO blood group and the incidence of ischemic heart disease. Br J Haematol 1994;88: in press.

13.   Meade TW, Howarth DJ, Cooper J, MacCallum PK, Stirling Y. Fibrinolytic activity and arterial disease. Lancet 1994;343:1442.

14.   Heinrich J, Balleisen L, Schulte H, Assmann G, van de Loo J. Fibrinogen and factor VII in the prediction of coronary risk. Results from the PROCAM study in healthy men. Arterioscler Thromb 1994;14:54-59.

15.   Miller GJ, Stirling Y, Esnouf MP, et al. Factor VII- deficient substrate plasma depleted of protein C raise the sensitivity of the factor VII bio-assay to activated

factor VII an international study. Thromb Haemost 1994;71:38-48.

16. Kario K, Skata T, Matsuo T, Miyata T. Factor VII in non-insulin-dependent diabetic patients with microalbuminuria. Lancet 1993;342:552.

17. Kario K, Matsuo T, Sakata T, Miyata T. Factor VII hyperactivity and ischemic heart disease. Lancet 1994;343:233.

18. Miller GJ. Personal communication.

19. Rosendaal FR, Varekamp I, Smit C, et al. Mortality and causes of death in Dutch haemophiliacs, 1973-86. Br J Haematol 1989;71:71-76.

20. Haines AP, Howarth D, North WRS, et al. Hemostatic variables and the outcome of myocardial infarction. Thromb Haemost 1983;50:800-803.

21. Resch KL, Ernst E, Matrai A, Paulsen HF. Fibrinogen and viscosity as risk factors for subsequent cardiovascular events in stroke survivors. Ann Intern Med 1992;177:371-375.

22. Qizilbash N, Jones L, Warlow C, Mann J. Fibrinogen and lipid concentrations as risk factors for transient ischemic attacks and minor ischemic strokes. BMJ 1991;303:605-609.

23. Banerjee AK, Pearson J, Gilliland EL, et al. A six year prospective study of fibrinogen and other risk factors associated with mortality in stable claudicants. Thromb Haemost 1992;68:261-263.

24. Wiseman S, Kenchington G, Dain R, et al. Influence of smoking and plasma factors on patency of femoropopliteal vein grafts. BMJ 1989;299:643-646.

CARDIOVASCULAR GENE THERAPY: POSSIBILITIES AND REALITIES

Victor J. Dzau, Ryuichi Morishita, and Gary H. Gibbons
Falk Cardiovascular Research Center
Division of Cardiovascular Medicine
Stanford University School of Medicine
300 Pasteur Drive
Stanford, California 94305
USA

In vivo gene transfer provides the opportunity of introducing genetic materials into the cardiovascular system, thereby altering gene expression and/or function. For several cardiovascular diseases, no effective therapy exists, for example, homozygote familial hypercholesterolemia, and restenosis after angioplasty. Gene therapy research may result in breakthrough treatment for these refractory diseases.

Gene-Transfer Techniques

For cardiovascular disease, somatic rather than germ line gene therapy holds much promise. Of the three methods of gene modification: gene replacement, gene correction, and gene augmentation (i.e. the addition of genetic material), gene augmentation is the most promising technique for modifying targeted cells in cardiovascular therapy. As the application of antisense technology *in vivo* is now feasible [1-3], blocking the expression of specific disease-causing genes *in vivo* is becoming an attractive possibility. Gene-transfer techniques appropriate for cardiovascular applications include: (1) viral-vector-mediated gene transfer, such as retrovirus, adenovirus, hemagglutinating virus of Japan (HVJ; also called Sendai virus); (2) liposomal gene transfer, such as the use of cationic liposomes (Lipofectin); and (3) reimplantation of cells modified *in vitro* (Table 1). However, *in vivo* methods currently available for cardiovascular gene transfer are limited by relatively low efficiency and potential toxicity.

Gene Transfer and Therapy for Cardiovascular Diseases

The vascular wall, heart, and liver have been target organs for cardiovascular gene therapy. The potential applications in cardiovascular therapy include the treatment of vascular disease

35

A.M. Gotto et al. (eds.), Multiple Risk Factors in Cardiovascular Disease, 35-41.

Table 1. Gene therapy for cardiovascular disease.

Indication	Target Gene
Familial hypercholesterolemia	Low density lipoprotein receptor
Atherosclerosis	High density lipoprotein
Hypercoagulable states	Tissue-plasminogen activator
Refractory diabetes mellitus	Insulin
Local Gene Therapy	
Restenosis after angioplasty	Cell-cycle regulatory gene
Transplant rejection	Leukocyte adhesion molecule
Transplant vasculopathy	Cytokine
Myocardial infarction:	
Cardiac remodeling;	Fibroblast growth factor
Angiogenesis	Transforming growth factor β
Myocarditis	Cytokine
Congenital heart disease	Myocyte differentiation factors
Thrombosis	Tissue-plasminogen activator
Glomerular diseases	Cytokine, cell-cycle regulatory gene
Aortic aneurysms	Protease

(restenosis, atherosclerosis), cardiac diseases (myocardial infarction, cardiac remodeling) and metabolic disorders (diabetes mellitus, hypercholesterolemia, hypertension).

Liver

The liver is an ideal organ for the transfection of genes whose products can be secreted into the circulation for systemic gene therapy. However, gene transfer into the liver has proven quite difficult because the cells are highly differentiated. Recent progress in gene-transfer methods using HVJ [4-7], adenovirus [8,9], retrovirus [10], and direct injection using the high-energy-microprojectile-bombardment method [11], or DNA-protein complexes [12-14] have yielded positive results. Using the HVJ method, Kaneda et al. [5] injected a human insulin gene into the rat portal vein and demonstrated transient gene expression and secretion of human insulin into the plasma.

Perhaps the most dramatic effect of liver gene transfer is in the therapy of familial hypercholesterolemia (FH), an inherited disease in humans caused by a deficiency of LDL receptors. *Ex vivo* transfer of a LDL-receptor-gene-protein complex (using poly-L-lysine) into hepatocytes reimplanted into the Watanabe heritable hyperlipidemic (WHHL) rabbit or infusion of the LDL receptor gene protein complex into its portal vein resulted in the temporary amelioration of hypercholesterolemia [12]. These results demonstrated the feasibility of somatic gene therapy for FH. Currently, a clinical trial is under way to examine the efficacy of LDL-receptor gene transfer in vivo for the treatment of homozygote FH patients. Thus, the liver is thought to be a target for gene therapy of inherited metabolic disorders affecting the cardiovascular system.

Vascular Wall

The vascular wall is an important organ for gene therapy. In 1989, Wilson et al. [15] and Nabel et al. [16] first demonstrated the feasibility of transfecting blood vessels with the reputer gene B galactosidase *in vivo*. A similar study was performed by Dichek et al. [17] using intravascular stents seeded with modified endothelial cells that had been transfected with the genes encoding β-Gal and human tPA. Direct physical transfer of genes into intact blood vessels *in vivo* has been reported using cationic liposomes (Lipofectin) as the DNA carrier [18-21]. However, the levels of expression of the transfected β-Gal and luciferase cDNAs were quite low.

We have employed HVJ-mediated gene transfer for gene delivery into the vessel wall. The HVJ method was efficient (up to 30% of the vessel wall showed SV40 T-antigen expression) without apparent toxicity and thus is suitable for *in vivo* gene transfer to blood vessels. The adenoviral gene-transfer method has also been tested and has resulted in successful gene transfer into blood vessels [22,23]. Recently, we have successfully transfected and expressed endothelial-type nitric oxide synthesis (ec-NOS) into injured rat carotid artery *in vivo*. We hypothesized that the restoration of nitric oxide production after vascular injury and endothelial denudation could result in the inhibition of VSMC proliferation and migration *in vivo*. Indeed, our data demonstrated that ec-NOS transfer inhibited neointimal lesion development suggesting that this approach may be useful for treating restenosis.

Another attractive strategy for gene therapy is the use of antisense oligonucleotides. Previously, we showed that antisense oligonucleotides against basic fibroblast growth factor (bFGF) and platelet-derived growth factor (PDGF) inhibited vascular growth *in vitro* [24,25]. Growth-factor induced cell proliferation involves the sequential activation of intracellular proteins that promote cell-cycle progression. Genes regulating cell-cycle progression are the final common pathway. We demonstrated that the combination of antisense oligonucleotides against cdc 2 kinase and proliferating cell nuclear antigen (PCNA) inhibited serum-stimulated VSMC growth [1]. Direct addition of antisense oligonucleotides against c-myb (oncogene), nonmuscle myosin heavy chains, and PCNA alone was also reported to inhibit VSMC replication [26,27].

Recently, the *in vivo* administration of antisense oligonucleotides against c-myb (at concentrations in excess of 150 μM), using pluronic gels applied to the adventitial layer, inhibited vascular smooth-muscle accumulation induced by angioplasty injury [2]. Unfortunately, this peri-adventitial polymer-delivery system is not a practical approach for the prevention of restenosis after percutaneous transluminal angioplasty in humans. The HVJ liposome method is an intraluminal molecular delivery system that has several advantages over the peri-adventitial polymer-delivery approach. Introducing oligonucleotides by the HVJ method substantially increases the efficiency of oligonucleotide uptake, and improves the stability of the oligonucleotides within intracellular compartments. Our recent data revealed that a single administration of antisense oligonucleotides against the PCNA and cdc 2 kinase genes (at a concentration of 15 μM) inhibited neointimal formation after angioplasty for at least up to four weeks after transfection [3]. Antisense to cyclin B and cdk2 kinase and other cell cycle regulatory gas has also been shown to be effective. Finally, we have recently used double standard DNA decoy to the transcriptional factor E2F that transactivates the expressions of c-myc, PCNA, cdk that mediate cell proliferation. Decoy E2F also inhibited neointimal hyperplasia in rat carotid artery in response to angioplasty injury. The use of *in vivo* transfer for therapy in humans will require the development of catheter-based drug-delivery systems that are compatible with the incubation times that are necessary for efficient gene transfer, yet are capable of maintaining tissue perfusion.We speculate that continued development of these methodologies will facilitate the use of gene transfer technology to characterize further the biological role of gene products activated in response to vascular injury, as well as providing new therapeutic agents for use in humans.

Heart

There has been little experience of *in vivo* gene transfer to the heart. Direct injection of DNA is the only way of gene transfer into the heart to date. Lin et al. [28] first reported the expression of β-Gal in cardiac myocytes *in vivo* for at least four weeks after direct injection into the left ventricle [28]. Direct injections of the alpha-myosin heavy chain gene and the reporter gene, luciferase, under the control of the alpha myosin heavy chain promoter also resulted in the regulated expression of these genes [29].

Successful gene transfer *in vivo* will pave the way for gene therapy of the heart. Healing and remodeling of the ventricle after myocardial infarction (MI) remains an important clinical problem. Some genes, for example transforming growth factor β (TGF-β) and myogenin, may enhance the healing and recovery of myocytes after injury associated with MI. The induction of neovascularization or angiogenesis is ischemic myocardium after coronary-artery occlusion *in vivo* using gene transfer may salvage myocardium at risk by enhancing the blood supply to the ischemic areas. Indeed, a single administration of bFGF to dog coronary artery reduced the infarct size after ischemia [30]. The future use of gene therapy will depend on the ability to deliver the genes by less invasive methods. For example, direct infusion into coronary arteries is a more practical and less injurious method.

Towards Clinical Applications

The first federally approved human gene-therapy protocol started on 14 September, 1990 for the treatment of patients with ADA deficiency [31-33]. Three years after the first approval, more than 18 active clinical studies of gene therapy are under investigation. In the cardiopulmonary field, two protocols (transfer of the LDL receptor to hepatocytes and the cystic fibrosis transmembrane conductance regulator to lung) have been approved. Their objectives are generally: (1) to evaluate the in vivo efficacy of gene-transfer methods; (2) to evaluate the safety of the gene-transfer method; and (3) to determine the possible therapeutic efficacy. Although there are still many unresolved issues, human gene therapy for cardiovascular disease is now a reality.

References

1.   Morishita R, Gibbons GH, Ellison KE, et al. Intimal hyperplasia after vascular injury is inhibited by antisense CDK2 oligonucleotides. J Clin Invest 1994;93:1458-1464.
2.   Simons M, Edelman ER, DeKeyser JL, Langer R, Rosenberg RD. Antisense c-myb oligonucleotides inhibit intimal arterial smooth muscle cell accumulation in vivo. Nature 1992;359:67-70.
3.   Morishita R, Gibbons GH, Ellison KE, et al. Single intraluminal delivery of antisense cdc2 kinase and proliferating-cell nuclear antigen oligonucleotides results in chronic inhibition of neointimal hyperplasia. Proc Nat Acad Sci USA 1993;90:8474-8478.
4.   Kaneda Y, Iwai K, Uchida T. Increased expression of DNA cointroduced with nuclear protein in adult rat liver. Science 1989;243:375-378.
5.   Kaneda Y, Iwai K, Uchida T. Introduction and expression of the human insulin gene in adult rat liver. J Biol Chem 1989;264:12126-12129.
6.   Kato K, Nakanishi M, Kaneda Y, Uchida T, Okada Y. Expression of hepatitis B virus surface antigen in adult rat liver. Co-introduction of DNA and nuclear protein by a simplified liposome method. J Biol Chem 1991;266:3361-3364.
7.   Kato K, Kaneda Y, Sakurai M, Nakanishi M, Okada Y. Direct injection of hepatitis B virus DNA into liver induced hepatitis in adult rats. J Biol Chem 1991;266:22071-22074.
8.   Gomez-Foix AM, Coats WS, Baque S, Alam T, Gerard RD, Newgard CB. Adenovirus-mediated transfer of the muscle glycogen phosphorylase gene into hepatocytes confers altered regulation of glycogen metabolism. J Biol Chem 1992; 267:25129-25134.
9.   Jaffe HA, Danel C, Longenecker G, et al. Adenovirus-mediated in vivo gene transfer and expression in normal rat liver. Nature Genet 1992;1:372-378.
10.   Ferry N, Duplessis O, Houssin D, Danos O, Heard JM. Retroviral-mediated gene transfer into hepatocytes in vivo. Proc Nat Acad Sci USA 1991;88:8377-8381.
11.   Williams RS, Johnston SA, Riedy M, DeVit MJ, McElligott SG, Sanford JC. Introduction of foreign genes into tissues of living mice by DNA-coated microprojectiles. Proc Nat Acad Sci USA 1991;88:2726-2730.

12. Wilson JM, Grossman M, Wu CH, Chowdhury NR, Wu GY, Chowdhury JR. Hepatocyte-directed gene transfer in vivo leads to transient improvement of hypercholesterolemia in low density lipoprotein receptor-deficient rabbits. J Biol Chem 1992;267:963-967.

13. Wilson JM, Grossman M, Cabrera JA, Wu CH, Wu GY. A novel mechanism for achieving transgene persistence in vivo after somatic gene transfer into hepatocytes. J Biol Chem 1992;267:11483-11489.

14. Wu GY, Wilson JM, Shalaby F, Grossman M, Shafritz DA, Wu CH. Receptor-mediated gene delivery in vivo. Partial correction of genetic analbuminemia in Nagase rats. J Biol Chem 1991;266:14338-14342.

15. Wilson JM, Birinyi LK, Salomon RN, Libby P, Callow AD, Mulligan RC. Implantation of vascular grafts lined with genetically modified endothelial cells. Science 1989;244:1344-1346.

16. Nabel EG, Plautz G, Boyce FM, Stanley JC, Nabel GJ. Recombinant gene expression in vivo within endothelial cells of the arterial wall. Science 1989;244:1342-1344.

17. Dichek DA, Neville RF, Zwiebel JA, Freeman SM, Leon MB, Anderson WF. Seeding of intravascular stents with genetically engineered endothelial cells. Circulation 1989;80:1347-1353.

18. Lim CS, Chapman GD, Gammon RS, et al. Direct in vivo gene transfer into the coronary and peripheral vasculatures of the intact dog. Circulation 1991;83:2007-2011.

19. Lynch CM, Clowes MM, Osborne WR, Clowes AW, Miller AD. Long-term expression of human adenosine deaminase in vascular smooth muscle cells of rats: a model for gene therapy. Proc Nat Acad Sciences USA 1992;89:1138-1142.

20. Nabel EG, Plautz G, Nabel GJ. Site-specific gene expression in vivo by direct gene transfer into the arterial wall. Science 1990;249:1285-1288.

21. Flugelman MY, Jaklitsch MT, Newman KD, Casscells W, Bratthauer GL, Dichek DA. Low level in vivo gene transfer into the arterial wall through a perforated balloon catheter. Circulation 1992;85:1110-1117.

22. Lemarchand P, Jones M, Yamada I, Crystal RG. In vivo gene transfer and expression in normal uninjured blood vessels using replication-deficient recombinant adenovirus vectors. Circ Res 1993;72:1132-1138.

23. Meidell RS, Gerard RD, Williams RS. The end of the beginning. Gene transfer into the vessel wall. Circulation 1992;85:1219.

24. Itoh H, Mukoyama M, Pratt RE, Gibbons GH, Dzau VJ. Multiple autocrine growth factors modulate vascular smooth muscle cell growth response to angiotensin II. J Clin Invest 1993;91:2268-2274.

25. Itoh H, Mukoyama M, Pratt RE, Dzau VJ. Specific blockade of basic fibroblast growth factor gene expression in endothelial cells by antisense oligonucleotide. Biochem Biophys Res Commun 1992;188:1205-1213.

26. Simons M, Rosenberg RD. Antisense nonmuscle myosin heavy chain and c-myb oligonucleotides suppress smooth muscle cell proliferation in vitro. Circ Res 1992;

70:835-843.
27. Speir E, Epstein SE. Inhibition of smooth muscle cell proliferation by an antisense oligodeoxynucleotide targeting the messenger RNA encoding proliferating cell nuclear antigen. Circulation 1992;86:538-547.
28. Lin H, Parmacek MS, Morle G, Bolling S, Leiden JM. Expression of recombinant genes in myocardium in vivo after direct injection of DNA. Circulation 1990;82: 2217-2221.
29. Kitsis RN, Buttrick PM, McNally EM, Kaplan ML, Leinwand LA. Hormonal modulation of a gene injected into rat heart in vivo. Proc Nat Acad Sci USA 1991; 88:4138-4142.
30. Yanagisawa-Miwa A, Uchida Y, Nakamura F, et al. Salvage of infarcted myocardium by angiogenic action of basic fibroblast growth factor. Science 1992; 257:1401-1403.
31. Thompson L. Gene therapy. Harkin seeks compassionate use of unproven treatments. Science 1992;258:1728.
32. Miller AD. Human gene therapy comes of age. Nature 1992;357:455-460.
33. Anderson WF. Human gene therapy. Science 1992;256:808-813.

TRIGLYCERIDES AND CORONARY HEART DISEASE: AN UPDATE

Michael H. Criqui
Department of Family and Preventive Medicine
University of California, San Diego
9500 Gilman Drive
La Jolla, California 92093-0607
USA

Introduction

Assessment of triglycerides as a risk factor for coronary heart disease (CHD) has posed some rather unique methodological problems [1]. These problems result from the close correlation of triglycerides with certain lipoproteins such as VLDL cholesterol (positive) and HDL cholesterol (inverse), its skewed distribution, its large intraindividual variation, its particle heterogeneity, its potential differential impact in various subgroups of its population, and its strong correlation with manifestations of the insulin-resistance syndrome [1]. Although some investigators believe triglycerides are not independent of total and/or HDL cholesterol as a risk factor for CHD [2], there have now been a number of studies showing an independent association for triglycerides [3-11].

A recent meta-analysis indicated a modest but statistically significant relative risk of triglycerides for cardiovascular disease in both sexes after multivariate adjustment for other risk factors including lipids and lipoproteins [12]. The relative risks per mmol of triglycerides (88.6 mg/dl) were 1.21 in men (CI 1.15-1.27) and 1.50 in women (CI 1.20-1.88).

This meta-analysis highlights that in population-based prospective studies triglycerides are a consistent predictor of cardiovascular risk, although the magnitude of the relative risks indicate that a rather substantial difference in triglyceride levels would be necessary to produce a doubling of risk; i.e. 422 mg/dl in men and 177 mg/dl in women.

The Lipid Research Clinics Follow-up Study

In the Lipid Research Clinics (LRC) follow-up study, a prospective population-based study of men and women, we evaluated the risk of triglycerides for CHD death using the natural log of triglycerides as the independent variable, to account for the skewed distribution of triglycerides [1]. The relative risks were per natural log unit of triglycerides, and thus the increment in triglycerides for a given relative risk was nonlinear and varied by the level of

A.M. Gotto et al. (eds.), Multiple Risk Factors in Cardiovascular Disease, 43-52.
© *1995 Kluwer Academic Publishers and Fondazione Giovanni Lorenzini.*

triglycerides. Nonetheless, comparison between the LRC study and the studies in the meta-analysis noted above showed good agreement.

The Effects of Triglycerides in Subgroups

In the LRC study, we also attempted to address previous reports that triglycerides were a stronger risk factor in certain subgroups; i.e. women, diabetics, and persons with low cholesterol.

WOMEN VERSUS MEN

The meta-analysis data suggested that both the univariate and multivariate relative risks were greater for women than for men [12]. The LRC data confirm the greater univariate risks for women but did not show a greater multivariate risk [1].

DIABETES

The meta-analysis did not address other subgroups. Triglycerides have been reported to be a stronger risk factor in diabetics [13-15]. The LRC study had insufficient numbers of diabetics to directly address this question. However, there were 694 men (16.8%) and 283 women (8.4%) with fasting plasma glucose (FPG) levels of 110 mg/dl or greater. There was no difference in the relative risk of triglycerides for CHD mortality in higher or lower strata of FPG.

Confounding by fasting plasma glucose. In addition to stratifying on FPG, we also considered FPG as a possible confounding variable, since higher levels of FPG, even in the nondiabetic range, have been shown to be a risk factor for CHD [16], and there was a strong positive association between FPG and triglycerides in the LRC study [17]. To our knowledge, no other population-based prospective study has considered FPG as a possible confounder when assessing the risk of triglycerides for cardiovascular disease. FPG was a strong and statistically significant predictor of CHD mortality in our population. In addition, it was a partial confounder for the triglycerides-CHD association, since after adjustment for FPG the Cox regression coefficient for the effect of triglycerides on CHD was reduced substantially in both men and women. We thus concluded that in considering the entire population, a substantial portion of the risk of triglycerides for CHD could be accounted for by elevated FPG levels.

HDL CHOLESTEROL, LDL CHOLESTEROL, AND AGE

Additional subgroup analyses involved strata of lipoprotein cholesterol levels. A study from France had reported a greater relative risk of triglycerides at lower total cholesterol levels [18]. Since total cholesterol is carried on 3 major subclasses of lipoproteins, HDL, LDL, and VLDL, which have differing associations with CHD, it was decided to look at subgroups by HDL and LDL cholesterol levels. Obviously, VLDL cholesterol strata were not considered since the VLDL cholesterol level faithfully reflects the triglyceride level. The National Cholesterol Education Program (NCEP) cutpoints for LDL (160 mg/dl) and HDL (35 mg/dl) were selected *a priori* [19].However, the cutpoint for HDL cholesterol in women had to be raised to 45 mg/dl to obtain adequate numbers for subgroup analysis. Since a previous report in men had indicated triglycerides were a risk factor for CHD at younger but not older ages [20], we also stratified on age.

The results of these subgroup analyses are shown in Table 1. For each subgroup, the number of subjects is given, along with the number and percent who died of CHD. For triglycerides, two relative risks are given. The first is adjusted for age, HDL cholesterol, LDL cholesterol, smoking, systolic blood pressure, body mass index, and postmenopausal estrogen use (in women). The second relative risk is additionally adjusted for FPG. For HDL cholesterol, only the relative risks adjusted for all the above variables including FPG are shown, since relative risks without FPG adjustment were essentially identical.

For men with HDL < 35 mg/dl, triglycerides were a highly significant risk factor for CHD death, while HDL cholesterol was unrelated. The relative risk for triglycerides was reduced somewhat after adjustment for FPG. At higher levels of HDL, triglycerides were unrelated to CHD death, while HDL became a highly significant protective factor. For LDL strata, we found a similar pattern, with triglycerides being highly predictive (and marginally significant even after adjustment for FPG) in the lower LDL strata, while HDL was unrelated to outcome. At higher levels of LDL, triglycerides were unrelated and HDL was strongly inversely related to outcome. Finally, both the triglyceride and HDL associations were present only in men aged < 70 years at baseline.

For women, findings in the HDL strata were equivocal. For LDL strata, the findings were strikingly similar to men. The age strata revealed that, like men, the association for triglycerides was limited to age < 70, but in contrast to men, the HDL association was stronger in the elderly.

These findings, taken together, suggest that a subgroup where triglycerides might be particularly useful in discriminating risk would be persons characterized by lower HDL, lower LDL, and middle-aged (as opposed to elderly). It should be pointed out that while triglycerides are a good predictor in the lower HDL strata which has a relatively high overall risk, the lower LDL and younger age strata, where it also predicts well, are at relatively low overall risk.

We are unaware of any other study which has examined such subgroups in a population-based study. However, Laakso et al. have recently reported stratified analyses in 313 patients with noninsulin dependent diabetes (NIDDM) followed 7 years for CHD events [21]. The results for HDL cholesterol and VLDL triglycerides are shown in Table 2. Cutpoints for the strata were LDL cholesterol 166 mg/dl and HDL cholesterol 43 mg/dl, and thus similar to the ones we employed in the LRC study.

Table 1. Relative risk for CHD death per natural log unit of triglycerides in strata of HDL cholesterol, LDL cholesterol, and age. The Lipid Research Clinics Follow-up Study.

	CHD Deaths N	(%)	RR TG_1	$(TG)_2$	RR HDL_2
Men					
HDL <35 mg/dl	41/893	(4.6)	1.86[++]	(1.44)	1.02
HDL ≥35 mg/dl	99/3236	(3.1)	1.05	(0.86)	0.73[+++]
LDL <160 mg/dl	56/2644	(2.1)	1.86[++]	(1.60[+])	0.98
LDL ≥160 mg/dl	84/1485	(5.7)	1.13	(0.94)	0.68[+++]
Age <70 years	121/3984	(3.0)	1.41[+]	(1.20)	0.71[+++]
Age ≥70 years	19/145	(13.1)	0.68	(0.40)	1.15
Women					
HDL <45 mg/dl	16/678	(2.4)	1.66	(1.46)	0.84
HDL ≥45 mg/dl	45/2698	(1.7)	1.30	(1.17)	0.91
LDL <160 mg/dl	24/2218	(1.1)	1.64	(1.53)	1.12
LDL ≥160 mg/dl	37/1158	(3.2)	1.08	(0.86)	0.67[+++]
Age <70 years	39/3187	(1.2)	1.85[+]	(1.61)	0.99
Age ≥70 years	22/189	(11.6)	0.38	(0.33)	0.74[+]

1 - adjusted for age, HDL, LDL, smoking, systolic blood pressure, body mass index, and replacement estrogen use (in women)

2 - adjusted for the above variables plus fasting plasma glucose

+ = p < .10
++ = p < .05
+++ = p < .01

* adapted from Criqui et al. [1]

Table 2. Unstandardized beta coefficients for the association of VLDL triglycerides and HDL cholesterol with CHD events in patients with noninsulin-dependent diabetes.

	CHD Events		Unstandardized Beta Coefficient	
	N	(%)	VLDL TG	HDL Chol
HDL ≤43 mg/dl	52/163	(31.9)	0.813[+]	-1.157
HDL >43 mg/dl	29/150	(19.3)	-0.125	-1.693
LDL ≤166 mg/dl	37/157	(23.6)	1.027[+]	-0.309
LDL >166 mg/dl	39/156	(25.0)	0.1816	-2.453[++]

+ p <.05
++ p <.01

* adapted from Laakso et al. [21]

The event rates in this group are several times higher than in the LRC study, since all subjects had NIDDM and all CHD events were counted, rather than just fatal events as in the LRC study. Nonetheless, a strikingly similar differential relationship of triglycerides and HDL to CHD across strata is seen. In the lower stratum of HDL, VLDL triglycerides were strongly and significantly related to CHD, whereas HDL cholesterol was not. In the upper HDL stratum, the association of HDL was stronger (albeit short of statistical significance), while VLDL triglycerides were unrelated to CHD. In the lower LDL stratum, VLDL triglycerides were significant and HDL was unrelated, while the reverse was true in the upper LDL stratum. The marked concordance of there results in patients with NIDDM and in the LRC population, the only two studies which have looked at the differential effects of triglycerides and HDL within HDL and LDL strata, suggests strongly that in subgroups of lower HDL or lower LDL, triglycerides may be an important independent risk indicator. Interestingly, such data also suggest that in such subgroups HDL cholesterol may not be an important risk indicator.

A recent clinical trial appears relevant to the finding that triglycerides are a good predictor at lower levels of LDL. Lovastatin therapy at 80 mg/day in patients with total cholesterol between 190 and 295 mg/dl, and triglycerides < 500 mg/dl, lowered the baseline average LDL of 156 mg/dl to an average of 86 mg/dl [22]. Lovastatin therapy produced regression in larger (≥ 50%) coronary stenoses but not in smaller lesions. On treatment, in multivariate analyses including multiple lipid and nonlipid risk factors, the predictors of progression in smaller lesions were limited to triglyceride-rich lipoproteins. Thus, these data again support the concept that triglycerides are an important risk indicator in a setting of lower levels of LDL cholesterol.

Particle Heterogeneity

It has been suggested that different kinds of triglycerides elevation may have differing prognostic significance: for example, lipoprotein phenotype IV is reported to be associated with increased CHD risk, but types I or V are not. Types I and V are rare, and in the LRC study there were only 39 subjects so characterized, and only one died of CHD [1]. A clinical trial has reported estrogen replacement therapy results in increased production of larger, triglyceride-rich VLDL, most of which was cleared directly from the circulation without conversion to small VLDL or LDL [23].

LDL particles are heterogeneous as well. Persons with increased levels of small, dense LDL particles (pattern B) are at reportedly increased risk of CHD [24]. However, the proportion of small, dense LDL particles is a direct function of the triglyceride level, and adjustment for triglyceride level eliminates much of the risk associated with pattern B, calling into question the independence of pattern B as a risk factor for CHD.

Hypercoagulability

Hypertriglyceridemia is associated with hypercoagulability. Elevated triglycerides have been associated with increased levels of fibrinogen and factor X [25], and with decreased fibrinolytic capacity due to increased levels of a rapid inhibitor of tissue-type plasminogen activator (PAI-1) [26]. In addition, gemfibrozil, which has a pronounced triglyceride lowering effect, also appears to potentiate fibrinolysis by direct diminution of synthesis of endogenous PAI-1 [27]. Thus, whether the triglycerides-CHD link reflects atherogenesis, thrombosis, or both, and the resultant therapeutic implications, are currently unclear and well deserving of further study.

Endothelial Dysfunction

Vasodilatation in human arteries in response to acetylcholine is endothelium dependent, and in hypercholesterolemia and/or hypertension vasodilatation may be reduced or vasoconstriction may occur [28]. Thus, endothelial dysfunction may be another pathway for biologic effects of risk factors, beyond atherogenesis and thrombosis. Kuhn et al. have reported an association between low HDL cholesterol and endothelial dysfunction in 20 men and 7 women undergoing angiography, and no association for total or LDL cholesterol [29]. Their results, however, were based on univariate correlation coefficients. The raw data for these 27 patients were presented in a table, and we reanalyzed the data with univariate correlations for the effects of HDL, LDL, and the natural log (ln) of triglycerides on endothelial dysfunction, and by multivariate analysis using multiple linear regression to simultaneously adjust for the potential confounding effects of age, gender, hypertension, diabetes, and cigarette smoking. As in the original manuscript, we analyzed the acetylcholine response in both smooth and diseased segments, but also separately evaluated the 20 of 27 patients who were men to look for a gender interaction. The results are shown in Table 3.

Table 3. Lipids and lipoproteins and response to acetylcholine*.

		Univariate Correlation Coefficient				Multivariate Regression Coefficients			
		Smooth Seg. r (p value)		Diseased Seg. r (p value)		Smooth Seg. b (p value)		Diseased Seg. b (p value)	
All subjects	LDL	-.02	(.92)	.05	(.86)				
N = 27	HDL	.59	(<.01)	.62	(.02)	+	(.51)	+	(.02)
(diseased=14)	lnTG	-.37	(.06)	-.40	(.16)	-	(.63)	-	(.09)
Men	LDL	.13	(.59)	.14	(.67)				
N = 20	HDL	.57	(<.01)	.55	(.08)	-	(.37)	+	(.14)
(diseased=11)	lnTG	-.44	(.05)	-.48	(.13)	-	(.23)	-	(.12)

* adapted from Kuhn et al. [29]

The univariate correlations show LDL cholesterol to be unrelated to coronary artery response, and thus LDL was not considered in multivariate analysis. In univariate correlations, HDL cholesterol was positively and significantly related to coronary artery size after acetylcholine in both smooth and diseased segments, and in all subjects as well as the subset of men. Ln triglycerides were inversely associated with coronary size in both smooth and diseased segments, and this relationship was somewhat stronger in the subset of men. In multivariate analysis, there was no association of HDL in smooth segments, but the inverse triglyceride association for smooth segments was suggestive in men. For diseased segments, both for all subjects and the subset of men, HDL and triglycerides appeared to have roughly equal and opposite relationships. Thus, both HDL and triglycerides may have independent effects of endothelial function, at least in diseased coronary artery segments, and this may be a new pathway for effects of these lipid variables on CHD.

Conclusion

The significance of triglycerides as a risk factor is difficult to assess. If the problematic nature of triglycerides is taken into account to the extent possible in study design and analysis, a somewhat more coherent picture emerges. Triglycerides appear to be an important independent risk factor in persons with lower HDL levels, lower LDL levels, and in the nonelderly. Not all triglyceride elevations are likely to be atherogenetic; smaller, denser VLDL particles may carry greater risk.

Triglyceride elevations are often associated with several other abnormalities such as low HDL cholesterol; central obesity; hyperinsulinemia and insulin resistance; glucose intolerance; hypertension; small, dense LDL; hypercoagulability; and endothelial dysfunction, a constellation which has been variously named Syndrome X [30] or the insulin resistance syndrome (IRS) [31]. In multivariate analyses, some associated variables such as lower HDL cholesterol and glucose intolerance appear to explain some but not all of the risk of triglycerides for CHD. Because of the strong correlation of these risk factors, it is tempting to look for a central underlying pathology, such as insulin resistance, or at least a critical associated variable, such as atherogenic dyslipidemia, so that intervention efforts could be focused. Such investigations are currently underway. For now, initial interventions should include diet and weight control, and exercise, which have been shown to simultaneously benefit most of the abnormalities in this syndrome. In addition, careful guidelines for managing dyslipidemia [19] and hypertension [32] have recently been updated.

References

1. Criqui MH, Heiss G, Cohn R, et al. Plasma triglyceride level and mortality from coronary heart disease. N Engl J Med 1993;328:1220-5.
2. Hulley SB, Rosenman RH, Bawol RD, Brand RJ. Epidemiology as a guide to clinical decisions: The association between triglyceride and coronary heart disease. N Engl J Med 1980;302:1383-9.
3. Pelkonen R, Nikkilä EA, Koskinen S, Penttinen K, Sarna S. Association of serum lipids and obesity with cardiovascular mortality. BMJ 1977;2:1185-7.
4. Glynn RJ, Rosner B, Silbert JE. Changes in cholesterol and triglyceride as predictors of ischemic heart disease in men. Circulation 1982;66:724-31.
5. Petersson B, Trell E, Hood B. Premature death and associated risk factors in urban middle-aged men. Am J Med 1984;77:418-26.
6. Aberg H, Lithell H, Selinus I, Hedstrand H. Serum triglycerides are a risk factor for myocardial infarction but not for agina pectoris: Results from a ten-year follow-up of Uppsala primary preventive study. Atherosclerosis 1985;54:89-97.
7. Carlson LA, Böttinger LE. Risk factors for ischaemic heart disease in men and women: results of the 19-year follow-up of the Stockholm Prospective Study. Acta Med Scand 1985;218:207-11.
8. Lapidus L, Bengtsson C, Linquist O, Sigurdsson JA, Rybo E. Triglycerides-main lipid risk factor for cardiovascualr disease in women? Acta Med Scand 1985;217:481-9.
9. Tverdal A, Foss OP, Leren P, Holme I, Lund-Larsen PG, Bjartveit K. Serum triglycerides as an independent risk factor for death from coronary heart disease in middle-aged Norwegian men. Am J Epidemiol 1989;129:458-65.
10. Welin L, Eriksson H, Larsson B, et al. Triglycerides a major coronary risk factor in elderly men: a study of men born in 1913. European Heart Journal 1991;12:700-4.
11. Bainton D, Miller NE, Bolton CH, et al. Plasma triglyceride and high density lipoprotein cholesterol as predictors of ischaemic heart disease in British men: The

Caerphilly and Speedwell Collaborative Heart Disease Studies. Br Heart J 1992;68:60-6.

12. Austin MA. Triglycerides and small, dense LDL as risk factors for coronary heart disease. 3rd International Symposium, Multiple Risk Factors in Cardiovascular Disease, Florence, Italy, July 6-9, 1994. Abstract.

13. West KM, Ahaja MMS, Bennett PH, et al. The role of circulating glucose and triglyceride concentrations and their interactions with other "risk factors" as determinants of arterial disease in nine diabetic population samples from the WHO multinational study. Diabetes Care 1983;6:361-9.

14. Janka HU. Five year incidence of major macrovascular complications in diabetes mellitus. Horm Metab Res Suppl 1985;15:15-9.

15. Fontbonne A, Eschwege E, Cambien F, et al. Hypertriglyceridaemia as a risk factor of coronary heart disease mortality in subjects with impared glucose tolerance or diabetes: Results from the 11-year follow-up of the Paris Prospective Study. Diabetologia 1989; 32:300-4.

16. Barrett-Connor E, Wingard DL, Criqui MH, Suarez L. Is borderline fasting hyperglycemia a risk factor for cardiovascular death? J Chron Dis 1984;37:773-9.

17. Cowan LD, Wilcosky T, Criqui MH, et al. Demographic behavioral, biochemical, and dietary correlates of plasma triglycerides: The Lipid Research Clinics Program Prevalence Study. Arteriosclerosis 1985;5:466-80.

18. Cambien F, Jacqueson A, Richard JL, Warnet JM, Ducimetiere P, Claude JR. Is the level of serum triglyceride a significant predictor of coronary death in "normocholesterolemic" subjects? A Paris prospective study. Am J Epidemiol 1986;124: 624-32.

19. Expert panel. Summary of the second report of the National Cholesterol Education Program (NCEP) Expert Panel on Detection, Evaluation, and Treatment of High Blood Cholesterol in Adults (adult treatment panel II). JAMA 1993;269:3015-23.

20. Benfante RJ, Reed DM, MacLean CJ, Yano K. Risk factors in middle-age that predict early and late onset of coronary heart disease. J Clin Epidemiol 1989;42:95-104.

21. Laakso M, Lehto S, Penttilä I, Pyörälä K. Lipid and lipoproteins predicting coronary heart disease mortality and morbidity in patients with non-insulin-dependent diabetes. Circulation 1993;88:1421-30.

22. Hodis HN, Mack WJ, Azen SP, et al. Triglyceride- and cholesterol-rich lipoproteins have a differential effect on mild/moderate and severe lesion progression as assessed by quantitative coronary angiography in a controlled trial of lovastin. Circulation 1994;90:42-9.

23. Walsh BW, Schiff I, Rosner B, Greenberg L, Ravnikar V, Sacks FM. Effects of postmenopausal estrogen replacement of the concentrations and metabolism of plasma lipoproteins. N Engl J Med 1991;325:1197-204.

24. Austin MA, Breslow JL, Hennekens CH, Buring JE, Willen WC, Krauss RM. Low-density lipoprotein subclass patterns and risk of myocardial infarction. JAMA 1988; 260:1917-21.

25.   Simpson HCR, Mann JI, Meade TW, CHakrabarti R, Stirling Y, Woolf L. Hypertriglyceridaemia and hypercoagulability. Lancet 1983;1:786-90.

26.   Hamsten A, Wiman B, de Faire U, Blombäck M. Increased plasma levels of a rapid inhibitor of tissue plasminogen activator in young survivors of myocardial infarction. N Engl J Med 1985;313:1557-63.

27.   Fujii S, Sobel BE. Direct effect of gemfibrozil on the fibrinolytic system: Dminution of synthesis of plasminogen activator inhibitor type I. Circulation 1992;85:1888-93.

28.   Lüscher TF. The endothelium and cardiovascular disease-a complex relation. N Engl J Med 1994;330:1081-3.

29.   Kuhn FE, Mohler ER, Satler LF, et al. Effects of high-density lipoprotein on acetylcholine-induced coronary vasoreactivity. Am J Cardiol 1991;68:1425-30.

30.   Reaven GM. Role of insulin resistance in human disease: Banting Lecture 1988. Diabetes 1988;37:1595-607.

31.   Haffner SM, Valdez RA, Hazuda HP, Mitchell BD, Morales PA, Stern MP. Prospective analysis of the insulin-resistance syndrome (Syndrome X). Diabetes 1992;41:715-22.

32.   The Fifth Report of the Joint National Committee on Detection, Evaluation, and Treatment of High Blood Pressure. National Institutes of Health, National Heart, Blood, Lung, and Blood Institute. NIH Publication no. 93-1088, 1993.

FACTORS CONTROLLING LIPOPROTEIN METABOLISM

Ephraim Sehayek and Shlomo Eisenberg
Institute of Lipid & Atherosclerosis Research
The Sheba Medical Center
Tel Hashomer 52621
ISRAEL

The metabolism of the two triglyceride-carrying lipoproteins, chylomicrons and very-low-density lipoproteins (VLDL), occurs in the plasma compartment, in close proximity to the endothelial cell layer and to tissue cells. Both lipoproteins transport triglycerides and cholesterol from sites of absorption (intestinal chylomicrons) and synthesis (hepatic VLDL) to sites of storage and utilization. The metabolism of the two lipoproteins is dependent on the normal triglyceride hydrolysis activity of lipoprotein lipases (LPL), enzymes situated on the luminal surface of endothelial cells in extra-hepatic tissues. The fatty acids are taken up by the tissues and a triglyceride-depleted particle, designated "remnant" lipoprotein is released back to the circulation. The fate of remnant lipoproteins differ between the two lipoproteins: chylomicron remnants are rapidly and irreversibly catabolized in the liver while at least part of the VLDL remnants continue to interact with lipases and are converted to LDL along the VLDL-IDL-LDL cascade. Hence, the circulating mass of the major atherogenic lipoprotein in human plasma, LDL, is determined to a considerable degree by the number of VLDL particles (apoB-100) that enter the plasma and the fraction of VLDL remnants that escape catabolism and complete the VLDL to LDL conversion cascade [1,2]. The rate of clearance of LDL from the plasma through the LDL-receptor pathway [3] determines LDL concentration only after the particles have been formed and at a relatively slow rate; several days, as compared to a few hours (or less), are necessary for the clearance of remnant particles. Elucidation of processes responsible for remnant catabolism, therefore, is a major challenge in lipoprotein research.

Lessons from human pathophysiology [4] and, more recently, from transgenic mice models [5] have unequivocally demonstrated that the catabolism of chylomicron remnants (apoB-48 containing lipoproteins) is dependent on the presence of functionally apoE molecules (E-3 and E-4) on the surface of the particles. The mechanisms involved with the clearance from plasma of VLDL remnants (apoB-100 containing lipoproteins) however are still obscure. Our studies in recent years attempted to elucidate, at least in part, the basic pathways that determine the interaction of the triglyceride-rich lipoproteins and their remnants with cellular receptors.

A.M. Gotto et al. (eds.), Multiple Risk Factors in Cardiovascular Disease, 53-60.
© 1995 Kluwer Academic Publishers and Fondazione Giovanni Lorenzini.

Role of Apolipoproteins

The major apoproteins of chylomicrons and VLDL are apoB (B-48 and B-100, respectively), apoCs and apoE. ApoA-I and apoA-IV are present in nascent chylomicrons and small amounts of other apoproteins may be associated with either lipoprotein. Both apoB-100 and apoE contain receptor-binding domains and exhibit high affinity binding to the LDL-receptor (LDL-R). ApoE also specifically binds to the LDL-receptor-related protein (LRP) [6] and perhaps the VLDL-receptor [7]. Yet, neither chylomicrons nor VLDL are taken up and degraded to an appreciable degree through receptor-dependent pathways in cell cultures that express lipoprotein receptors. Of interest, enrichment of VLDL and chylomicrons with exogenous apoE-3 (recombinant or plasmatic) causes a many-fold increase of binding, internalization, and degradation of the lipoproteins [8], indicating that apoE on chylomicrons and VLDL can mediate receptor recognition. These observations led us to test the possibility that endogenous apoE in triglyceride-rich particles is not adequately available for interaction with cellular receptors but may become exposed during the metabolic cascade of the lipoproteins. A natural approach to test that possibility was to determine the effects of lipolysis on the ability of VLDL and chylomicrons to interact with cellular receptors. The investigations were carried out with human plasma lipoproteins, and demonstrated that *in vitro* lipolysis indeed increases by many times the uptake and degradation of the lipoproteins [9,10]. The unique finding in the study was that the lipolysis process "exposes" the unreactive endogenous apoE molecules associated with the VLDL. If the VLDL contains apoE-3 or E-4 (but not E-2), a specific apoE-dependent interaction of the particles with cellular receptors, predominantly the LDL-R, occurs. The mechanism(s) responsible for "activation" of unreactive apoE molecules have not been fully elucidated but are, at least in part, due to conformational change of apoE at the surface of the lipoprotein. Another contributing mechanism is deletion of apoCs, molecules that were shown to inhibit apoE-dependent interactions of lipoproteins with the LDL-R [11] and LRP [12] in cultured cells.

The data described above led us to suggest that a single mechanism regulates triglyceride transport, remnant catabolism, and LDL synthesis along the VLDL-IDL-LDL cascade [9] (Figure 1). In newly secreted VLDL (and chylomicrons), apoB and apoE are oriented such that their receptor binding domains are unexposed while the apoC molecules (predominantly C-II) are fully active. The lipoprotein particles therefore interact avidly with lipoprotein lipases on endothelial cells and deliver triglycerides to peripheral tissues (TG transport, Figure 1). Catabolic events are rare. With the progression of lipolysis however, the receptor binding domain of apoE becomes exposed, apoC molecules are deleted the lipoprotein acquires the properties of a "remnant" and now can interact with cellular receptors (remnant removal, Figure 1).

Remnants that interact with receptors are irreversibly catabolized while others complete the cascade and form LDL. It is only when LDL is formed that apoB-100 (in VLDL) becomes fully reactive and is removed from the circulation at a relatively slow rate by the LDL receptor. A similar initial sequence of events has been found by us for human

Regulation of TG-Transport, Remnant Removal and LDL Catabolism along the Apo B-100 Cascade

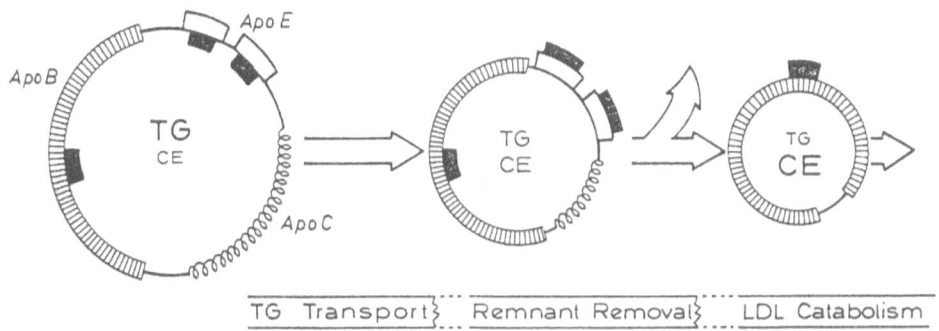

Figure 1. Regulation of triglyceride transport, remnant catabolism, and LDL formation along the apoB-100 (VLDL→IDL → LDL) cascade. Reproduced from the Journal of Clinical Investigation (1991;88:553-560) by copyright permission of the Rockefeller University Press.

chylomicrons [10]. However, the smaller apoB-48 perhaps does not allow the conversion of chylomicron remnants to LDL and allows many apoE molecules to become associated with the particle. The excessive enrichment of the chylomicron remnants with apoE undoubtedly contributes to their rapid and complete clearance from the plasma.

Role of Heparin Sulfate

Triglyceride hydrolysis in chylomicrons and VLDL by lipoprotein lipase, as described above, appears to result in two exceedingly important metabolic events: transport of triglycerides to tissues and transformation of the particles to remnants. Lipoprotein lipase yet appears to have at least two additional functions in lipoprotein metabolism. The first is binding of lipoproteins to heparin sulfate on cell surfaces and extracellular matrix [13] and the second, is binding to the LRP [14]. Interestingly, both functions are shared by apoE, a protein that binds to heparin sulfate and to the LRP. Studies in our laboratory focused mainly on lipoprotein lipase.

In our initial study [13], we investigated the ability of LPL to bind a variety of human plasma lipoproteins to cell surfaces and extracellular matrix (ECM) and the possible metabolic consequences of the binding phenomenon. Binding of all human plasma lipoproteins (chylomicrons, VLDL, IDL, LDL, and HDL) was enhanced by 10- to 100-fold by lipoprotein lipase. This effect was observed with all cell types investigated, including normal and LDL-receptor negative human skin fibroblasts, Chinese hamster ovary (CHO) cells, and hepG-2 cultures. LPL-enhanced binding was abolished by treating cells and ECM with heparinize and was not observed in mutant CHO cells that are heparin sulfate deficient. The enhanced binding was independent of the catalytic activity of the enzyme and could be detected with low LPL concentrations, 15-150 ng/ml, similar to the concentration of circulating LPL before or after heparin injection to human subjects. Two observations deserve a special attention. The first is the effect of binding of lipoproteins (LDL) to heparansulfate on the uptake and degradation of the lipoprotein by the LDL-receptor, and the second, the dependence of this effect on the degree of expression of the LDL receptor. In a series of experiments we observed a 50%-150% enhanced uptake and degradation of LDL in the presence of lipoprotein lipase that is abolished when the cells are treated with heparinize. A similar observation was made with wild type and mutant heparin-sulfate-deficient CHO cells (unpublished). In other experiments, we found that the enhanced catabolism of LDL in cells could be reduced by down-regulating the LDL receptor activity and that only minimal effects were found in LDL-R negative cells. These dramatic differences of uptake and degradation of LDL were observed in spite of similar effects of LPL on binding of the lipoprotein to heparin sulfate. Thus, the enhancement of LDL uptake and degradation was dependent on interaction of the lipoprotein with the receptor while the binding to heparin sulfate reflected the concentration of the heparin sulfate molecules on the cell surface. Whether other lipoproteins, especially those that are taken up through apoE-dependent mechanisms behave similarly to LDL, remains to be established (see below).

The studies described above elucidated a new mechanism that may play an important role in lipoprotein metabolism and perhaps in processes that lead to the initiation and progression of atherosclerosis. The mechanism is shown graphically in Figure 2. The hypothesis is that lipoprotein lipase binds to lipoproteins through its lipid binding domain and to heparin sulfate through its heparin binding domain. Thus, the enzyme forms a "bridge" between the lipoproteins and the cell surface heparin sulfate. Lipoprotein lipase is normally bound to heparin sulfate and binds lipoproteins. Some lipoproteins (predominantly remnant particles) may carry lipoprotein lipase attached to their outer coat and become anchored to free heparin sulfate molecules on cell surfaces. Regardless of the binding route, once lipoproteins are attached to heparin sulfate and therefore are concentrated in close proximity to the cell surface, the particles are transferred at an enhanced rate to cellular receptors. Binding to the receptor, cellular uptake, and proteolytic degradation of the particles however takes place only when proper exposure of biologically reactive receptor binding domains of apoB or apoE occurs. It is this last property of the heparin sulfate pathway that is possibly responsible for the targeting of lipoprotein particles to specific tissues, e.g. the liver.

Role of Cellular Receptors

The concepts described above do not support the view that binding of lipoproteins to heparin sulfate is sufficient to initiate an "heparin sulfate dependent catabolic pathway." On the contrary, our data indicate that while binding to heparin sulfate may be responsible

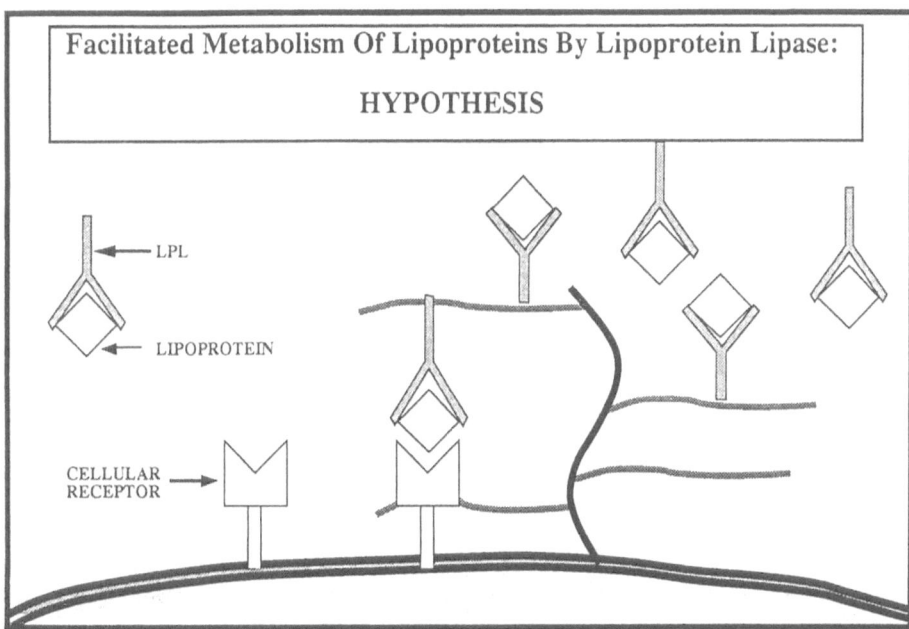

Figure 2. Lipoprotein lipase-mediated binding of lipoproteins to heparin sulfate on cell surfaces facilitates their uptake and degradation by cellular receptors.

for sequestration of lipoproteins in specific sites, very few particles, if any become irreversibly catabolized together with the heparin sulfate molecule. Similar considerations must be applied to other molecules that can form a "bridge" between lipoproteins and heparin sulfate, in particular apoE. For example, while apoE-2 retains the ability to bind lipoproteins to heparin sulfate [15], its lack of proper interaction with receptors causes inability of the particles to undergo irreversible catabolism. We have recently explored the relationships between binding to heparin sulfate and receptor-dependent uptake and degradation of lipoproteins and of molecules involved with lipid metabolism by using several different approaches.

In a series of studies we wished to learn the role of heparin sulfate in the metabolism of the lipoprotein lipase enzyme protein (unpublished). To this end, radioiodinated bovine milk LPL was used and the investigations were carried out with several cell types (normal and LDL-R negative human skin fibroblasts, hepG-2 cells, and wild type and mutant heparin-sulfate-deficient CHO cells) and under a variety of experimental conditions. All cell types including LDL-R negative fibroblasts avidly bound LPL and the binding was followed by internalization and proteolytic degradation of the enzyme in the lysosomal compartment. Treatment of the cells with heparinize decreased LDL binding and degradation by 60-70%. Similar findings were recorded when sulfation of glycosaminoglycans was prevented, or when mutant heparin-sulfate-deficient CHO cells were investigated. Interestingly, chondroitin sulfate could not replace heparin sulfate and treatment of the cells with chondroitinase had no effect on the binding and degradation of the enzyme. Heparin, even in very low concentrations (1 μg/ml) had however a considerably more dramatic effect and abolished the binding and degradation to values very close to background, less than 10% of untreated cells. These observations, we believe, point to the presence in cells of two pathways that are responsible for LPL uptake and degradation. The first pathway is dependent on the presence of heparin sulfate, and the second reflects the presence on cell surfaces of another molecule that can bind and degrade LPL in a heparin-dependent reaction. That other pathway is perhaps the LRP, a receptor protein that can bind LPL. Noteworthy, the data indicates that while heparin sulfate can be regarded as a "receptor" that mediates LPL uptake and degradation in a variety cells, this same pathway can not, or is very inefficient, in the process of clearance of lipoproteins even when bound to heparin sulfate through a LPL (or apoE) bridge.

Finally, we attempted to clarify the relationships between binding of lipoproteins to heparin sulfate via LPL and their subsequently enhanced receptor-mediated cellular uptake and degradation. These investigations were carried out in cultured endothelial cells derived from bovine cornea or aorta. The studies utilized LDL, VLDL, and apoE-enriched VLDL. Similar to the previous observations, endothelial cells demonstrate a dramatic enhanced binding of the lipoproteins to heparin sulfate when bovine milk LPL is added to the culture medium. The binding process then is followed by enhanced uptake and proteolytic degradation. Both the enhanced binding and degradation reactions are inhibited by pretreatment of the cells with heparinize or in the presence of 1 μg/ml of sodium heparin. Also in agreement with previously reported results, the uptake and degradation reactions reflected the degree of regulation of the LDL receptor, and were low in down regulated cells and high in subconfluent cultures. Because the study included experiments with VLDL and apoE-rich VLDL, it was possible to assess the contribution of apoE alone, of LPL alone and of a combination of apoE and LPL on the enhanced VLDL uptake and degradation. Metabolism, that was enhanced several fold, was seen with either apoE-3 alone or LPL alone as reported in our previous experiments. Unexpectedly. however, synergism between the two occurred and resulted in uptake and degradation values that were 2-3-fold higher than the combined effect of apoE and LPL alone. Next we studied the effects of monoclinal antibodies (Mab C-7, directed against the LDL-R; 1D7, directed against the receptor binding domain of apoE-3; and 4G3, directed against the receptor binding domain of apoB-100) on the basal and enhanced uptake and degradation of LDL and VLDL. Mab C-7 blocked completely the basal activity of LDL but only partially (50-60%) the enhanced activity. With VLDL, the antibody had only partial (30-60%) blocking effect. Monoclinal 1D7 blocked almost completely the metabolism of VLDL and 4G3 had a marginal additional effect. We concluded from the study that the LDL-R was the predominant, but not the only, receptor responsible for the enhanced metabolism of LDL and VLDL in the cells, and that receptor binding domains were absolutely required for the enhanced cellular metabolism of LDL and VLDL, at least in endothelial cells.

Conclusions

Data reported during the last few years have unequivocally showed that the control of lipoprotein uptake and degradation by cells is considerably more complex than previously believed. It now appears that several interacting reactions are involved in the process and evidence is accumulating that defects in any one of these reactions may severely affect the optimal metabolic cascade. Apoproteins E and B-100 and their proper-exposure; lipoprotein lipase activity and "bridging" effects; binding of lipoproteins through LPL and apoE to cell surface heparin sulfate and enhanced delivery of the particles to receptors; and finally a crucial role for receptors, most probably the whole family of the LDL-R (LDL-receptor, VLDL-receptor, and LRP) in the process, should be considered. Our data and that reported by other investigators [16,17] have began to elucidate the interactions and consequence of these four reactions, the many proteins that are involved with the processes that control lipoprotein metabolism, their cellular interactions, and the initiation/progression of atherosclerosis.

References

1. Eisenberg S, Bilheimer DW, Lindgren FT, Levy RI. On the metabolic conversion of human plasma very low density lipoprotein to low density lipoprotein. Biochim Biophys Acta 1973;326:361-377.

2. Eisenberg S, Sehayek E. Remnant catabolism. Nutr Metab Cardiovasc Dis 1993;3:102-104.

3. Brown MS, Goldstein JL. A receptor-mediated pathway for cholesterol homeostasis. Science 1986;232:34-47.

4. Mahley RW, Angelin B. Type III hyperlipoproteinemia: Recent insights into the genetic defect of familial dysbetalipoproteinemia. Adv Int Med 1984;29:385-411.

5. Plump AS, Smith JD, Hayek T, et al. Severe hypercholesterolemia and atherosclerosis in apoprotein E-deficient mice by homologous recombination in ES cells. Cell 1992;71:343-353.

6. Beisiegel U, Weber W, Ihrke G, Herz J, Stanley KK. The LDL-receptor-related protein, LRP, is an apolipoprotein E-binding protein. Nature 1989;341:162-164.

7. Sakai J, Hoshino A, Takahashi S, et al. Structure, chromosome location, and expression of the human very low density lipoprotein receptor gene. J Biol Chem 1994;269:2173-2182.

8. Eisenberg S, Friedman G, Vogel T. Enhanced metabolism of normolipidemic human plasma very low density lipoprotein in cultured cells by exogenous apolipoprotein E-3. Arteriosclerosis 1988;8:480-487.

9. Sehayek E, Lewine-Velvet U, Chajek-Shaul T, Eisenberg S. Lipolysis exposes unreactive endogenous apoprotein E-3 in human and rat very low density lipoprotein. J Clin Invest 1991;88:553-560.

10. Arnon R, Sehayek E, Vogel T, Eisenberg S. Effects of exogenous apo E-3 and of cholesterol-enriched meals on the cellular metabolism of human chylomicrons and

their remnants. Biochim Biophys Acta 1991;1085:336-342.

11.   Sehayek E, Eisenberg S. Mechanisms of inhibition by apolipoprotein C of apolipoprotein E-dependent cellular metabolism of human triglyceride-rich lipoproteins through the low density lipoprotein receptor pathway. J Biol Chem 1991;266:18259-18267.

12.   Kowal RC, Herz J, Weisgraber KH, Mahley RW, Brown MS, Goldstein JL. Opposing effects of apolipoproteins E and C on lipoprotein binding to low density lipoprotein receptor-related protein. J Biol Chem 1990;265:10771-10779.

13.   Eisenberg S, Sehayek E, Olivecrona T, Vlodavsky I. Lipoprotein lipase enhances binding of lipoproteins to heparan sulfate on cell surfaces and extracellular matrix. J Clin Invest 1992;90:2013-2021.

14.   Chappell DA, Fry GL, Waknitz MA, Iverius PH, Williams SE, Strickland DK. The low density lipoprotein receptor-related protein/α2-macroglobulin receptor binds and mediates catabolism of bovine milk lipoprotein lipase. J Biol Chem 1992;267:25764-25767.

15.   Ji ZS, Fazio S, Mahley RW. Variable heparan sulfate proteoglycan binding of apolipoprotein E variants may modulate the expression of type III hyperlipoproteinemia. J. Biol Chem 1994;13421-13428.

16.   Ji ZS, Brecht JB, Miranda RD, Hussain MM, Innerarity TL, Mahley RW. Role of heparan sulfate proteoglycans in the binding and uptake of apoprotein E-enriched remnant lipoproteins by cultured cells. J Biol Chem 1993;268:10160-10167.

17.   Chappell DA, Inoue I, Fry GL, et al. Cellular catabolism of normal very low density lipoproteins via the low density lipoprotein receptor-related protein/α_2-macroglobulin receptor is induced by the C-terminal domain of lipoprotein lipase. J Biol Chem 1994;269:18001-18006.

APOLIPOPROTEINS IN THE TREATMENT OF VASCULAR AND NONVASCULAR DISEASE

Cesare R. Sirtori
Center E. Grossi Paoletti, Institute of Pharmacological Sciences
University of Milan
Via Balzaretti 9
20133 Milan
ITALY

Introduction

Apolipoproteins are attractive molecules for potential use in therapeutics; they are quite stable and water soluble, and can bind at the same time lipids and other chemicals. Some apolipoproteins can also interact with cell receptors, either regulating cholesterol biosynthesis, or possibly removal. A therapeutic use of apolipoproteins may not be strictly linked to their lipid binding properties. In some cases, apolipoprotein segments have been proposed for clinical use; in other, complexes of apolipoproteins with other circulating proteins (e.g., immunoglobulins) may provide a potentially useful tool. Some of the possible or future uses of apolipoproteins in a variety of clinical fields will be examined. They range from human fertilization, to the treatment of gout, neurodegenerative disorders, obesity, acquired immunodeficiency syndrome, endotoxin shock, and finally prevention and possibly treatment of arterial disease.

Activation of Sperm Motility

In vitro fertilization studies have clearly indicated that human serum is superior both to seminal plasma and follicular fluid in supporting motility of human spermatozoa. The major sperm activating capacity in serum was previously found to be mediated by a fraction with a molecular weight (MW) of about 250 kD [1]. More recently, this complex was described as containing albumin, apolipoprotein AI, and immunoglobulin heavy and light chains [2]. Boiling destroys the activity, thus suggesting that the complex acts as a macromolecule. At specific concentrations, sperm motility is increased, and so is the ATP content of sperm. The mechanism by which the sperm activating protein (SPAP) induces sperm activation is unknown. Judging from the small amounts of SPAP required for activation, a likely hypothesis may be that of a receptor-mediated or enzyme linked mechanism. Since the

A.M. Gotto et al. (eds.), Multiple Risk Factors in Cardiovascular Disease, 61-73.
© 1995 *Kluwer Academic Publishers and Fondazione Giovanni Lorenzini.*

effect on ATP content is not of a similar extent as that on sperm motility, it is not clear whether SPAP affects motility via an increase of ATP content. Recent structural studies show that the plausible structure of SPAP places one molecule of apo AI between the two arms of the Fab portion of an IgG molecule [3]. Immunofluorescence studies in human spermatozoa indicate a direct interaction of SPAP with the lower part of the sperm head. Use of SPAP is postulated both for diagnostic and therapeutic purposes in human fertilization.

Gout and Inflammatory Conditions

Gout is characterized by increased levels of uric acid in plasma, consequent either to excess production or reduced excretion. The resulting pathological condition is arthritis, mainly at the lower extremities (toe), with crystal formation and abundant inflow of polymorpho-nuclear (PMN) leukocytes. Treatment of gout is of a preventive nature, either using drugs increasing urate excretion or, more often, inhibiting biosynthesis (allopurinol).

Apolipoprotein E (apo E), a relatively basic protein, can bind urate crystals *in vitro*, in cultured PMNs [4]. The effects of apo E might not be only of a chemical nature, but may also involve lymphocyte maturation, up to the formation of active cells. Prior observations linked a subfraction of LDL to an immunoregulatory property of these lipoproteins. LDL_{in} can in fact inhibit lymphocyte immortalization, a prerequisite for lymphoid tumor development [5]. As a result of later studies, apo E, or possibly a modified form, was identified as being responsible for these immunoregulatory properties [6]. These observations, pertaining to the immunoregulatory effect of apo E, may be pertinent to its possible use in inflammatory disorders, ranging from gouty arthritis (where the lipid binding properties would not be in play), up to progressive lupus erythematosus, rheumatoid arteritis, or even the control of graft rejection.

Neurodegenerative Disorders

Degenerative disorders of the nervous system, both at the central or peripheral level, may be the result of trauma, infectious diseases, or part of a generalized condition of the central nervous system (CNS). Injured mammalian peripheral nerves release a soluble protein of MW 37 kD [7], the secretion of which increases dramatically after injury, accounting for up to 5% of total secretory proteins. This protein, identified as apo E, is produced by macrophages surrounding the injured nerve.

In the last two years, the interest in apo E, particularly in apo E polymorphism in the etiology of Alzheimer's disease (AD) has grown tremendously. Retrospective studies have clearly shown that subjects carrying the E4 isoform of apo E are at considerably enhanced risk of the late-onset form of the disease [8]. Studies on the mechanism of this putative association have been less enlightening. Laboratory evidence indicates that, differently from the E2 and E3 isoforms, apo E4 can bind β-amyloid more tightly, thus resulting in an enhanced β-amyloid deposition, the classic pathologic sign of AD, or else in a delayed removal of the E-β-amyloid complex [9].

Aside from these basic and clinical observations, the recognition of apo E release from injured nerves has led to a number of investigations, in order to examine the possibility that this might not be only a consequence of tissue damage, but also a mechanism for repair. Released apo E is recognized by high affinity receptors, with characteristics of the B, E receptors [10]. Receptor/mediated uptake is elevated in growing neuronal cells, in particular growth cones, thus possibly providing an additional, local source of lipid for myelin regeneration [11]. Quantitative evaluation of accumulated apolipoproteins in regenerating nerves shows that apo D and E are increased over 500 and 250-fold, respectively, 3 weeks after injury, versus minimal increases of apo A-I and apo A-IV (both, probably, reaching the nerve from plasma) [12]. Cholesterol released from injured nerves becomes associated with apo E-containing lipoproteins, thus becoming available for local reutilization [13]. This finding is of particular significance, in view of the fact that regenerating nerves synthesize very little cholesterol. Very recently, Nathan et al. [14] showed that the E3 isoform is more effective in inducing nerve regeneration versus the E4.

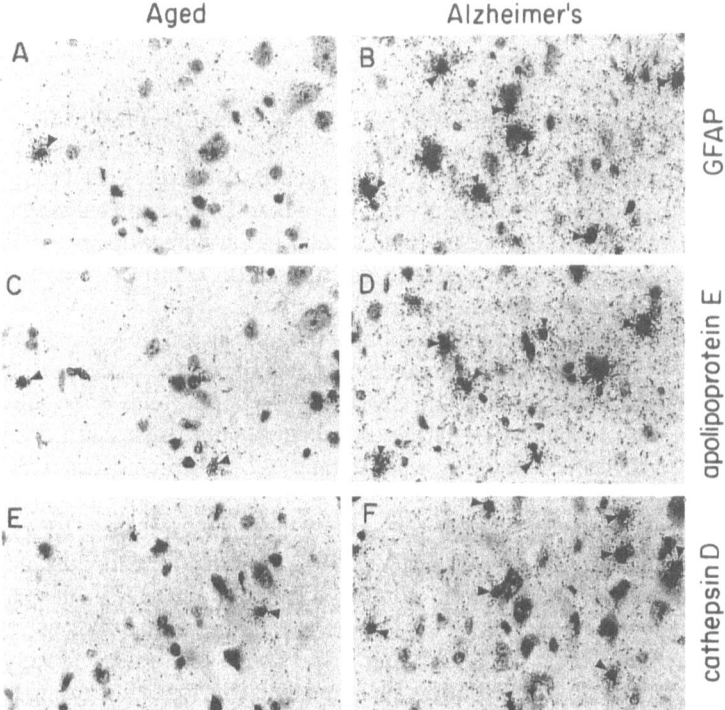

Figure 1. In situ hybridization of glial fibrillar acid protein (GFAP), apo E and cathepsin D (CD) mRNAs in brains from control and Alzheimer's patients [15].

Marked increases of apo E expression have been described in astrocytes from brains of Alzheimer's patients and scrapie-infected mice [15], both characterized by focal or diffuse neural degeneration, accompanied by extensive myelin changes (Figure 1). No clear evidence, has been provided, up to now, as to the nature of the increased apo E (E4 or also other isoforms?).

Nevertheless, this observation provides a very exciting clue to a possible management of early β-amyloid accumulation. It is well established that, at least in *in vitro* systems, apo E2 or E3 can compete with E4 for β-amyloid binding, thus providing a possible tool to reduce β-amyloid accumulation in Alzheimer's [9], eventually reverting some of the initial changes in patients with the so called "age associated memory impairment" [16]. On the other hand, very recently, Whitson et al. [17] have indicated that rabbit apo E (isoform undefined) can by itself protect against the neurotoxicity of the Aβ amyloid peptide.

Apo E is produced in large quantities after nerve injury (be it acute or chronic, as in AD) and is stored in lipoprotein particles, interacting with high affinity receptors in regenerating nerve. The hypothesis of therapeutic use of apo E in cases of neuronal injury, has never been tested either in experimental animals or in man.

Obesity

Excess body weight is an extremely frequent abnormality in the Western world: not less than 20-30% of adults have a body mass index in excess of 30% of desirable levels. In addition, treatment of obesity has proven most elusive. By everybody's experience there has been little change in the prospective of "treatment": not more than 20% of treated obese patients can maintain a reduced body weight, versus 40% of patients for whom treatment failed and a further 40% with a short- or long-term relapse. For this reason, any treatment, be it dietary or pharmacological, is looked upon with interest.

Apolipoprotein A-IV, a structural component of chylomicrons (CM), may play a role in the catabolism of triglyceride rich lipoproteins and also in reverse cholesterol transport. Apo A-IV may be rapidly displaced from CM by other lipoproteins upon entering the circulation [18]. The output of apo A-IV into intestinal lymph increases markedly as a result of lipid feeding [19] and is not mediated by lipid uptake into the enterocytes or by changes in cellular triglyceride content.

The initial suggestion that increased apo A-IV levels in mesenteric lymph may act as a physiological signal for satiation and that apo A-IV might be an important factor in satiation after fatty meals [20] has been supported by clear changes in the patterns of feeding, drinking, and ambulation in rats after single A-IV doses of 60-200 μg infused IV via a chronic indwelling right atrial catheter. Apo A-IV suppresses food intake by decreasing meal size without changing intervals between meals (speed of eating or latency to the first meal after infusion) [21]. The effect is dose dependent and lasts for 3 hours after the infusion.

While these findings support the hypothesis that apo A-IV may act as a physiological signal for satiety after a lipid meal, more recently a central effect of the apolipoprotein was suggested by a comparative effect of infusions into the third ventricle versus IV doses. As low as 1 μg/rat infused into the ventricle suppressed food intake close to 50% and at 4 μg food intake is almost totally suppressed [22]; similar results can be achieved by IV doses around 100-200 μg (Figure 2). The hypothesis that apo A-IV may have regulatory mechanisms in food intake is supported by the observation that obese hyperlipoproteinemic Zucker rats have a two-fold higher hepatic A-IV gene expression versus lean controls, thus indicating some derangement in the synthesis of the apolipoprotein in body weight abnormalities [23]. Whether this finding can provide indications to a potential use of apo A-IV in reducing food intake in man needs further evaluation.

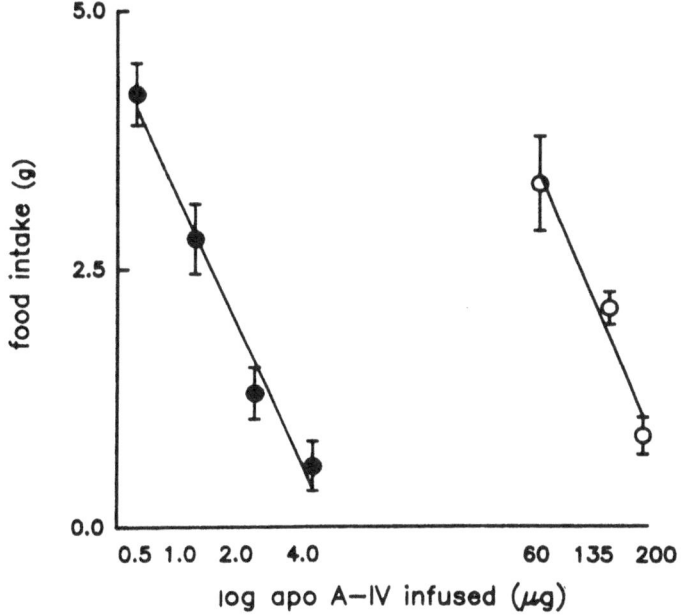

Figure 2. Suppression of food intake by infusion of apo A-IV, into the third ventricle (●) or IV (○) [22].

Acquired Immunodeficiency Syndrome (AIDS) and Endotoxin Shock

Apolipoproteins, particularly apo A-I, may have found an unexpected role in the management of AIDS and also of shock due to bacterial endotoxins. In these two conditions, the amphipathic helixes of A-I may, in fact, interact with phospholipids on the surface of either the virus or the endotoxin, in this way potentially reducing clinical consequences.

AIDS, a rapidly diffusing immunological disorder, is related to an infection with a retrovirus (HIV), specifically affecting helper T-lymphocytes (T4) [24]. AIDS is characterized by an asymptomatic period, followed by a full blown disease, associated with diffuse tissue damage, high frequency of infectious complications and, in some cases, development of characteristic tumors (Kaposi sarcomas). The HIV infection leads to cytopathic effects, characterized by the formation of multinucleated syncytia, followed by cell fusion. This effect is mediated by the intracellular cleavage of the envelope glycoprotein gp160 to a gp120-gp41 complex, transported to the plasma membrane. After cleavage, a new hydrophobic amino terminus is exposed on gp41, mediating fusion of the envelope with cell membranes. Interruption of the process of viral cell fusion can reduce viral replication and syncytium formation in a number of systems [25]. In model membrane systems, agents stabilizing the membrane bilayer have also been shown to inhibit membrane fusion [26].

Among agents with a high affinity for membrane bilayers, amphipathic helical peptides offer an attractive option for the prevention of syncytium formation. Recent reports have indicated the presence of potential amphipathic helical domains in the HIV envelope glycoprotein. Proteins with a high content of amphipathic helices may interact with the system, thus affecting cell fusion. Among the numerous proteins with amphipathic α-helices there are lipid associating polypeptide hormones (β-endorphin and calcitonin), novel antimicrobial agents, such as magainins and cecropins, as well as type I and type II (IFN-γ) interferons [27]. Apo A-I was suggested to possibly play a role in HIV infections, due to a clear effect on the Herpes simplex virus-induced cell fusion at physiological (1 μM) concentrations [28]; a similar preventive effect on HIV induced syncytium formation was also shown [27]. The possible mechanism(s) of inhibition of HIV-induced membrane fusion by the amphipathic helices of the apolipoprotein are shown in Figure 3A.

Figure 3B also reports the possible mechanism of apo A-I in protecting against endotoxin shock [29]. This frequent clinical condition, resulting from a release of endotoxins from Gram- bacteria, leads to death in 30-80% of cases due to septic shock (30). HDL provide a natural component of plasma, known to neutralize endotoxin *in vitro*, and high plasma HDL concentrations can protect mice against endotoxin *in vivo*; transgenic animals with two-fold elevations of plasma HDL show an improved survival rate compared to low HDL mice; IV infusions of HDL almost totally protect mice from endotoxin shock [29].

Atherosclerosis Treatment

In addition to being certainly involved in the determination of atherosclerotic lesions, apolipoproteins may possibly serve as therapeutic tools for arterial plaque removal. Two apolipoproteins have been designated as potentially effective in atherosclerosis prevention/reversal. Studies with apo E have been focused on the clearance of VLDL or remnant particles, and on the regression of arterial lesions in the Watanabe heritable hyperlipidemic (WHHL) rabbit. The hypothetical beneficial effect of apo A-I is based on studies on atherosclerosis regression, induced by HDL or by isolated A-I or A-I Milano infusions; these latter may be available as extractive or recombinant apolipoproteins.

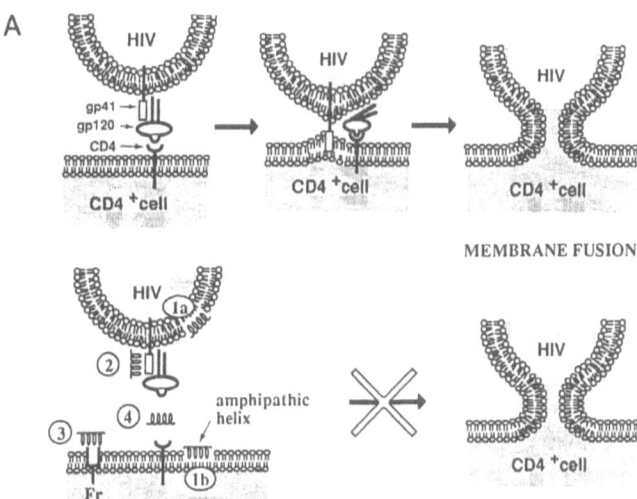

Figure 3A. Model of possible sites of inhibition of HIV-induces membrane fusion by the amphipathic helices of apo A-I [27].

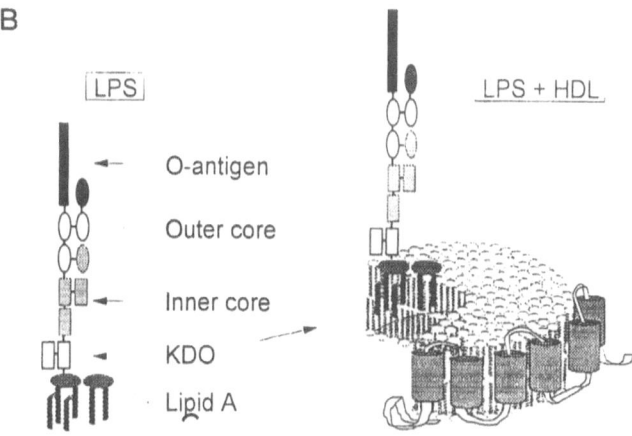

Figure 3B. Hypothesis on the interaction of bacterial lipopolysaccaride (LPS) with HDL in the prevention of endotoxin shock [29]. Similar activities versus the AIDS virus and Gram- endotoxin have been shown for synthetic amphipathic analogues of apo A-I. Twenty-two aminoacid residue synthetic peptides, corresponding to the helical domains of apo A-I or 18-residue long model amphipathic peptides show a similar activity as HDL versus the cytopathic effects of HIV [31]. In the case of endotoxin, the activity of an 18 aminoacid peptide seems to be as effective, when incorporated into liposomes, as the whole lipoprotein [29].

Apo E

The use of apo E for improving lipoprotein metabolism was suggested, based on the affinity of apo E containing lipoproteins for liver cell membranes, responsible for the uptake of dietary cholesterol by way of CM remnants [32]. The CM-remnant receptor, distinct from the LDL receptor, has been recently identified as a multifunctional membrane component, i.e. also mediating the uptake of α-2 macroglobulin, lipoprotein lipase, PAI-1, and others [33].

Yamada et al. [34] tested the hypothesis that injections of apo E in WHHL rabbits could improve remnant clearance, in this way reducing cholesterolemia. By infusing approximately 30 mg apo E per rabbit, a plasma cholesterol reduction of 8.3% by 1 hour and of 19% after 3 hours was observed; reduced levels could be maintained for up to 8 hours after the injection. Cholesterol was reduced primarily in VLDL and intermediate density lipoproteins during the first 2 hours, followed by a reduction in LDL later on.

Mahley et al. [35] with an infusion of apo E (70 mg) to cholesterol fed rabbits, achieved a 20-40% acute reduction of plasma cholesterol within 2-3 hours. The addition of apo E to ^{14}C-cholesterol labelled CM also resulted in an accelerated clearance, with an enhanced uptake, occurring primarily in the liver. The major findings of these studies [34, 35] are summarized in Figure 4.

More recently, Yamada et al. [36] reported the results of a chronic treatment in WHHL rabbits with thrice-weekly injections of apo E (30 mg per rabbit). This study clearly indicates that repeated injections of the apolipoprotein for 8.5 months may result in a dramatic reduction (-40%) of the lesions.

Apo A-I/HDL

The beneficial effects of elevated HDL levels against arterial lipid deposition are well substantiated and have suggested testing the activity of whole HDL or apolipoprotein fractions on arterial lipid deposits, mainly in cholesterol-fed rabbits. In a first study by Badimon et al. [37] the lipoprotein plasma fraction, isolated at density (d) 1.063 to 1.25 gml (HDL-VHDL) was administered to rabbits receiving a 0.5% cholesterol-rich diet for 8 weeks. Lipoproteins (50 mg of protein) were given once weekly IV throughout the period of cholesterol feeding. Treatment did not lead to any marked changes in plasma lipid/lipoprotein distribution. However, aortic sudanophilia was markedly reduced in the HDL-VHDL treated group (15.2% of fatty streak involvement, versus 38.6% in vehicle treated controls), and the cholesteryl ester content of aortas from treated animals went down from 10.9 ± 2.6 mg/g to 4.5 ± 0.6 mg/g of tissue (p < 0.03). In a follow-up study [38], the authors investigated the potential of d > 1.125 lipoproteins to induce regression in rabbits with established lesions. Arterial disease was induced by feeding a 0.5% cholesterol-rich diet for 60 days (group 1). Another group of animals was maintained on the same diet for 90 days (group 2), whereas a third group was fed the cholesterol diet for 90 days, but received in addition 50 mg of HDL-VHDL protein per week during the last 30 days (group 3). At the end of the study aortic atherosclerosis involvement was $34 \pm 4\%$ in

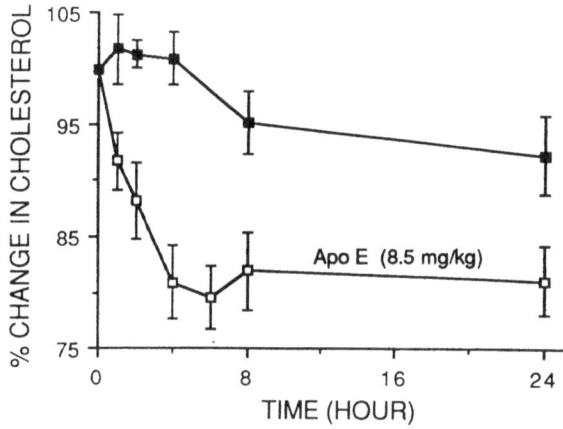

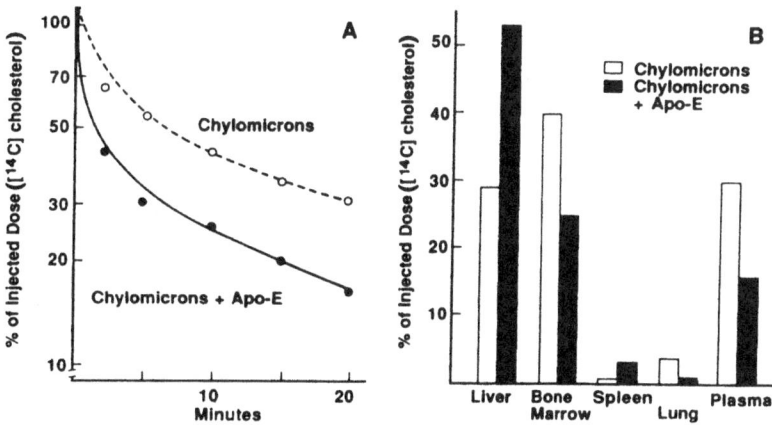

Figure 4. Major findings in studies on the acute infusions of apo E. In the upper panel [34], the acute infusion of apo E in WHHL rabbits determines a significant, although transient, reduction of cholesterolemia. In the lower panel, the infusion of apo E (70 mg) to cholesterol fed rabbits resulted in an accelerated clearance of chylomicrons (A) and also in an enhanced uptake of chylomicron cholesterol in the liver (B) [35].

group 1, 38.8 ± 5% in group 2 and 17.8 ± 4% in group 3 (p < 0.005). Aortic lipid deposition was also significantly reduced in group 3, compared to group 1 (studied only at 60 days) and group 2. These studies suggest that HDL may not only inhibit disease progression, but also reduce established atherosclerotic lesions.

The responsible component of HDL was, at first the object of debate. Components aside of apo A-I might have been responsible (apo E, the cholesteryl ester transfer protein, or possibly others). However, a definitive clue to the identification of apo A-I as the responsible component came from a study showing that mice, transgenic for human apo A-I [39], are extremely resistant to the induction of atherosclerotic lesions by a high fat diet. In addition, HDL exert a prostacyclin stabilizing property [40], attributed to apo A-I and apo A-I itself shows direct fibrinolytic activity in *in vitro* models [41].

The definitive support to a direct activity of apo A-I in inhibiting atherosclerosis progression/stimulating regression, has come from a number of studies using either apo HDL isolated from plasma [42], or recombinant apo A-I obtained in different vectors. The most significant data have come, however, from the use of a recombinant dimer of apo AI-Milano (AI-M). AI-M is a natural mutant of apo A-I (Cys for Arg at position 173) apparently associated to a reduced risk of arterial disease [43]. Very recent kinetic studies have indicated that the dimer of apo AI-Milano (AI-M/AI-M) exhibits a prolonged permanence in plasma [44], thus suggesting a more useful therapeutic potential versus AI-M itself or the wild type AI. In addition, other data suggest that the AI-M dimer may show a potent direct fibrinolytic activity, in the presence or absence of tPA. These observations have prompted direct evaluations in animals, both in cholesterol fed rabbits undergoing peripheral angioplasty, as well as in animals with a carotid constriction according to the model of Booth et al. [45]. In both of these models, 5 injections of the AI-M dimer, evenly spaced before and after the procedures, resulted in a more than a 50% reduction of lesion development. These findings provide a direct support to the hypothesis that the AI-M dimer may prove a potent tool for direct intervention on initial or established lesions at major arterial sites.

Acknowledgements

Supported by the Consiglio Nazionale delle Ricerche of Italy (P.F. Ingegneria Genetica).

References

1. Akerlöf E, Fredricsson B, Gustafson O, et al. Serum factors stimulate the motility of human spermatozoa. Int J Androl 1987;10:124-130.
2. Akerlöf E, Jörnvall H, Slotte H, Pousette A. Identification of apolipoprotein AI and immunoglobulin as components of a serum complex that mediates activation of human sperm motility. Biochemistry 1991;30:8986-8990.
3. Pousette A, Leijonhufvud PK, Akerlöf E. Purification, structure and partial characterization of the major sperm activating protein complex in human serum. Scand J Clin Lab Invest 1993;213:39-44.

4.   Terkeltaub RA, Dyer CA, Martin J, Curtiss LK. Apolipoprotein (Apo) E inhibits the capacity of monosodium urate crystals to stimulate neutrophils. J Clin Invest 1991;87:20-26.

5.   Chisari FV, Curtiss LK, Jensen FC. Physiologic concentrations of normal human plasma lipoproteins inhibit the immortalization of peripheral B lymphocytes by Epstein-Barr virus. J Clin Invest 1981;68:329-336.

6.   Pepe MG, Curtiss LK. Apolipoprotein E is a biologically active constituent of the normal immunoregulatory lipoprotein, LDL-In. J Immunol 1986;136:3716-3723.

7.   Skene JHP, Shooter EM. Denervated sheath cells secrete a new protein after nerve injury. Proc Natl Acad Sci USA 1983;80:4169-4173.

8.   Corder EH, Saunders AM, Strittmatter WJ, et al. Gene dose of apolipoprotein E type 4 allele and the risk of Alzheimer's disease in late onset families. Science 1993; 261:921-923.

9.   Strittmatter WJ, Weisgraber KH, Huang D, et al. Binding of human apolipoprotein E to βA4 peptide: isoform-specific effects and implications for late-onset Alzheimer'disease. Proc Natl Acad Sci 1993;90:8098-8102.

10.   Pitas RE, Boyles JK, Lee SH, Foss D, Mahley RW. Astrocytes synthesize apolipoprotein E and metabolize apolipoprotein E-containing lipoproteins. Biochim Biophys Acta 1987;917:148-161.

11.   Ignatius MJ, Shooter EM, Pitas RE, Mahley RW. Lipoprotein uptake by neuronal growth cones in vitro. Science 1987;236:959-962.

12.   Boyles JK, Notterpek LM, Anderson LJ. Accumulation of apolipoprotein in the regenerating and remyelinating mammalian peripheral nerve. J Biol Chem 1990;265:17805-17815.

13.   Goodrum JF. Cholesterol from degenerating nerve myelin becomes associated with lipoproteins containing apolipoprotein E. J Neurochem 1991;56:2082-2086.

14.   Nathan BP, Bellosta S, Sanan DA, Weisgraber KH, Mahley RW, Pitas RE. Differential effects of apolipoprotein E3 and E4 on neuronal growth *in vitro*. Science 1994;264:850-852.

15.   Diedrich JF, Minnigan H, Carp RI, et al. Neuropathological changes in scrapie and Alzheimer's disease are associated with increased expression of apolipoprotein E and cathepsin D in astrocytes. J Virol 1991;65:4759-4768.

16.   Rebeck GW, Reiter JS, Strickland DK, Hyman BT. Apolipoprotein E in sporadic Alzheimer's disease. Allelic variation and receptor interactions. Neu. 1993;11:575-580.

17.   Whitson JS, Mims MP, Strittmatter WJ, Yamaki T, Morrissett JS, Appel SH. Attenuation of the neurotoxic effect of Aβ amyloid peptide by apolipoprotein E. Biochem Biophys Res Comm 1994;199:163-170.

18.   Weinberg RB, Spector MS. Human apolipoprotein A-IV: Displacement from the surface of triglyceride-rich particles by HDL_2 associated C-apoproteins. J Lipid Res 1985;26:26-37.

19.   Hayagashi H, Nutting DF, Fujimoto K, Cardelli JA, Black D, Tso P. Transport of lipid and apolipoproteins A-I and A-IV in intestinal lymph of the rat. J Lipid Res

1990; 31:1613-1625.

20.   Fujimoto K, Cardelli JA, Tso P. Increased apolipoprotein A-IV in rat mesenteric lymph after lipid meal acts as a physiological signal for satiation. Am J Physiol 1992; 262:41002-41006.

21.   Fujimoto K, Machidori H, Iwakiri R, et al. Effect of intravenous administration of apolipoprotein A-IV on patterns of feeding, drinking and ambulatory activity of rats. Brain Res 1993; 608:233-237.

22.   Fujimoto K, Fukagawa K, Sakata T, Tso P. Suppression of food intake by apolipoprotein A-IV is mediated through the central nervous system in rats. J Clin Invest 1993;91:1830-1833.

23.   Strobl W, Knerer B, Gratzl R, Arbeiter K, Lin-Lee Y-C, Patsch W. Altered regulation of apolipoprotein A-IV gene expression in the liver of the genetically obese Zucker rats. J Clin Invest 1993;92:1766-1773.

24.   Robey WG, Safai B, Oroszlan S, et al. Characterization of envelope and structural gene products of HTLV-III with sera from AIDS patients. Science 1985;228:1402-1405.

25.   Richardson CD, Choppin PW. Oligopeptides that specifically inhibit membrane fusion by paramyxoviruses: Studies on the site of action. Virology 1983;131:518-532.

26.   Epand RM. Virus replication inhibitory peptides inhibit the conversion of phospholipid bilayers to the hexagonal phase. Biosci Rep 1986;6:647-653.

27.   Owens RJ, Anantharamaiah GM, Kahlon JB, Srinivas RV, Compans RW, Segrest JP. Apolipoprotein A-I and its amphipathic helix peptide analogues inhibit human immuno-deficiency virus-induced syncytium formation. J Clin Invest 1990;86:1142-1150.

28.   Srinivas RV, Birkedal B, Owens RJ, Anantharamaiah GM, Segrest JP, Compans RW. Antiviral effects of apolipoprotein A-I and its synthetic amphipathic peptide analogs. Virology 1990;176:48-57.

29.   Levine DM, Parker TS, Donnelly TM, Walsh A, Rubin AL. In vivo protection against endotoxin by plasma high density lipoprotein. Proc Natl Acad Sci 1993; 90:12040-12044.

30.   Bone RC. The pathogenesis of sepsis. Ann Int Med 1991;115:457-469.

31.   Srinivas RV, Venkatachalapathi YV, Rui Z, et al. Inhibition of virus-induced cell fusion by apolipoprotein A-I and its amphipathic peptide analogs. J Cell Biochem 1991;45:224-237.

32.   Hussain MM, Mahley RW, Boyles JK, Fainaru M, Brecht WJ, Lindquist PA. Chylomicron-chylomicron remnant clearance by liver and bone marrow in rabbits. Factors that modify tissue-specific uptake. J Biol Chem 1989;264:9571-9582.

33.   Nykjaer A, Bengtsson-Olivecrona G, Lookene A, et al. The α_2-macroglobulin receptor/low density lipoprotein receptor-related protein binds lipoprotein lipase and β-migrating very low density lipoprotein associated with the lipase. J Biol Chem 1993;268:15048-15055.

34.   Yamada N, Shimano H, Mokuno H, et al. Increased clearance of plasma cholesterol

after injection of apolipoprotein E into Watanabe heritable hyperlipidemic rabbits. Proc Natl Acad Sci USA 1989;86:665-669.

35. Mahley RW, Weisgraber KH, Hussain MM, et al. Intravenous infusion of apolipoprotein E accelerates clearance of plasma lipoproteins in rabbits. J Clin Invest 1989;83:2125-2130.

36. Yamada N, Inoue I, Kawamura M, et al. Apolipoprotein E prevents the progression of atherosclerosis in Watanabe heritable hyperlipidemic rabbits. J Clin Invest 1992;89:706-711.

37. Badimon JJ, Badimon L, Galvez A, Dische R, Fuster V. High density lipoprotein plasma fractions inhibit aortic streaks in cholesterol-fed rabbits. Lab Invest 1989;60:455-461.

38. Badimon JJ, Badimon L, Fuster V. Regression of atherosclerosis lesions by high density lipoprotein plasma fraction in the cholesterol-fed rabbit. J Clin Invest 1990;1234-1241.

39. Rubin EM, Krauss RM, Spangler EA, Verstuyft JG, Clift SM. Inhibition of early atherogenesis in transgenic mice by human apolipoprotein AI. Nature 1991;353:265-267.

40. Aoyama T, Yui Y, Morishita H, Kawai C. Prostaglandin I_2 half-life regulated by high density lipoprotein is decreased in acute myocardial infarction and unstable angina pectoris. Circulation 1990;81:1784-1791.

41. Saku K, Ahmad M, Glas-Greenwalt P, Kashyap ML. Activation of fibrinolysis by apolipoproteins of high density lipoproteins in man. Thromb Res 1985;39:1-8.

42. Beitz J, Beitz A, Antonov IV, Misharin AY, Mest HJ. Does a HDL injection reduce the development of serum hyperlipidemia and progression of fatty streaks in cholesterol fed rabbits? Prostagland Leukotr Ess Fatty Acids 1992;47:149-152.

43. Franceschini G, Vecchio V, Gianfranceschi G, Magani D, Sirtori CR. Apolipoprotein AI_{Milano}. Accelerated binding and dissociation from lipids of a human apolipoprotein variant. J Biol Chem 1985;260:16321-16325.

44. Roma P, Gregg RE, Meng MS, et al. In vivo metabolism of a mutant form of apolipoprotein A-I, apo A-I_{Milano}, associated with familial hypoalphalipoproteinemia. J Clin Invest 1993; 91:1445-1452.

45. Booth RFG, Martin JF, Honey AC, Hassall DG, Beesley JE, Moncada S. Rapid development of atherosclerotic lesions in the rabbit carotid artery by perivascular manipulation. Atherosclerosis 1989;76:257-268.

EXPLORATIONS OF POST PRANDIAL LIPIDS IN A CASE OF HOMOZYGOUS APO B45.2

Bernard Jacotot, Alain Piolot, Marise Ayraut-Jarrier, Nicole Lemort, Claude Martin, Sylvie Braschi, Frances Yen, and Bernard Bihain.
Unité INSERM 391 et Service de Médecine Interne
Hôpital Henri Mondor
94000 Créteil
FRANCE

Introduction

Hypobetalipoproteinemia is a rare disease, with autosomic dominant transmission characterized by a low plasma concentration or an absence of apolipoprotein (apo)B and reduced plasma levels of VLDL-cholesterol (VLDL-C) and LDL-cholesterol (LDL-C) [1-3]. The disease is due to a mutation of the apo-B gene, responsible for a truncated apo-B which is detected in the patient's lipoproteins. Heterozygous patients are asymptomatic and present LDL-C plasma levels comprising between 20 and 60 mg/dl. In the lipoproteins of these patients, it is possible to find the two isoforms of apo-B observed in a normal subject: apo-B100 and apo-B48, as well as the truncated apo-B. The exceptional homozygous cases have a LDL-C level below 10 mg/dl and clinical manifestations, such as fat and liposoluble vitamin malabsorption, mental retardation, ataxia, and acanthocytosis of red blood cells [4,5].

Routine examination of a 48-year-old woman revealed severe hypocholesterolemia (70 mg/dl), a very low apo-B level (0.10 mg/dl), the absence of LDL in lipoprotein electrophoresis profiles, and the absence of apo-B100 and apoB48 [6].

These abnormalities were completely asymptomatic; the clinical exam yielded strictly normal results. There was no malabsorption; the plasma levels of vitamin A and of vitamin E were normal. The apo-B present in the plasma was a truncated apo-B45.2, resulting from a mutation on exon 26 of the apo-B gene (transversion T→A on the nucleotide 6368). This mutation converts TYR 2053 to a premature stop-codon [7].

Taking into account the important role of the apo-B48 and the apo-B100 in the triglyceride-rich (TG-rich) lipoprotein metabolism, we studied the postprandial lipoprotein metabolism in this case where these two forms of apoB were absent.

A.M. Gotto et al. (eds.), Multiple Risk Factors in Cardiovascular Disease, 75-79.
© 1995 *Kluwer Academic Publishers and Fondazione Giovanni Lorenzini.*

Methods

The study of postprandial lipoprotein metabolism was performed after an oral fat load in the hypobetalipoproteinemic patient (MS) and in a healthy control subject (LFW) with the same sex, age and body mass index.

After 12 hours of fasting, a venous catheter was installed in the forearm. After twenty minutes, a blood sample was obtained and designated as the fasting sample. The patient then ingested a test meal within 15 minutes, comprising of 1,000 kcal with 50% lipids, 30% carbohydrates, 20% proteins, and 100,000 units of vitamin A esters. The blood samples were taken at the following times after the meal was consumed: 1 hour, 2 hours, 3 hours, 4 hours, 6 hours, 8 hours, 12 hours, and 24 hours. During this period, there was no alimentary intake; only water was ingested. Triglycerides (TG) were analyzed by enzymatic method (kit Boeringher, Mannheim). Retinyl-palmitate (RP) was assayed, after extraction by hexane, by HPLC, according to De Ruyter and De Leenher [8]. These assays were performed: 1) on the whole plasma, 2) on the chylomicron fraction (obtained by plasma centrifugation at 18,000 rpm (6.10^5 g.mn, 30 min, 10°C), and 3) on the fraction remaining after removal of chylomicrons.

Results

After meal consumption, the TG concentration (Figure 1) reached a peak 2 times both in the patient and in the control: 1) the first peak that was small at t=1 hour and 2) the second peak that was at t=6 hours. This second peak was higher in the patient (MS) than in the control (LFW). TG of the chylomicron fraction was two-fold higher in MS than in LFW, with a delay in its disappearance in MS. The area under the curve was greatly increased in MS as compared with LFW. The reduction of chylomicron clearance was also apparent when compared the ratio of chylomicron TG/whole plasma TG (Table 1). Although the plasma RP peak occurred 8 hours after the meal for both subjects, the RP concentrations (of whole plasma and chylomicron free fraction) were much higher in MS (4-fold the control values) (Figure 2).

Discussion

The observation reported here is exceptional because it concerns a totally asymptomatic homozygous truncated apo-B case. The rare case of homozygous truncated apo-B reported elsewhere presented neurological symptoms, as well as fat and vitamin malabsorption [4,9]. However, in this study two cases of apo-87 from the same family were asymptomatic.

In these cases, apo-48 was present in the plasma lipoproteins. On the other hand, apo-B87 and apo-B100 were somewhat nearby. In patient MS, the premature stop of apo-B synthesis at the codon 2035 allowed the production of apo-B45.2; however, neither apo-B48 nor apo-B100 could be synthesized. Interestingly, the carboxy-terminal portion of the apo-B missing in patient MS comprises the binding site reported for the apo-B,E membrane receptor.

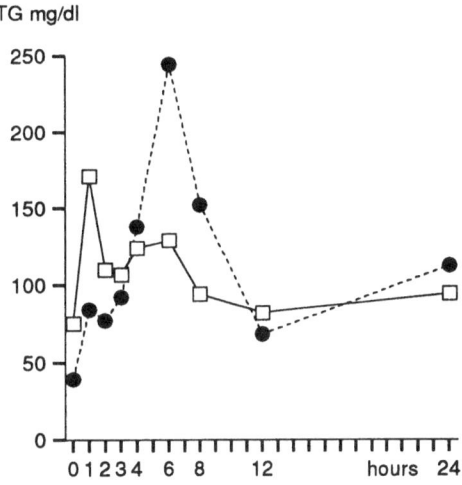

Figure 1. Plasma triglycerides after fat load test.
□=LWF; ●=MS.

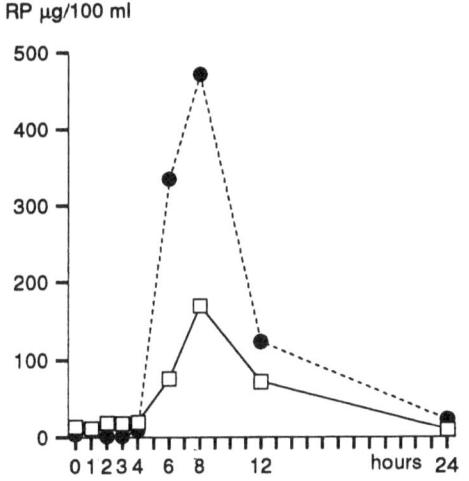

Figure 2. Plasma retinyl palmitate after fat and vitamin A load test.
□=LWF; ●=MS.

Table 1. Chylomicrons TG/whole plasma TG ratio in lipoproteins after fat load test.

Hours	0	1	2	3	4	6	8	12
Chylomicrons TG / whole plasma TG								
M.S.	0.26	0.44	0.38	0.28	0.33	0.38	0.27	0.09
L.F.W.	0.08	0.37	0.12	0.13	0.19	0.25	0.13	0.037

The study of postprandial metabolism of TG and vitamin A confirms that intestinal lipid absorption is adequate in our patient. Chylomicrons were increased, suggesting a normal production of intestinal apo-B45.2, which replace the normal apoB-48 in the chylomicrons. The chylomicron and remnant catabolism seems slower in patient MS, compared to the control. This could be explained by a reduction of the chylomicron hydrolysis, as well as a delay in the removal of their remnants from the plasma. These results could indicate that the 100 AA fragment lacking in the apo-B-45.2 is critical for the postprandial lipoprotein catabolism.

Moreover, this observation shows that a subject having practically no LDL, can live normally. The LDLs originating from the intravascular catabolism of VLDL have two major functions: a) by their binding with LDL-receptors, they provide cholesterol to cells and contribute to the intracellular cholesterol regulation [10] and, b) by lipid exchanges with HDL, they participate in the reverse transport of cholesterol to the liver [11]. The absence of LDL in patient MS most likely induces compensatory mechanisms allowing the maintenance of correct lipid homeostasis. Moreover, the absence of LDL, or the low levels observed in other members of the MS family (heterozygous cases), gives some protection against atherosclerosis lesions.

References

1.   Gabelli C. The lipoprotein metabolism of apolipoprotein B mutants. Curr Opin Lipidol 1992;3:208-214.
2.   Young SG. Recent progress in understanding apolipoprotein B. Circulation 1990;82:1574-1594.
3.   Linton MF, Farese RV Jr, Young SG. Familial hypobetalipoproteinemia. J. Lipid Res 1993;34:521-541.
4.   Malloy MJ, Kane JP, Hardman DA, Hamilton RL, Dalal KB. Normotriglyceridemic abetalipoproteinemia. Absence of the B-100 apolipoprotein. J Clin Invest 1981;67:1441-1450.
5.   Hardman DA, Pullinger CR, Hamilton RL, Kane JP, Malloy MJ. Molecular and metabolic basis for the metabolic disorder normotriglyceridemic abetalipo-proteinemia. J Clin Invest 1991;88:1722-1729.
6.   Ayrault-Jarrier M, Piolot A, Lemort N, et al. Absence of apolipoproteins B100 and

B48 in a 48 year old female in perfect health. Metabolic exploration of first case of apo B45.2 homozygote. In preparation.

7. Young SG, Bihain B, Flynn LM, Sanan DA, Ayrault-Jarrier M, Jacotot B. Asymptomatic homozygous hypobetalipoproteinemia associated with apolipoprotein B 45.2. Hum Molecular Gen 1994;3:741-744.

8. De Ruyter MCM, De Leenher AP. Simultaneous determination of retinol and retinyl esters in serum or plasma by reversed phase high performance liquid chromatography. Clin Chem 1978;24:1920-1923.

9. Gabelli C, Martini S, Bilato C, Bertolini S, Corti MC, Crepaldi G, Baggio G. Apolipoprotein B mutants: Impact on low density lipoprotein levels and metabolism. In: Stein O, Eisenberg S, Stein Y, editors. Atherosclerosis IX. Tel Aviv: R & L Creative Comm Ltd, 1992:243-250.

10. Brown MS, Goldstein JL. A receptor mediated pathway for cholesterol homeostasis. Science 1986;232:34-47.

11. Miller GJ, Miller NE. Plasma high density lipoprotein cholesterol and development of ischaemic heart disease. Lancet 1975;1:16-19.

APOLIPOPROTEIN E BINDING AND HEPATIC LIPASE-MEDIATED CATABOLISM MAKE ALTERNATE PATHWAYS IN THE METABOLISM OF INTERMEDIATE LIPOPROTEIN PARTICLES: OBSERVATION IN PATIENTS WITH HEPATIC LIPASE DEFICIENCY

Akira Yamamoto, Yasuyuki Ikeda, Zenta Tsutsumi, Atsuo Mori, Atsuko Takagi, and Motoo Tsushima*
Department of Etiology and Pathophysiology
National Cardiovascular Center Research Institute
*Department of Medicine
National Cardiovascular Center Hospital
Suita, Osaka 565
JAPAN

Introduction

The metabolism of triglyceride-rich lipoprotein particles (chylomicrons and VLDL) is initiated by the hydrolysis of triglyceride by lipoprotein lipase. In *in vitro* studies, where a sufficient amount of apolipoprotein C-II (apo C-II) is provided, the hydrolysis continues near the terminal state until almost all triglyceride is degraded. However, in the circulation of the living body, a considerable amount of intermediate metabolites, that is, so-called remnants or intermediate density lipoproteins (IDL) are present, in addition to LDL, the end product of VLDL.

The increase of such intermediate particles takes place in some pathological states related to atherosclerotic vascular diseases. It has been speculated that the intermediate lipoprotein particles or the remnant are metabolized by 1) the clearance through LDL receptors or so-called remnant receptors mediated by the specific affinity binding of apolipoprotein E (apo E) to the receptors, and 2) by further degradation of lipid components by hepatic lipase, which is present on the cell surface of sinusoidal endothelium. However, in contrast to lipoprotein lipase, the physiological function and the major target of the catalytic activity of hepatic lipase have not yet been clearly identified. Patients with hepatic lipase deficiency seem to be an important model for understanding the physiological role of this enzyme. But only a few families with this disease have been reported [1-4], and available data are not sufficient because hyperlipoproteinemia is strongly modified by nutrition and the presence of other hereditary factors or underlying metabolic diseases.

Recently, we found a patient with severe depletion of hepatic lipase in postheparin

A.M. Gotto et al. (eds.), Multiple Risk Factors in Cardiovascular Disease, 81-87.

plasma (PHP) and could identify the site of mutation in this lipase gene. Besides this case, we have experienced several patients with this enzyme deficiency, which was suspected to be due to the hereditary predisposition. In this presentation, we would like to report the specific feature of plasma lipoprotein lipid composition in hepatic lipase deficiency and discuss the role of this enzyme in the metabolism of triglyceride-rich lipoproteins and its relation to the apo E-mediated metabolism of intermediate lipoprotein particles.

Materials and Methods

We have screened about 500 patients with hyperlipoproteinemia, who have visited our National Cardiovascular Center Hospital, for lipoprotein lipase and hepatic lipase in PHP by use of a newly developed assay system [5]. Enzyme protein mass was assayed by sandwich enzyme immunoassay using two different mouse antihuman lipoprotein lipase or antihuman hepatic lipase monoclonal antibodies, each recognizing a different epitope of the enzyme protein. Enzyme protein mass levels were expressed as Δ lipoproptein lipase (LPL) and Δ hepatic (triglyceride) lipase (HTGL), the difference of postheparin from preheparin levels. The value of each enzyme protein mass in PHP showed a good correlation with the value of the enzyme activity, which was measured by a selective immunoinactivation assay, also developed in our laboratory [6].

The proband with complete deficiency in hepatic lipase was a 49-year-old male. Other two male patients aged 48 and 67 showed a marked reduction of the enzyme (327 and 162 ng/ml; less than 25% of the average in the normal control). Fifteen healthy male volunteers aged 39 ± 9 years (HTGL mass 1456 ± 469 ng/ml, serum triglyceride 150 mg/dl or less, and cholesterol 250 mg/dl or less) and 4 male patients with type IV hyperlipoproteinemia according to the WHO standards aged 39 ± 11 years (HTGL mass in normal range, serum triglyceride 302 ± 81 mg/dl, cholesterol 250 mg/dl or less) were used as controls for this study. We selected only males, because hepatic lipase is affected by estrogen and the value in PHP varies with age in females.

Results

HOMOZYGOUS HEPATIC LIPASE DEFICIENCY AND LIPOPROTEIN LIPID COMPOSITION

The proband MS with a complete deficiency in hepatic lipase in his PHP had a missense mutation in exon 2 of the hepatic lipase gene. All his children, including three sons and one daughter, showed heterozygosity for this mutation by the restriction enzyme fragment analysis of the hepatic lipase gene, although their serum lipid levels were in normal range. A 222 base pair band of normal hepatic lipase gene was divided into two smaller bands (188 and 34 base pair bands) in the proband, and all his children showed 222 and 188 bands.

The most impressive laboratory finding was the appearance of blood serum; it was not turbid like type IV hyperlipoproteinemia even if serum triglyceride was as high as 320 mg/dl. Lipid analysis of lipoprotein fractions obtained by ultracentrifugation showed that the increased triglyceride distributed mainly in LDL (105 mg/dl) and HDL (80 mg/dl) fractions. Density gradient ultracentrifugation revealed a peak of LDL, which showed a deviation into a lighter range (from d=1.059 of the control to 1.032) and the treatment of this patient's LDL with hepatic lipase resulted in the shift of this peak into the normal range. The average size of LDL particles of the proband (24.1 nm) was within the normal range (24.03 ± 0.34 nm).

The increase in IDL fraction was not so remarkable and the VLDL triglyceride did not show an increase compared to the samples from healthy controls. Agarose gel electrophoresis of VLDL of the proband did not show a broad β band peculiar to type III hyperlipoproteinemia and the ratio of VLDL-cholesterol to triglyceride (0.21) was within the normal range (Table 1).

Table 1. Lipids in blood serum and in the VLDL fraction in patients with different types of hypertriglyceridemia.

Subject	1 MS	2 SN	3 NM	4 TT
Phenotype	HL-deficiency	type IV	type III	Normal
Serum-TG	320 mg/dl	374	381	136
Serum-ch	204	214	246	187
VLDL-TG	90	260	280	90
VLDL-ch	19	66	115	16
VLDL-ch/TG	0.21	0.25	0.41	0.18

CORRELATION OF THE LIPID COMPONENT OF SERUM LIPOPROTEIN FRACTIONS WITH HEPATIC LIPASE MASS IN PHP

The lipoprotein lipid composition was analyzed in patients with hepatic lipase deficiency, those with Type IV hyperlipoproteinemia, and the normal controls and the correlation with hepatic lipase mass in PHP was studied. The increase in IDL was found in both hepatic lipase deficiency and Type IV hyperlipoproteinemia and there was no significant difference in its lipid and apolipoprotein composition of IDL between these two types of hypertriglyceridemia.

The ratio of triglyceride to apo B in LDL fraction was calculated as a measure of triglyceride content of the LDL particle. It was obviously high in the patients with hepatic lipase deficiency, but there was no difference between the patients with Type IV hyperlipoproteinemia and the normolipidemic healthy volunteers. Hepatic lipase mass in PHP inversely correlated with LDL-triglyceride with a high correlation coefficient. The correlation became much stronger when the ratio of LDL-triglyceride to apo B ratio was used as a parameter in place of LDL-triglyceride. There was also a significant correlation between hepatic lipase mass in PHP and HDL-triglyceride. (Ikeda, Y. et al., Multiple Risk Factors in Cardiovascular Disease, Proceedings of the 2nd International Symposium on Multiple Risk Factors in Cardiovascular Disease, Churchill-Livingstone, Tokyo, in press).

LOCALIZATION OF HEPATIC LIPASE IN THE LIVER

It has been thought that hepatic lipase is localized on the vascular surface of the sinusoidal endothelium. Recently Ikeda and Takaichi succeeded in taking an electron micrograph with immunochemical staining using specific antibody and showed the localization of this enzyme on the surface of hepatocytes facing the Disse's space. Although some of the gold-labelled enzyme was detected on the surface of the sinusoidal endothelium facing Disse's space, the density was much smaller than on the hepatocytes. Hepatic lipase is originally synthesized in and transferred to the surface of hepatocytes. As the size of triglyceride-rich LDL, the most suitable substrate of this enzyme, is much smaller than chylomicrons and VLDL, it is reasonable that the enzyme is present on the surface of hepatocytes instead of sinusoidal endothelium.

Discussion

Our present results on the change in lipoprotein lipid composition are consistent with the results of our basic study on the kinetics of the enzymology on lipoprotein lipase and hepatic lipase (Tsutsumi, Z. et al. in preparation). Lipoprotein lipase was very active in metabolizing triglyceride in chylomicrons, VLDL, and IDL, while hepatic lipase more readily hydrolyzed triglyceride in LDL and HDL than lipoprotein lipase. Hepatic lipase essentially can affect all lipoproteins in the blood stream. However, it differs from lipoprotein lipase in the strength of its action. Hepatic lipase mainly works on triglyceride-rich LDL and HDL *in vivo*, and strongly affects the triglyceride content of LDL and HDL.

Recently Clay et al. compared the lipoprotein composition in humans and rabbits and mentioned that rabbit lipoproteins were relatively enlarged, enriched in triglyceride, and depleted of cholesteryl esters [7]. They incubated the lipoprotein in the presence of hepatic lipase and found that both HDL and LDL reduced their size as the enzyme degraded triglyceride in these lipoproteins. The results of our present investigation essentially agreed with their results and suggest that those people with hepatic lipase deficiency are susceptible to hyperlipidemia when they eat a high-fat diet.

It has been suggested by Havel and Yamada that there are two kinds of VLDL particles; one with apo E in addition to apo B as major constitutional apoproteins and the other with apo B and no apo E [8]. Evidence has accumulated showing that apo E functions as a mediator for lipoprotein binding to the cell surface receptors: 1) the apo E concentration on lipid particles increases their affinity to the cell surface [9]; 2) the injection or overexpression of apo E enhances the clearance of VLDL [10]; and 3) those with apo E2 allele have higher VLDL-triglyceride and IDL levels with a lower LDL compared to those with E3 and E4 [11].

Lipoprotein lipase can almost completely hydrolyze triglyceride in VLDL and convert it into triglyceride-rich LDL if enough apo C-II is provided. But apo C-II tends to bind to the surface of lipid particles of larger size [12] and, therefore, the possibility for lipoprotein lipase to attack triglyceride-rich particles in the circulation seems to be limited. When apo E- concentration is high as in the cases of type III hyperlipoproteinemia, intermediate lipoproteins derived from VLDL become apo E and cholesterol-rich in the presence of cholesteryl ester transfer protein (CETP) and less liable to the degradation by lipoprotein lipase, leading to the accumulation of IDL and β-VLDL. The peculiar feature of the hepatic lipase deficiency is an increase of triglyceride in HDL and LDL fractions. In the proband of this study with a complete deficiency in hepatic lipase, the increase of triglyceride was almost limited to LDL and HDL fractions and the blood serum was not turbid. Although there was also an increase in IDL to some extent, the intermediate lipoprotein particles were not as cholesterol-rich as β-VLDL.

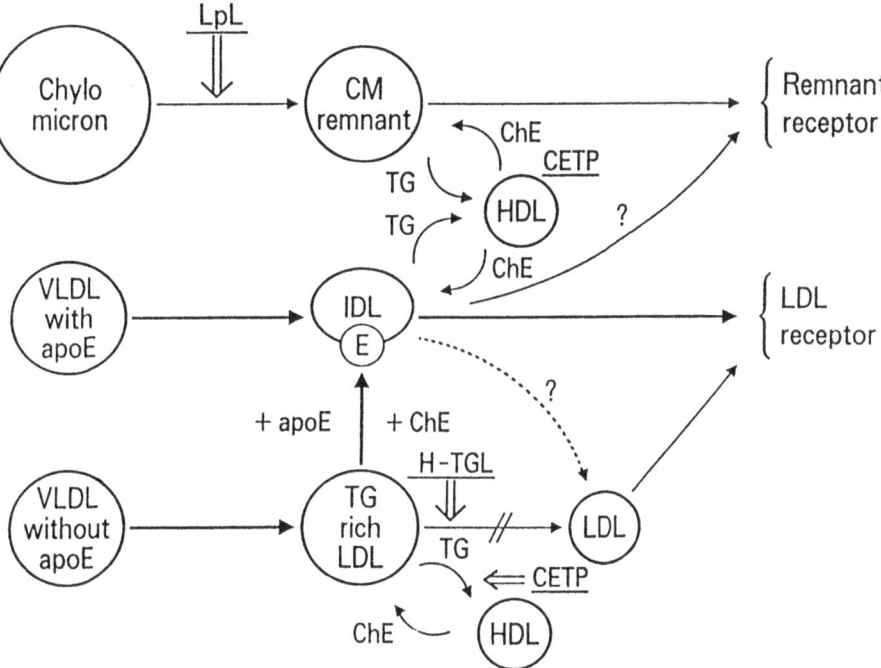

Figure 1. Metabolism of triglyceride-rich lipoproteins.

The fate of the triglyceride-rich LDL in hepatic lipase deficiency is still not clear. As HDL is also triglyceride-rich, the efficiency of the action of CETP should be reduced and the conversion of triglyceride-rich LDL into IDL-like particles should be limited.

One of the physiological functions of hepatic lipase seems to be in increasing the efficiency of the transport of cholesteryl esters from HDL to VLDL and intermediate lipoproteins by reducing the triglyceride concentration in HDL. In this case, apo E-mediated uptake plays a role in the uptake of intermediate lipoproteins into hepatocytes when enough apo E is provided. But, at the same time, hepatic lipase affects the metabolism of LDL. When apo E concentration in Disse's space is low, triglyceride-rich LDL and IDL are hydrolyzed by hepatic lipase and the reaction products could be taken up by hepatocytes if LDL-receptors are fully expressed. Therefore, apo E-mediated uptake and the hydrolyses by hepatic lipase make alternative pathways of the metabolism of intermediate metabolites of triglyceride-rich lipoproteins and also LDL (Figure 1).

References

1. Carlson LA, Holmquist L, Nilsson-Ehle P. Deficiency of hepatic lipase activity in post-heparin plasma in familial hyper-α-triglyceridemia. Acta Med Scand 1986;219:435-47.

2. Hegele RA, Little JA, Vezina C, et al. Hepatic lipase deficiency. Clinical, biochemical and molecular genetic characteristics. Arterioscl Thromb 1993;13:720-28.

3. Yamamura T, Sudo H, Matsuzawa Y, Yamamoto A. Familial hyperlipoproteinemia showing an interconversion between type III and V with a trait of xeroderma pigmentosum. Med J Osaka Univ 1979;30:5-14.

4. Auwerx JH, Babirak SP, Hokamson JE, et al. Coexistance of abnormalities of hepatic lipase and lipoprotein lipase in a large family. Am J Hum Genet 1990;46:470-77.

5. Ikeda Y, Takagi A, Ohkaru Y, et al. A sandwich-enzyme immunoassay for the quantification of lipoprotein lipase and hepatic lipase in post-heparin plasma using monoclonal antibodies to the corresponding enzymes. J Lipid Res 1990;31:1911-24.

6. Ikeda Y, Takagi A, Yamamoto A. Purification and characterization of lipoprotein lipase and hepatic triglyceride lipase from human postheparin plasma: Production of monospecific antibody to the individual lipase. Biochim Biophys Acta 1989;1003:254-69.

7. Clay MA, Hopkins GJ, Ehnholm CP, Barter PJ. The rabbit as an animal model of hepatic lipase deficiency. Biochim Biophys Acta 1989;1002:173-81.

8. Yamada N, Shames DM, Stoudemire JB, Havel RJ. Metabolism of lipoproteins containing apolipoprotein B-100 in blood plasma of rabbits: Heterogeneity related to the presence of apolipoprotein E. Proc Natl Acad Sci USA 1986;83:3479-83.

9. Funahashi T, Yokoyama S, Yamamoto A. Association of apolipoprotein E with the low density lipoprotein receptor: Demonstration of its co-operativity on lipid microemulsion particles. J Biochem (Tokyo) 1989;105:582-87.

10.   Yamada N, Shimano H, Mokuno H, et al. Increased clearance of plasma cholesterol after injection of apolipoprotein E into Watanabe heritable hyperlipidemic rabbits. Proc Natl Acad Sci USA 1989;86:665-69.

11.   Mahley RW. Apolipoprotein E: Cholesterol transport protein with expanding role in cell biology. Science 1988;240:622-30.

12.   Tajima S, Yokoyama S, Kawai Y, Yamamoto A. Behavior of apolipoprotein C-II in an aqueous solution. J Biochem (Tokyo)1982;91:1273-79.

NEW ASPECTS OF THE PHARMACOLOGY OF DIHYDROPYRIDINE CALCIUM ANTAGONISTS

Théophile Godfraind, Olivier Feron, Nicole Morel, Salvatore Salomone, and Maurice Wibo
Laboratoire de Pharmacologie
Université Catholique de Louvain, FARL 5410
1200 Bruxelles
BELGIUM

Introduction

Classical calcium antagonists belong to different chemical families: the diphenylpiperazines, the dihydropyridines, the diphenylalkylamines, and the benzothiazepines. Therefore, in the 1960's a question often raised was: "How could such diverse drugs show similar pharmacological properties?" The response is indicated by recent molecular biology studies showing that distinct sites on the α_1 subunit of L-type calcium channels interact with calcium channel modulators. The question which is raised now is the following: "Are there pharmacological differences among the new dihydropyridine derivatives?"

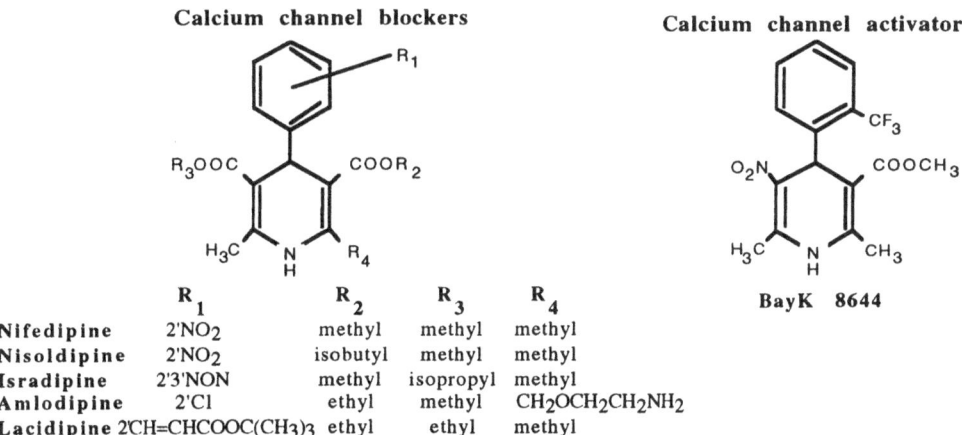

Calcium channel blockers

Calcium channel activator

BayK 8644

	R₁	R₂	R₃	R₄
Nifedipine	2'NO2	methyl	methyl	methyl
Nisoldipine	2'NO2	isobutyl	methyl	methyl
Isradipine	2'3'NON	methyl	isopropyl	methyl
Amlodipine	2'Cl	ethyl	methyl	CH2OCH2CH2NH2
Lacidipine	2'CH=CHCOOC(CH3)3	ethyl	ethyl	methyl

Figure 1. Structures of 1,4-dihydropyridine calcium channel modulators discussed in this paper.

A.M. Gotto et al. (eds.), Multiple Risk Factors in Cardiovascular Disease, 89-96.

Figure 1 illustrates the chemical structures showing dissimilarities which do not seem to be so important. However, when examining the effect of various dihydropyridines in several isolated preparations, different pharmacological profiles may be delineated considering: the characteristics of the drug; the properties of the tissue; and the characteristics of the stimulus.

This paper deals with a discussion of some of those factors, mainly in the cardiovascular field. In this presentation, examples of drug characteristics will be discussed, namely their voltage-dependency and its relation to vascular selectivity (in the case of nisoldipine) and their interaction with storage sites located close to L-calcium channels allowing a pseudo-irreversible interaction with the inactivated state of the channel (in the case of lacidipine). It will be shown that tissue-specific and development-regulated expression of calcium channel α_1 subunit isoforms might be involved in tissue selectivity. We will also show that abnormalities of calcium channels in arteries from hypertensive animals may increase their sensitivity to calcium channel modulators.

Diversity of Calcium Channels and of Calcium Antagonists Binding Sites

Calcium channels may be identified by combined electrophysiological and pharmacological techniques. Tsien and colleagues [1] identified different channels which they called L, T, and N according to their sensitivity to membrane potential variation and to their kinetics of inactivation. Other channels have been identified in the central nervous system. Cardiac and smooth muscle α_1 proteins are homologous and are splicing products of the type 2 calcium channel gene (CaCh2) which is distinct from the CaCh1 gene encoding the skeletal α_1 subunit [1]. Although they constitute a heterogenous chemical group, all calcium antagonists interact with the α_1 subunit of the L-type calcium channel. Diebold et al. [2] have reported in the rat heart that the α_1 subunit gene generates developmentally regulated isoforms IVS3A and IVS3B. Recently, those isoforms have been expressed in CHO cells [3]. We have quantified the splicing events in different tissues [4]. cDNA fragments encoding a representative region of the L-type calcium channel α_1 subunit of different tissues were amplified by polymerase chain reaction (PCR). In the region of the third (S3) and fourth (S4) transmembrane segments, we observed primary structure variations corresponding to alternative splicing phenomenons. We perfected the RT-PCR method (polymerase chain reaction from reverse transcribed mRNA) to determine the amount of the different splice variants in various tissues and species and their ontogeny. In the mutually exclusive alternative splicing of the IVS3 segment, there is a prevalence of one isoform (IVS3B) with, however, important discrepancies in the amount of both trancripts according to the nature of the tissue studied. We also observed in rat brain that the proportion of isoform IVS3B increased in function of maturation and aging. Furthermore, we reported that a 33 bp-cassette located in the loop between IVS3 and IVS4 is ubiquitously proned to splicing but rarely excluded from the gene product, except at the embryonic and early postnatal stage of development.

The localization of the binding sites for calcium antagonists on the cell membrane has been explored by radioligand and by electrophysiological experiments. The binding sites of dihydropyridines are located at the external surface of the cell membrane as indicated by the observations that charged dihydropyridines or related drugs (such as the quaternary ammonium compound pinaverium) have access to their receptors when given extracellularly [5,6]. On the other hand, D600, the derivative of verapamil, is active from the inside of the cardiac cell [7], but there is good evidence that diltiazem is bound extracellularly [8].

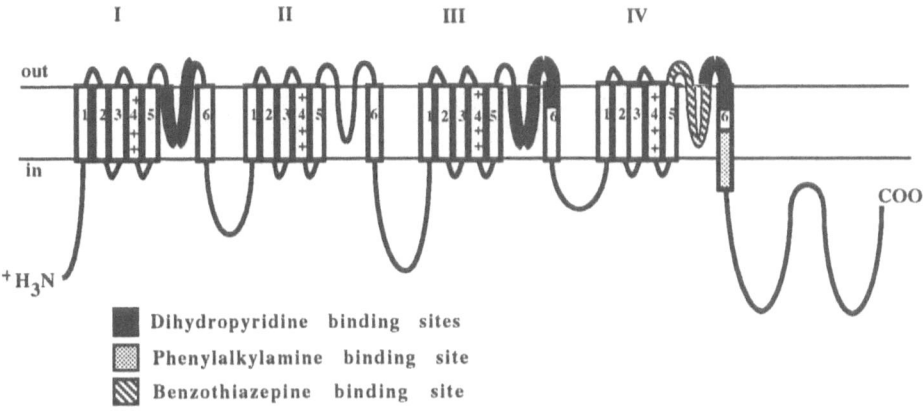

Figure 2. Location of calcium antagonist binding sites.

Catterall et al. [9] have further localized the molecular areas of dihydropyridine binding in antibody mapping experiments, and have obtained evidence for the extracellular orientation of the site. Their experiments indicate that the core of the dihydropyridine binding site is constituted, in part, by the transmembrane segment IIIS6, specifically labelled with isradipine (PN 200-110). Extracellular segments of the α_1 subunit located between transmembrane segments S5 and S6 of repeat I and IV [10] constitute other sites for drug binding and are located close to segment IIIS6 in the folded structure of the α_1-subunit. When the three-dimensional structure of the 1,4-dihydropyridine receptor is considered, possible interactions can be predicted between calcium channel modulators. Figure 2 illustrates the location of those binding sites including phenylakylamine binding sites localized by Striessnig et al. [11] and the benzothiazepine binding site studied by Watanabe et al. [12].

Pharmacodynamic Differences among Dihydropyridines

Comparison of calcium antagonist effects on vascular and on cardiac contraction has revealed that the ratio of IC_{50} values estimated respectively in isolated heart and in isolated vessels varies according to the molecule tested. *In vitro* mechanical studies on human tissues (arterial and cardiac preparations) have shown that the cardiovascular ratio is near 1 for diltiazem and verapamil, is equal to 14 for nifedipine, but to 1555 for nisoldipine. However, radioligand studies in membrane preparations have not shown that the affinity of nisoldipine differs markedly in cardiac and vascular membranes [13].

The inhibitory action of lacidipine, isradipine, and nisoldipine on contractions evoked by a depolarizing stimulus in arteries is characterized by a marked time-dependency, in which inhibition increases slowly after depolarization to attain a steady state value. This inhibitory pattern has not been observed with nifedipine, verapamil and diltiazem [13,14,15,16]. Preincubation of arteries with calcium antagonists in a solution which slightly depolarized the vessel, increased the inhibition of arterial contraction by nisoldipine but not by verapamil, diltiazem, or nifedipine, the increased inhibition of nisoldipine returned to predepolarization value when the preparations were transferred to normal physiological solution. The kinetics of inhibition of contraction in depolarized arteries followed the kinetics of binding to isolated membranes, indicating that the interaction of some dihydropyridines with the calcium channel conformation evoked by depolarization occurs during the stimulation of the intact artery and is responsible for the characteristic pattern of the contraction recorded in the presence of the calcium channel blocker [14,16].

The combination of voltage- and time-dependency contributes to the tissue selectivity of nisoldipine which may thus be related to tissue differences in the modulation of calcium channels. The slow time-course of the association of nisoldipine with its receptors in depolarized tissues might account for its comparatively low potency in cardiac muscle as compared with vascular smooth muscle. Taking into account the observation that the rate of association to the 1,4-dihydropyridine receptor in isolated membranes and the rate of inhibition of contraction in intact depolarized tissue follow a similar pseudo-first-order kinetics, it is easy to show that the drug concentration required for a given level of receptor occupancy is inversely related to the time of depolarization [17,18]. Assuming that, in first approximation, IC_{50} in depolarized tissue corresponds to 50% occupation of the receptor and that this occupation in human myocardial tissue is achieved by the end of systolic depolarization, that is 0.2 sec, the corresponding depolarization time in coronary arteries should be 0.2 times 1555 (the IC_{50} ratio mentioned above), that is 5.2 min, which is the time required to fully activate the smooth muscle. Clearly, the higher potency of nisoldipine in coronary arteries is mainly attributable to the longer duration of the depolarizing stimuli to which they are submitted. Further studies are required in order to characterize the role of L-type channel isoforms in tissue selectivity.

Lacidipine is known to have a long lasting inhibitory effect both *in vivo* and *in vitro* [19]. We have shown that inhibition by lacidipine of smooth muscle contraction persisted in depolarizing solution, even in the absence of the drug, whereas the action of isradipine was fully reversible (Figure 3) [16].

In radioligand experiments performed with membranes enriched in L-type calcium channels, we observed that the interaction of lacidipine with calcium channels was reversible and that the dissociation from the receptors followed a monoexponential kinetics, with a $t_{1/2}$ of 27 minutes, as compared to 11.7 minutes for isradipine. We could relate the persistent action of lacidipine in a drug-free solution to a storage site of lacidipine occurring in a cellular compartment characterized by membranes poor in cholesterol, different from the plasma membrane. The relation between this compartment and the dihydropyridine binding sites, which are accessible from the aqueous phase, still needs to be defined.

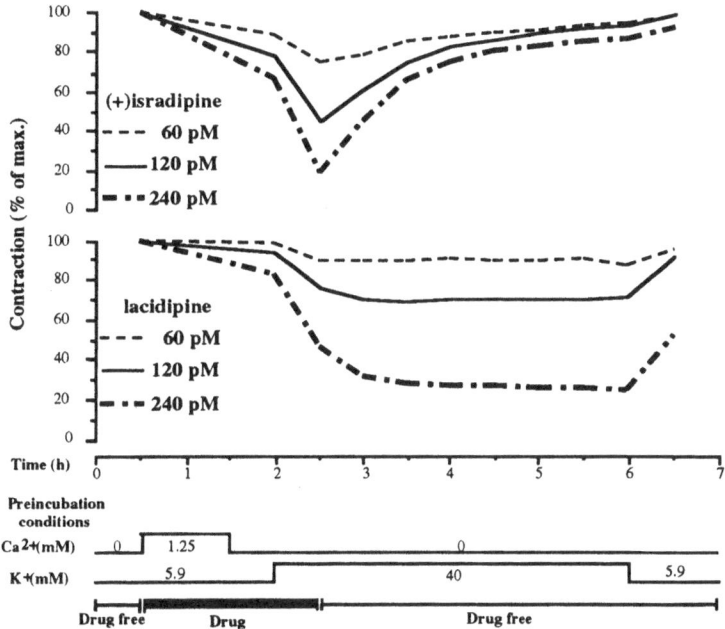

Figure 3. Reversal of (+)isradipine and lacidipine inhibition of K⁺-contraction of rat aorta, in drug-free Ca²⁺-deprived solutions. Ordinate scale: response to 100 mM K⁺-solution (containing 1.25 mM Ca²⁺) pulse of 2 min expressed as % of controls; abscissa scale: experimental time (h). Notice the increase of inhibition after preincubation in 40 mM K⁺-solution and its reversal after preincubation in physiological solution (5.9 mM K⁺). (Modified from ref. 16)

Influence of Age and Pathological Factors

Some characteristics of the tissue are also important in the sensitivity to the action of calcium antagonists. Neonatal hearts are more sensitive to the negative inotropic effect of calcium antagonists than adult hearts. We showed that in the neonatal heart, calcium channels controlling the contraction are mainly localized in the peripheral sarcolemma, whereas in the adult heart, most of the channels are associated with the junctional areas of T-tubules, in close vicinity to the terminal cisternae of sarcoplasmic reticulum from which the activator calcium originates [20]. It is known that the ontogenetic development of the cardiac contractile function is controlled by thyroid hormones. Therefore we have recently examined the influence of thyroid hormone on the postnatal development of excitation-contraction coupling. Newborn rats were made hypo- or hyperthyroid and several key constituents directly or indirectly involved in calcium signalling were investigated in membrane fractions from ventricular tissue collected on day 21. Hypo- and hyperthyroidism moderately decreased the myocardial density of 1,4-dihydropyridine and ryanodine receptors. The localisation of L-type channels was similar in hyperthyroid animals and in controls, i.e. mainly in junctional structures, whereas in hypothyroid rats, most 1,4-dihydropyridine receptors were associated with nonjunctional sarcolemma, as in newborn rats. Differences in subcellular localization were correlated with functional changes of calcium signalling and contractility [21].

Vessels from hypertensive animals are hypersensitive to vasoconstrictors but the reason is unknown. We reported that calcium channels in arteries of hypertensive animals exhibit an abnormally prolonged activation after withdrawal of the depolarizing stimulus that may be the cause of the increase in peripheral resistance. After a careful bioassay, we observed that long-term administration of some 1,4-dihydropyridines at dosages which significantly reduced blood pressure in hypertensive (SHR) rats, did not change the blood pressure of normotensive (WKY) rats, an indication for a specific action of calcium channel blockers as antihypertensive and not simply vasodilator agents, which is consistent with the observation that they are powerful remodelling agents able to suppress cardiac hypertrophy of hypertensive animals [22,23].

We also studied changes in contractile response and 1,4-dihydropyridine receptors occupation after such chronic administration of 1,4-dihydropyridines. We observed that the occupation of calcium channels by 1,4-dihydropyridines given per os was more marked in SHR than in WKY, resulting in different responses between the two strains. This observation was consistent with the higher affinity for calcium channel modulators we observed in SHR arteries *in vitro* when compared to WKY arteries. We also noticed that SHR arteries were more depolarized than WKY arteries and showed that this difference in sensitivity may be related to interaction kinetics with the receptors and might explain why the reduction of blood pressure by calcium antagonists is much more pronounced in hypertensives than in normotensives [23].

Several humoral factors have been proposed to play a role in the development of hypertension. An interesting observation we made is that low (threshold) concentrations of endothelin can sensitize vascular smooth muscle cells to the effects of various vasoconstrictor agonists [24]. Hypertension is associated with a hypersensitivity to the Ca^{2+} channel activator Bay K 8644, we investigated the effect of the endothelin ET_A receptor antagonist, BQ-123, on the contractions induced by Bay K 8644 in aorta from spontaneously hypertensive (SHR) and normotensive (WKY) rats. BQ-123 (1 µM) decreased the sensitivity to Bay K 8644 of aorta of SHR down to that of WKY. This observation is consistent with a role for endothelin in hypertension although the concentration estimated in hypertensive tissues is probably not sufficient to evoke an effect in resistance arteries, but endothelin could act as a growth factor and be responsible for hypertrophy in the cardiovascular system [25].

Concluding Remarks

In this paper we have shown that some calcium channel blockers of the dihydropyridine family exhibit different patterns of activity, although they all interact with the same molecular areas on the a_1 subunit of L-type calcium channel. Even if the pioneer proposition of blockade of calcium entry as a mechanism of drug action [26,27] is still sound, important pharmacodynamic differences may result from differences in calcium channel isoform profile and subcellular localization which are dependent on tissular and developmental factors. Finally, the sensitivity of a given tissue to the action of a given calcium channel blocker may be influenced by pathological conditions like hypertension.

References

1. Zhang JF, Randall AD, Ellinor PT, Horne WA, Sather WA, Tanabe T, Schwarz TL, Tsien RW. Distinctive pharmacology and kinetics of cloned neuronal Ca^{2+} channels and their possible counterparts in mammalian CNS neurons. Neuropharmacology 1993;32:1075-1088.
2. Diebold RJ, Koch WJ, Ellinor PT, et al. Mutually exclusive exon splicing of the cardiac calcium channel α_1 subunit gene generates developmentally regulated isoforms in the rat heart. Proc Natl Acad Sci USA 1992;89:1497-1501.
3. Welling A, Kwan YW, Bosse E, Flockerzi V, Hofmann F, Kass RS. Subunit-dependent modulation of recombinant L-type calcium channels: molecular basis for dihydropyridine tissue selectivity. Circ Res 1993;73:974-980.
4. Feron O, Octave JN, Christen MO, Godfraind T. Quantification of two splicing events in the L-type calcium channel α_1 subunit of intestinal smooth muscle and other tissues. Eur J Biochem 1994;222:195-202.
5. Kass RS, Arena JP, Chin S. Block of L-type calcium channels by charged dihydropyridines. Sensitivity to side of application and calcium. J Gen Physiol 1991;98:63-75.
6. Feron O, Wibo M, Christen MO, Godfraind T. Interaction of pinaverium (a quaternary ammonium compound) with 1,4-dihydropyridine binding site in rat ileum smooth muscle. Br J Pharmacol 1992;105:480-484.
7. Hescheler J, Pelzer D, Trube G, Trautwein W. Does the organic calcium channel blocker D600 act from inside or outside on the cardiac cell membrane? Pflügers Arch 1982;393:287-291.
8. Hering S, Savchenko A, Strubing C, Lakitsch M, Striessnig J. Extracellular localization of the benzothiazepine binding domain of L-type Ca^{2+} channels. Molec Pharmacol 1993;43:820-826.
9. Catterall WA, Striessnig J. Receptor sites for Ca^{2+} channel antagonists. Trends Pharmacol Sci 1992;13:256-262.
10. Kalasz H, Watanabe T, Yabana H, et al. Identification of 1,4-dihydropyridine binding domains within the primary structure of the α_1 subunit of the skeletal muscle L-type calcium channel. FEBS Lett 1993;331:177-181.
11. Striessnig J, Murphy BJ, Catterall WA. Dihydropyridine receptor of L-type Ca^{2+} channels: identification of binding domains for $[^3H](+)$-PN200-110 and $[^3H]$azidopine within the α_1 subunit. Proc Natl Acad Sci USA 1991;88:10769-10773.
12. Watanabe T, Kalasz H, Yabana H, et al. Azidobutyryl clentiazem, a new photoactivatable diltiazem analog, labels benzothiazepine binding sites in the α_1

subunit of the skeletal muscle calcium channel. FEBS Lett 1993;334:261-264.

13. Godfraind T, Salomone S, Dessy C, Verhelst B, Dion R, Schoevaerts J-C. Selectivity scale of calcium antagonists in the human cardiovascular system (based on in vitro studies). J Cardiovasc Pharmacol 1992;20(Suppl.5):S34-S39.

14. Wibo M, De Roth L, Godfraind T. Pharmacologic relevance of dihydropyridine binding sites in membranes from rat aorta: kinetic and equilibrium studies. Circ Res 1988;62:91-96.

15. Godfraind T, Dessy C, Salomone S. A comparison of the potency of selective L-calcium channel inhibitors in human coronary and internal mammary arteries exposed to serotonin. J Pharmacol Exp Ther 1992;263:112-122.

16. Salomone S, Godfraind T. Radioligand and functional estimates of the interaction of the 1,4-dihydropyridines, isradipine and lacidipine, with calcium channels in smooth muscle. Br J Pharmacol 1993;109:100-106.

17. Wibo M. Mode of action of calcium antagonists: voltage-dependence and kinetics of drug-receptor interaction. Pharmacol Toxicol 1989;65:1-8.

18. Godfraind T. Importance of kinetic parameters for the tissue selectivity of calcium antagonists. Biochem Pharmacol 1992;43:55-56.

19. Micheli D, Collodei A, Semeraro C, Gaviraghi G, Carpi C. Lacidipine: a calcium antagonist with potent and long-lasting antihypertensive effects in animal studies. J Cardiovasc Pharmacol 1990;15:666-675.

20. Wibo M, Bravo G, Godfraind T. Postnatal maturation of excitation-contraction coupling in rat ventricle in relation to the subcellular localization and surface density of 1,4-dihydropyridine and ryanodine receptors. Circ Res 1991;68:662-673.

21. Wibo M, Kolar F, Zheng L, Godfraind T. Dihydropyridine and ryanodine receptors in developing heart: influence of thyroid status. J Mol Cell Cardiol 1994;26:LXII.

22. Godfraind T, Kazda S, Wibo M. Effects of a chronic treatment by nisoldipine, a calcium antagonistic dihydropyridine, on arteries of spontaneously hypertensive rats. Circ Res 1991;68:674-682.

23. Morel N, Godfraind T. The antihypertensive action of the calcium antagonist amlodipine in relation with calcium channels ocupation in arteries. J Cardiovasc Pharmacol 1994;24:524-533.

24. Godfraind T, Mennig D, Morel N, Wibo M. Effect of endothelin-1 on calcium channel gating by agonists in vascular smooth muscle. J Cardiovasc Pharmacol 1989;13(Suppl.5):S112-S117.

25. Morel N, Godfraind, T. The endothelin ET_A receptor antagonist, BQ-123, normalizes the response of SHR aorta to Ca^{2+} channel activator. Eur J Pharmacol 1994;252:R3-R4.

26. Godfraind T, Polster P. Etude comparative de médicaments inhibant la réponse contractile de vaisseaux isolés d'origine humaine ou animale. Thérapie 1968; 23:1209-1220.

27. Godfraind T, Kaba A. Blockade or reversal of contraction induced by calcium and adrenaline in depolarized arterial smooth muscle. Br J Pharmacol 1969;36:549-560.

MEMBRANE INTERACTION OF LIPOPHILIC DIHYDROPYRIDINES AS NEW MECHANISMS FOR VASCULAR PROTECTION

Giovanni Gaviraghi and David Trist
Glaxo Research Laboratories
Via Fleming 4
37135 Verona
ITALY

Introduction

1,4-Dihydropyridines (DHPs) are calcium entry blockers which have proved to be important antihypertensive agents. These compounds all seem to bind to plasma membrane voltage operated calcium channels (VOCs), the consequence of which is to reduce the transport of calcium through these channels causing a relaxation of smooth muscles [1]. Following the classification of Spedding and Paoletti [2], DHPs can be considered as class 1A antagonists, that is they all seem to bind to a specific site on the L-type VOC.

Whilst DHPs share many common chemical features (see Figure 1), they express both pharmacological and physicochemical differences.

With the advent of second generation DHPs a slightly different classification can be envisaged. On kinetic criteria DHPs can be divided as outlined in Figure 2. The early DHPs, such as nifedipine have a fast onset and tend to be short-acting. Whereas, the more recent molecules, such as lacidipine and amlodipine, have a much slower onset, are long-acting and show more lipophilicity. For example, the log P for lacidipine is 5.4, whereas, the value for nifedipine is considerably lower at 2.2.

It is now known that DHPs can differ widely in their potency, selectivity, and duration across a number of different muscle preparations and in animal models of hypertension. In particular, the effect of these compounds in models of vascular damage varies considerably. The three compounds shown in Figure 1 can be used to demonstrate these points.

Vascular Protection in Hypertensive Models

A highly lipophilic molecule such as lacidipine demonstrates a number of advantageous characteristics not seen with other DHPs. Not only does the lipophilicity help explain its antihypertensive profile of high potency, long duration of action, vascular selectivity, and

A.M. Gotto et al. (eds.), Multiple Risk Factors in Cardiovascular Disease, 97-103.
© 1995 *Kluwer Academic Publishers and Fondazione Giovanni Lorenzini.*

slow onset of activity, but it may be a critical factor in vascular protection as seen in models related to hypertension and atherosclerosis [3-6].

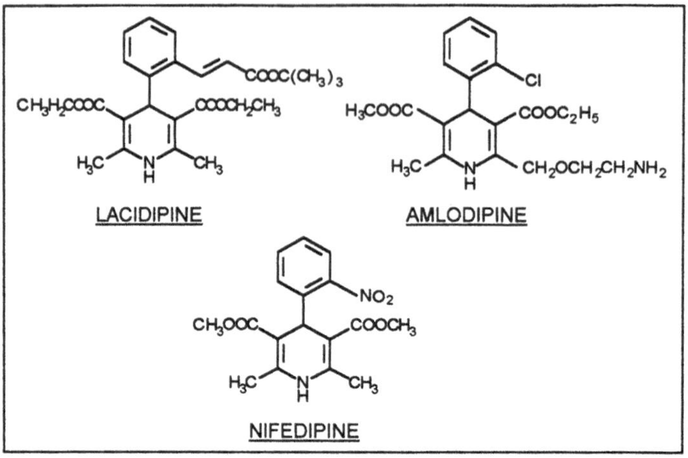

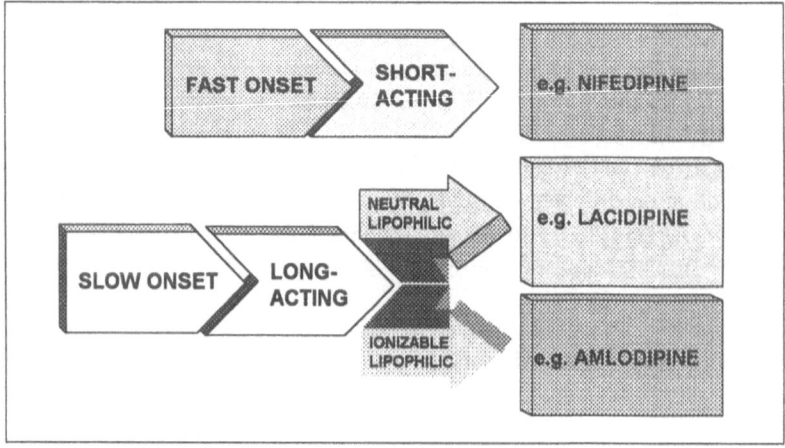

Figure 1. The structures of lacidipine, amlodipine and nifedipine, three 1,4-Dihydropyridines.

Figure 2. A kinetic classification of 1,4-Dihydropyridines.

Vascular protection could be defined as the capacity to inhibit or delay the development of arterial lesions [5]. These include changes in endothelial permeability, changes in smooth muscle proliferation, accumulation of connective tissue, and calcinosis.

The protective properties seen by DHPs can be ascribed to an antihypertensive activity. This has been clearly demonstrated for both lipophilic and less lipophilic molecules in animal models where excessive hypertension leads to both mortality and vascular and organ damage [3,4,7]. Unlike the less lipophilic DHPs, lacidipine has shown a vascular protective activity in hypertensive models at doses that do not block the development of hypertension (0.1-1.0 mg/kg, p.o., once daily) [4]. Thus, in the salt-loaded Dahl-S rat 0.3 mg/kg completely protects against mortality and damage to vessels such as the mesenteric artery [3]. In the stroke-prone SHR the same dose of lacidipine also protected against mortality and, importantly, abolished the damage to the brain and kidneys, two organs at risk in this animal model. Thus, other mechanisms need to be invoked to explain how a molecule like lacidipine protects against a deleterious calcium overload and maintains arterial endothelial and smooth muscle function.

Mechanism of Action of Lacidipine

The large log P for lacidipine translates experimentally into a high partition $K_{p(mem)}$ in model membrane systems. Thus, Herbette and his colleagues [8,9] have shown that lacidipine partitions much more than any other DHP into myocardial, phosphatidylcholine, multilamellar, membrane vesicles (MLV). A $K_{p(mem)}$ as high as ~136,000 can be achieved for lacidipine. The distribution of amlodipine and nifedipine is much less ($K_{p(mem)} = 21,300$ and 3,000, respectively). Not only does the lipophilic nature of lacidipine mean a large partition, but it also seems to determine where in the membrane the molecule resides. Small-angle x-ray scattering has revealed that the location of lacidipine is about 7 Å from the center of the membrane bilayer. Other DHPs, with less lipophilicity, are typically 12-16 Å from the center [10].

To explore further the contribution that lipophilicity makes to the mechanism of action of lacidipine, a series of experiments were carried out in rabbit basilar artery (RBA) following an initial observation by Salomone and Godfraind [11]. These authors showed that, whereas in depolarizing medium the relaxation of rat aorta due to lacidipine was only slowly reversed, in physiological medium the effect could be washed out. Therefore a protocol was designed to demonstrate the permanence of the lacidipine effect. RBA was depolarized with 60 mM KCl and when a sustained contraction was achieved the DHP was added. Figure 3A shows the effect upon adding nifedipine to the bath. The onset of relaxation was rapid and when achieved the tissue was washed with physiological medium for 30 minutes. After this time, a second depolarization exhibited a sustained contaction similar to that before the addition of nifedipine. Therefore, it seems that nifedipine has been very rapidly washed from the tissue. An identical experiment was performed using amlodipine instead of nifedipine (Figure 3B). The only difference was that the washout period was extended to 60 minutes. In this case, the expected slow onset of action was seen [12] but, like nifedipine, its effect was washed away in physiological medium. In the third experiment, lacidipine was added to the tissue (Figure 3C). The onset of action was slow, as expected [13], but the washout profile was completely different compared to the other two DHPs. Upon the second depolarization there was an initial contraction followed by an immediate relaxation, even though there was no compound in the bathing medium. Thus, lacidipine has a permanence not shown by either amlodipine or nifedipine.

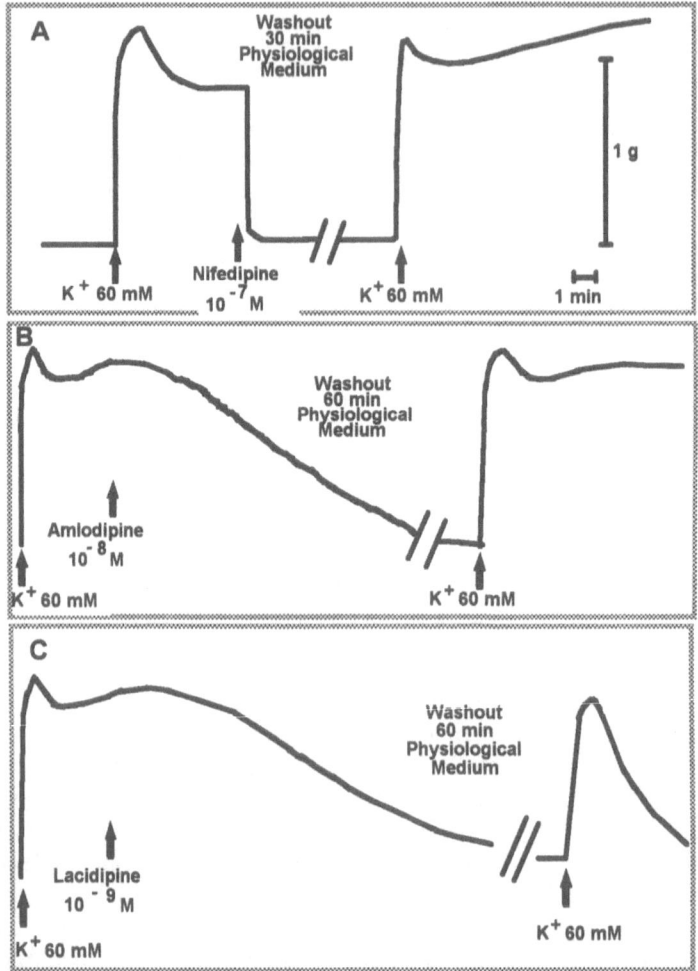

Figure 3. The Washout of 1,4-Dihydropyridines from Rabbit Basilar Artery.

Each trace is representative of four similar experiments. RBA was depolarized with 60 mM KCl and then either nifedipine 10^{-7}M (panel A), amlodipine 10^{-8}M (panel B) or lacidipine 10^{-9}M (panel C) were added. After a constant relaxation had been obtained, the tissues were washed with physiological medium (4.8 mM KCl) for either 30 or 60 minutes and them rechallenged with 60 mM KCl. For both nifedipine and amlodipine a sustained contraction was obtained. However, for lacidipine the initial contraction was immediately followed by a further relaxation. The magnitude of the contraction and the time interval shown in panel A are applicable to the other two panels.

The above results, might be interpreted in terms of a three-compartment model in series. This model is outlined in Figure 4 and tries to summarize the data obtained from the physicochemical studies as well as the experiments in RBA. It suggests that lacidipine enters the plasma membrane to a depth of 7 Å from the center. With time, lacidipine increases in the membrane until the proximate lipid adjacent to the VOC has sufficient concentration to form a reservoir. It is now known that the VOC exists in at least three states; resting, open, and inactive [14]. The channel is thought to spontaneously inactivate during depolarization. The evidence suggests that DHPs, like lacidipine, interact preferentially with the inactive state [14,15]. Thus, on depolarization, lacidipine can interact with its binding site on the inactive state of the channel. Upon repolarization, the channel returns to the resting state and the equilibrium for lacidipine is towards the reservoir in the lipid. Because of its position in the membrane lacidipine washes out slowly so that on subsequent depolarization the DHP is able to interact again with the channel as it inactivates.

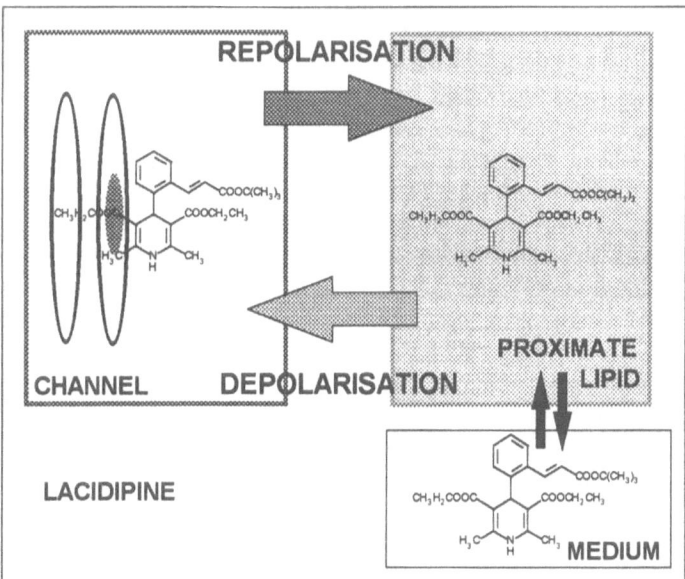

Figure 4. A compartmental model to explain the mechanism of action of lacidipine.

Conclusion

Although the structure of DHP CEBs may seem similar, their pharmacology and physicochemical properties are very diverse. In particular, lipophilic DHPs such as lacidipine exhibit a high partition into the membrane allowing the expression of a high potency on voltage-operated calcium channels. This membrane partitioning property explains the long duration of action of lacidipine and its slow onset of relaxation of arterial smooth muscles. In addition, vascular selectivity can be hypothesized to be, in part, due to different partitioning across different membranes.

Vascular protection by lacidipine at doses that are not maintaining a constant 24-hour blood pressure reduction can be explained in terms of the same mechanism that is hypothesized for its permanence of action. That is, the permanence of lacidipine in the membrane might be able to reset the intracellular calcium levels lower by titrating out inactivated channels. However, other mechanisms such as antioxidant properties can not be excluded.

References

1. Triggle DJ. Calcium channel drugs: antagonists and activators. ISI Atlas Pharmacol 1987;1:319-324.
2. Spedding M, Paoletti R. Classification of calcium channels and the sites of action of drugs modifying channel function. Pharmacol Rev 1992;44:363-376.
3. Cristofori P, Terron A, Micheli D, Bertolini G, Gaviraghi G, Carpi C. Vascular protection of lacidipine in salt-loaded Dahl-S rats at nonsustained antihypertensive doses. J Cardiovasc Pharmacol 1991; 7(Suppl.4):S75-S86.
4. Gaviraghi G, Godfraind T. New insight into the vascular properties of lacidipine. In: Paoletti R, editor. Comprehensive approach to cardiovascular care with a new calcium antagonist. Dordrecht, The Netherlands: Kluwer Academic Publishers and Fondazione Giovanni Lorenzini, 1993:11-15.
5. Weinstein DB. Protective effects of calcium channel antagonists in experimental models of atherogenesis and vascular disease. In: Laragh JH, Brenner BM, editors. Hypertension: Pathophysiology, diagnosis and management. New York: Raven Press, 1990:511-519.
6. Soma MR, Corsini A, Paoletti R, Bernini, F. Calcium antagonists in atherosclerosis: Focus on lacidipine. Research and Clinical Forums 1993;16:43-51.
7. Fleckenstein A, Fleckenstein-Grün G, Frey M, Zorn J. Future directions in the use of calcium antagonists. Am J Cardiol 1987;57:177B-187B.
8. Herbette LG, Gaviraghi G, Tulenko TN, Mason RP. Molecular interaction between lacidipine and biological membranes. J Hypertension 1993;11(Suppl.1):S13-S19.
9. Herbette LG, Gaviraghi G, Dring RJ, Briggs LJ, Mason RP. Interactions of lacidipine and other calcium channel drugs with biological membranes: A structural model for receptor/drug binding utilizing the membrane bilayer. In: Paoletti R, Godfraind T, Vanhoutte PM, editors. Calcium antagonists, pharmacology and clinical research. Dordrecht, The Netherlands: Kluwer Academic Publishers and Fondazione Giovanni Lorenzini, 1993;3:15-23.
10. Herbette LG, Mason PE, Gaviraghi G, Tulenko TN, Mason RP. The molecular basis for lacidipine's unique pharmacokinetics: optimal hydrophobicity results in membrane interactions that may facilitate the treatment of atherosclerosis. J

Cardiovasc Pharmacol 1994;23(Suppl.5):S16-S25.

11.   Salomone S, Godfraind T. Radioligand and functional estimates of the interaction of the 1,4-dihydropyridines, isradipine and lacidipine, with calcium channels in smooth muscle. Br J Pharmacol 1993;109:100-106.

12.   Giacometti A, Micheli D, Gaviraghi G, Trist DG. Quantification of the calcium antagonism of lacidipine by kinetic analysis. J Pharmacol Exptl Therap. 1994;269:424-429.

13.   Micheli D, Collodel A, Semeraro C, Gaviraghi G, Carpi C. Lacidipine: A calcium antagonist with potent and long-lasting antihypertensive effects in animal studies. J Cardiovasc Pharmacol 1990;15:666-675.

14.   Hess P, Lansman JB, Tsien RW. Different modes of Ca channel gating behaviour favoured by dihydropyridine Ca agonists and antagonists. Nature (Lond.) 1984;311:538-544.

15.   Cerbai E, Cavalcabo PD, Masini I, Visentin S, Giotti A, Mugelli A. Cardiac electrophysiologic effects of a new calcium antagonist, lacidipine. J Cardiovasc Pharmacol 1990;15:604-609.

MECHANISMS OF FREE RADICAL OXIDATIONS AND VASCULAR DAMAGE: PROTECTIVE EFFECT OF DIHYDROPYRIDINES

Fulvio Ursini
Department of Chemistry
Via del Cotonificio 108
33100 Udine
ITALY

Introduction

The most known pharmacological effects of Ca^{2+} antagonists or, more precisely, Ca^{2+} channel modulators, are related to the high affinity interaction with the α-1 subunit of the voltage dependent L-type Ca^{2+} channel. Nevertheless, dihydropyridines do interact with several other cellular structures, thus opening the possibility of therapeutic approaches different from hypertension [1].

Remarkably, in several models of atherosclerosis, all phases of the experimental disease appear to be influenced by Ca^{2+} antagonists [2,3], the protective effect of which is distinct from lowering blood pressure but may be applied directly to the prevention of atherosclerotic plaque development. This protective effect has been attributed to a decreased atherogenicity of LDL, suppression of foam cell generation, inhibition of platelet functions, chemotaxis, matrix protein synthesis and cellular proliferation, and eventually to the protection of the endothelium, thus delaying cell death [4-6]. Interestingly, several of these effects, although taking place on cells which do not express calcium channels, are calcium dependent, such as chemotaxis, proliferation and cytokine secretion [7,8]. On the other hand, it has been suggested that LDL containing oxidized lipids promotes the series of events, ultimately leading to plaque formation [9] and several aspects of atherogenesis, often related to cellular response to an injury (e.g. secretion of cytokines, proliferation, migration and margination of specific cell lines) [10-12], and are attributed to oxidants.

A complex scenario, therefore, could be envisaged where the damage brought about by oxidations (maybe free radical mediated) and protection by antioxidants (or free radical scavengers) are associated through a key role played by calcium. As a matter of fact, epidemiological and experimental studies support the hypothesis that antioxidants actually protect against spontaneous and experimental disease [13,14] and an antioxidant effect has been described for several cardiovascular drugs [15,16].

A.M. Gotto et al. (eds.), Multiple Risk Factors in Cardiovascular Disease, 105-108.

Antioxidant Effect Versus Calcium Antagonist Effect

In the framework of a study on lacidipine, a new potent dihydropyridine calcium antagonist, showing a high vascular protective activity in salt loaded Dahl-S and stroke prone rats, which could be only partially accounted for by the calcium antagonist activity, a possible mechanistic relationship between antioxidant protection and effects on calcium homeostasis has been identified.

The antioxidant activity of lacidipine has been studied by independently evaluating three aspects of the antioxidant effect: 1) the reactivity with a stable radical; 2) the rate constants for the reaction with peroxy radicals; 3) and the inhibition of peroxidation of rat cortex membranes [17]. Among these tests, the first gives an account for the possibility of a redox interaction between lacidipine and a free radical; the second offers a quantitative evaluation of the key antioxidant reaction (allowing a comparison with other chain breaking antioxidants); and the third quantifies the inhibition of peroxidation, which depends on the rate constant of the reaction with peroxy radicals, and the actual concentration of the antioxidant in membranes. Results indicated that lacidipine in a homogeneous solvent can undergo a one-electron redox transition by reacting with free radicals, although the rate constant for the interaction with peroxy radicals is five-hundred times lower than that of trolox (a soluble vitamin E analogue) used as reference. On the other hand, the difference between the antioxidant effect of lacidipine and vitamin E in membranes was much lower (within less than one order of magnitude). This was apparently due to the lipophilicity of the drug and, possibly, to the localization in membranes where free radical chain reaction takes place.

In a second set of experiments it has been shown that the calcium influx in smooth muscle cells, induced by hydrogen peroxide was prevented both by dihydropyridines and typical antioxidants such as trolox and diphenylparaphanylendiamine [18]. The calcium homeostasis impairment was sustained after removal of the oxidant and was repaired only by disulphide reducing agents, thus suggesting that hydrogen peroxide produces an oxidation of thiols in the membrane (possibly in the voltage-dependent channel), which is prevented both by antioxidants and calcium channel blockers and repaired by disulphide reducing agents. Remarkably, for this effect lacidipine was more active than typical antioxidants (ID_{50} 14×10^{-9} and 62×10^{-9} M for lacidipine and trolox, respectively).

Taken together the results of the two sets of experiments indicate that antioxidants can play a calcium antagonist effect and calcium antagonists undergo a redox transition compatible with an antioxidant effect. The higher efficiency of lacidipine than trolox in preventing calcium influx, while the opposite is true for the antioxidant capacity, is apparently due to the specificity of the dihydropyridine binding to structures where the redox transition takes place.

Thiol Redox Transitions, Intracellular Homeostasis and Cellular Activation

The concept that a thiol-disulfide redox transition affects calcium fluxes, resulting from the above discussion on the voltage-dependent channel, is not new. From the toxicological side

side it has been reported that the oxidative stress affects thiol-disulphide transitions and eventually calcium homeostasis, the modulation of which shift cellular responses from proliferation to apoptosis to death [19]. Moreover, it has been reported that calcium release from sarcoplasmic reticulum is activated by specific thiols oxidation [20] and that thiol oxidation increases the affinity of IP_3 receptor [21]. Recently, it has been also reported that the voltage sensor of the mitochondrial permeability transition pore is modulated by the redox state of thiols [22].

Taken together, these observation provide a rationale for the hypothesis that dihydropyridines exert their pharmacological effect by reducing an intermediate of the thiol disulphide transition (possibly the sulphothiolate anion radical), thus preventing the conformational change of the channel or the pore, eventually leading to the calcium flux. This mechanism would account for the overlap between calcium antagonist activity and the antioxidant effect.

The proposed chemistry of the interaction between dihydropyridines and thiols undergoing oxidation would contribute to the understanding of the molecular mechanism of the pharmacological effect of dihydropyridines, in terms of the relevant mechanism of cell biology.

References

1. Zernig G. Widening potential for Ca^{2+} antagonists: Non-L-type Ca^{2+} channel interaction. TIPS 1990;11:38-44 .

2. Bond MG, Purvis C, Mercuri M. Antiatherogenic properties of calcium antagosists. J Cardiovasc Pharmacol 1991;17(Suppl.4):87-92.

3. Oparil S, Calhoun G. The calcium antagosists in 1990s. Am J Hypertens 1991;4:396S-405S.

4. Henry PD. Calcium channel blockers and atherosclerosis. J Cadiovasc Pharmacol 1990;16(Suppl.1):12S-15S.

5. Sowers JR. Calcium channel blockers and atherosclerosis. Am J Kidney Dis 1990;16 (Suppl.1):3S-9S.

6. Orekhof AN, Tertov VV, Lysiakishev AA, Ruda MY. Use of cultured atherosclerotic cells for investigation of antiatherosclerotic effect of anipamil and other calcium antagonists. J Hum Hypertens 1991;5:425-430.

7. Schmitz G, Hankowitz J, Kovacs EM. Cellular processes in atherogenesis: Potential targets of calcium channel blockers. Atherosclerosis 1991;88:109-132.

8. Metha JL, Nicolini FA, Donnelly WH, Nichols WW. Platelet, leucocyte, endothelial interactions in coronary artery disease. Am J Cardiol. 1992;69:8B-13B.

9. Steinberg D, Parthasarathy S, Carew T, Khoo J, Witztum J. Beyond cholesterol. Modification of low density lipoprotein that increases its atherogenicity. New Engl J Med 1989;320:915-924.

10. Quinn MT, Parthasarathy S, Fong LG, Steinberg D. Oxidatively modified low density lipoproteins: A potential role in recruitment and retention of monocyte/macrophages during atherogenesis. Proc Natl Acad Sci 1987;84:2995-

2998.

11.   Berliner JA, Territo MC, Sevanian A, Ramin S, Kin JA, Esterson M, Fogelman AM.
       Minimally modified LDL stimulates monocyte endothelial interaction. J Clin Invest
       1990;85:1260-1266.

12.   Rajavashisth TB, Andalibi A, Territo MC, Berliner JA, Navab M, Fogelman AM,
       Lusis AJ: Induction od endothelial cell expression of granulocyte and macrophage
       colony stimulation factors by modified low-density lipoproteins. Nature 1990;344:
       254-257.

13.   Gey KF, Puska P, Jordan P, Moster UK. Inverse correlation between plasma vitamin
       E and mortality from ischemic heart disease in cross-cultural epidemiology. Am J
       Clin Nutr 1991;53:326S-334S.

14.   Bjorkhem I, Heriksson-Freyschuss A, Breuer O, Diczflausy U, Berglund L,
       Heriksson P. The antioxidant butylated hydroxy toluene protects against
       atherosclerosis. Arterioscler Thrombos 1991;11:15-22.

15.   Weglicki, WB, Mak, IT, Simic MG. Mechanisms of cardiovascular drugs as
       antioxidants. J Mol Cell Cardiol 1990;22:1199-1208.

16.   Mak IT, Weglicki B. Comparative antioxidant activities of propanolol, nifedipine,
       verapamil and diltiazem against sarcolemmal membrane lipid peroxidation. Circ Res
       1990;66:1449-1452.

17.   van Amsterdam F Th M, Roveri A, Maiorino M, Ratti E, Ursini F. Lacidipine: A
       dihydropyridine calcium antagonist with antioxidant activity. Free Rad Biol Med
       1992;12:183-187.

18.   Roveri A, Coassin M, Maiorino M, Zamburlini A, van Amsterdam F Th M, Ratti E,
       Ursini F. Effect of hydrogen peroxide on calcium homeostasis in smooth muscle
       cells. Arch Biochem Biophys 1992;297:265-270.

19.   Nicotera P, Dypbukt JM, Rossi AD, Manzo L and Orrenius S. Thiol modification
       and cell signalling in chemical toxicity. Toxicol Lett 1992;64:565-567.

20.   Salama G, Abramson JJ, Pike GK. Sulphydryl reagents trigger Ca^{2+} release from the
       sarcoplasmic reticulum of skinned rabbit psoas fibres. J Physiol London 1992;454:
       389-420.

21.   Hilly M, Pietri-Rouxel F, Coquil JF, Guy M, Maugler JP. Thiol reagents increase the
       affinity of the inositol 1,4,5 triphosphate receptor. J Biol Chem1993;268:16488-
       16494.

22.   Petronilli V, Costantini P. Scorrano L, Colonna R, Passamonti S, Bernardi P. The
       voltage sensor of the mitochondrial permeability transition pore is tuned by the
       oxidation reduction state of vicinal thiols. J Biol Chem 1994;269:16638-16642.

LIPOPHILIC DIHYDROPYRIDINES: NEW OPPORTUNITIES FOR PREVENTION OF ATHEROSCLEROSIS

Rodolfo Paoletti
Institute of Pharmacological Sciences
University of Milan
Milan
ITALY

Atherogenesis involves several mechanisms including: endothelial damage, lipid accumulation in the intimal tissue of the arterial vessel, smooth muscle cell proliferation and migration from the medial layer to the intimal layer of the artery, and the synthesis and accumulation of proteoglycans and other components of the extracellular matrix [1]. Several growth factors including cytokines and vasoactive molecules are also involved in the atherosclerotic lesion formation [1]. These factors can be synthesized by the different cell types involved in the atherosclerotic process. The main cell types present in the atheroma are arterial smooth muscle cells and macrophages originating from circulating monocytes [1]. Knowledge of the basic mechanisms involved in the pathophysiology of atherosclerosis offers a new rational for developing agents with a direct antiatherosclerotic activity. Pharmacological treatment of atherosclerosis may be directed to the control of the processes of atherogenesis occurring in the arterial wall.

The direct antiatherosclerotic effects of calcium antagonists have been known for more than 10 years. Henry et al. [2] have observed that nifedipine was able to inhibit atheroma formation induced by a cholesterol-rich diet in rabbits. This antiatherosclerotic effect was independent of blood pressure reduction and hypercholesterolemia. However, very high dosages of first-generation agents, e.g., nifedipine or verapamil, have had to be used possibly because of their short duration of action [3]. The introduction of new lipophilic calcium antagonists provide molecules with more potent antiatherosclerotic activity than prototypes [4]. These drugs may have effective antiatherosclerotic activity of clinical importance. This review summarizes the available data on the direct antiatherosclerotic activity of the lipophilic second-generation dihydropyridine-derivative lacidipine.

Effect of Lacidipine on Smooth Muscle Cells

During the formation of atherosclerotic lesions, smooth muscle cell proliferation begins in

A.M. Gotto et al. (eds.), Multiple Risk Factors in Cardiovascular Disease, 109-115.
© 1995 *Kluwer Academic Publishers and Fondazione Giovanni Lorenzini.*

the medial layer, followed by migration and further proliferation into the intima of the arterial wall [1]. Calcium channel blockers may inhibit myocyte migration and proliferation both *in vivo* and *in vitro* [5, 6]. Verapamil has been shown to reduce proliferation of smooth muscle cells cultured from rabbit and bovine aorta [7], and a similar effect has been demonstrated in primary cultures of subendothelial intimal cells isolated from atherosclerotic lesions of human aorta [8]. "In vivo" animal studies have shown that flunarizine and verapamil reduce intimal proliferation in rabbit carotid arteries stimulated with electrical impulses [9].

Our results indicate that lacidipine reduces myocyte proliferation in cell culture (Table 1) [10]. An inhibitory effect was also observed on the migration of arterial myocytes (data not shown).

Table 1. Effect of lacidipine and verapamil on [³H]thymidine incorporation in rat aorta smooth muscle cells

Drugs		[³H] Thymidine Uptake (% of control)
Verapamil	50 μM	79
Lacidipine	5 μM	83
"	10 μM	77
"	20 μM	71

[³H]thymidine was added to the incubation medium along with the reported concentration of drugs. The incorporation was evaluated after 48 hours of incubation: each point is the mean of triplicate dishes. Control value 72.5 ± 7.8 (cpm/plate x 10^{-3}) $\pm$ SD.
* $p < 0.05$ (Student's t-test)
Data from [10].

The mechanism by which calcium channel blockers affect the growth of smooth muscle cells is unknown. Cytosolic free calcium is required for the cell division cycle and calcium channel blockers could effect cell proliferation by modulating calcium homeostasis. However, this hypothesis has not been tested. Whatever the mechanism, calcium channel blockers have an apparent selectivity for arterial myocyte growth, since the drugs markedly reduced the incorporation of thymidine into aortic DNA in balloon-catheterized rats and rabbits without affecting DNA synthesis in other proliferating tissues [11].

In order to further characterize the antiproliferative activity of lacidipine, we have studied the effect of this drug on the hyperplasia induced by perivascular manipulation of hypercholesterolemic rabbit carotid artery. The carotid intimal hyperplasia is induced by the surgical insertion of silastic collar around one carotid [12,13]. The effectiveness of the periarterial insertion of the collar in inducing intimal carotid thickening was assessed in 10 hypercholesterolemic rabbits (positive control group) [14]. In these animals a marked increase in intimal thickness was evident in the carotids with collar, whereas the sham operated arteries showed no thickening of the intima either in positive control or drug-treated rabbits. The mean value of the intima/media (I/M) ratio in the collar arteries was twenty-fold greater than that observed in the sham.

Lacidipine did not modify plasma cholesterol after the 14-day experimental time. In treated animals lacidipine limited in a dose-dependent manner the increase of the I/M ratio when compared with the mean value of the positive control group. Differences versus positive control were statistically significant. This *in vivo* observation confirms the direct effect of lacidipine on smooth muscle cell migration and/or proliferation.

Effect of Lacidipine on Macrophages

Macrophages are derived from circulating monocytes and are the main lipid-loaded cells in the lesions. The mechanism by which they accumulate lipoprotein cholesterol and develop into foam cells depends mainly upon receptor-mediated processes, involving the so-called "scavenger receptor" that recognizes chemically and biologically modified low density lipoprotein (LDL), such as acetyl LDL and oxidized LDL [15,16]. The scavenger receptor, unlike the LDL receptor, is not subject to feed-back regulation, and the result is a massive accumulation of cholesterol in cells. Cholesterol accumulates in macrophages in esterified form by a process involving the enzymes acyl-coenzyme A-cholesterol acyltransferase (ACAT) which catalyzes the cholesterol esterification in cytoplasm [17]. Arterial myocytes migrate from the media layer and proliferate in the intima layer under the influence of various mitogens; both migration and proliferation are critical events in the development of atheromatous plaques [1]. *In vitro* studies using cell cultures have indicated that calcium channel blockers of various classes are active in modulating several of the processes involved in atherogenesis [18,19]. Cell-culture methods have been used extensively to investigate the possible mechanisms by which active compounds may affect atherogenesis [20-23]. Calcium antagonists have been shown to modulate LDL cholesterol metabolism in cells in culture [18]. Verapamil stimulates the receptor-mediated metabolism of LDL [24], thus contributing to an increase in LDL metabolism in the arterial wall. Verapamil analogues, diltiazem, amlodipine, and SIM 6080 [4,25,26], also stimulate LDL uptake. On the other hand, most dihydropyridine derivatives and flunarizine are inactive [27]. Verapamil, but not diltiazem [28], was shown to inhibit cholesterol esterification induced by β-very-low-density lipoprotein in rabbit alveolar macrophages. Schmitz and co-workers [29] reported that nifedipine partially inhibits cholesterol esterification in macrophages previously loaded with cholesterol, but not when the drug is simultaneously incubated with acLDL. Etinjin and Hajjar [30] reported that nifedipine was unable to inhibit ACAT activity in rabbit arterial smooth muscle cells. In contrast, Daugherty et al. [28] found that nifedipine was able to inhibit cholesterol esterification induced by β-very-low-density lipoprotein. We ourselves were unable to observe any major effect of nifedipine on cholesterol esterification in mouse peritoneal macrophages and J774 macrophage-like permanent cell line [31].

Our results indicate that lacidipine, like verapamil and progesterone, an ACAT inhibitor, affects intracellular cholesterol homeostasis by fully inhibiting acetyl LDL cholesterol esterification (Table 2) [10]. An inhibitory effect was observed at concentrations as low as 3 mmol/l (data not shown). Verapamil is known to have a major effect on cellular lipid metabolism by inhibiting cholesterol hydrolysis in lysosomes [18]. This action indirectly reduces cholesterol esterification, but paradoxically leads to a reduction in the free-to-esterified cholesterol ratio, due to the accumulation in lysosomes of cholesterol esters transported by lipoproteins. In cells stimulated by 25-hydroxycholesterol [32] and in cholesteryl ester-preloaded cells, verapamil has less effect and becomes inactive in cell-free homogenate [31,33]. Preliminary data obtained in our laboratory have indicated that this is not the case for lacidipine, which appears to act by directly inhibiting ACAT activity. Nifedipine has no effect on cholesterol esterification in macrophages (Table 2).

Table 2. Comparison of lacidipine, verapamil, nifedipine and progesterone effect on cholesterol esterification in mouse peritoneal macrophages.

Drugs			[^{14}C]oleate incorporation into cholesteryl ester (% of control)
Control		+ acLDL	100.0
Lacidipine	50 μM	+ "	0.4
Verapamil	50 μM	+ "	0.7
Nifedipine	50 μM	+ "	89.9
Progesterone	30 μM	+ "	2.1

Means of triplicate dishes. The cells were preincubated in Dulbecco's minimum essential medium containing 0.1% fatty-acid-free albumin and each drug for 2 hours. Monolayers underwent a second incubation (5 hours) in the presence of acLDL (50 mg/ml), the [^{14}C]oleate-albumin complex, and each drug. Control value 1555.2 ± 77.4 (ng/mg cell prot x h) ± SD.
Data from [10].

The vascular protection of lacidipine is further supported by the interesting data recently published by Gaviraghi and Godfraind [34] obtained in stroke-prone spontaneously hypertensive rats (SHR-SP). In these experiments once-a-day administration of lacidipine prevented in a dose-dependent manner the mortality in 1% of the salt-loaded stroke-prone SHR. This was accomplished without a major effect on the blood pressure in those rats. Neither macro- nor microscopic cerebral lesions were observed in rats treated with lacidipine at 0.3 and 1 mg/kg. On the contrary, all untreated animals had died. Marked hypertrophy, necrosis and occlusions of renal arterioles, generative changes of tubules and glomeruli, were detected in untreated animals. In salt-loaded SHR-SP treated for six months with lacidipine at 1 mg/kg, normal histological appearance of renal structure was maintained. This vasoprotective action of low doses of lacidipine could be ascribed to its potent and long-lasting calcium antagonist activity. The accelerated mortality of salt-loaded SHR-SP appears to be associated with an increase in plasma lipid peroxides, which is inhibited by lacidipine. The antioxidant activity of lacidipine might contribute to its tissue protection action [35].

In conclusion the available results suggest that lipophilic calcium antagonists like lacidipine may represent a potential effective class of antiatherosclerotic agents.

References

1. Ross R. The pathogenesis of atherosclerosis: A perspective for the 1990s. Nature 1993;362;801-809.
2. Henry PD, Bentley KI. Suppression of atherogenesis in cholesterol-fed rabbit treated with nifedipine. J Clin Invest 1981;68;1366-1369.
3. Fleckenstein A, Frey M, Zorn J, Fleckenstein-Grun G. Calcium, a neglected key factor in hypertension and arteriosclerosis. Experimental vasoprotection with calcium antagonists or ACE inhibitors. In: Laragh J, Brenner B, editors. Hypertension: Pathophysiology, diagnosis and management. New York: Raven Press, Ltd., 1990;471-509.
4. Paoletti R, Bernini F. A new generation of calcium antagonists and their role in atherosclerosis. Am J Cardiol 1990;66:28H-31H.
5. Jackson CL, Bush RC, Bowyer DE. Mechanism of antiatherogenic action of calcium antagonists. Atherosclerosis 1989;80;17-26.
6. Nomoto A, Mutoh S, Hagihara H, Yamaguchi I. Smooth muscle cell migration induced by inflammatory cell products and its inhibition by a potent calcium antagonist, nilvadipine. Atherosclerosis 1988;72;213-219.
7. Stein O, Halperin G, Stein Y. Long term effects of verapamil on aortic smooth muscle cells cultured in the presence of hypercholesterolemic serum. Arteriosclerosis 1987;7;585-592.
8. Orekhov AN, Tertov VV, Khashimov KA, Kudryashov SA, Smirnov VN. Antiatherosclerotic effects of verapamil in primary culture of human aortic intimal cells. J Hypertens 1986;4;S153-S155.
9. Betz E. The effect of calcium antagonists on intimal cell proliferation in atherogenesis. Ann NY Acad Sci 1988;522;399-410.

10.   Bernini F, Corsini M, Raiteri M, Soma MR, Paoletti R. Effects of lacidipine on experimental models of atherosclerosis. J Hypertens 1993;11(Suppl.3);S61-S66.

11.   Jackson CL, Bush RC, Bowyer RE. Inhibitory effect of calcium antagonists on balloon catheter-induced arterial smooth muscle cell proliferation and lesion size. Atherosclerosis 1988;69;115-122.

12.   Booth RGF, Martin JF, Honey AC, Hassall DG, Beesley JE, Moncada S. Rapid development of atherosclerotic lesions in the rabbit carotid artery induced by perivascular manipulation. Atherosclerosis 1989;76;257-268.

13.   Soma MR, Donetti E, Parolini C, et al. HMGCoA reductase inhibitors: In vivo effects on intimal carotid thickening in rabbits. Arterioscler Thromb 1993;13;571-578.

14.   Soma MR, Donetti E, Parolini C, et al. Effect of lacidipine on the carotid intimal hyperplasia induced by cuff injury. J Cardiovasc Pharmacol 1994;23(Suppl.5):S71-S74.

15.   Brown MS, Goldstein JL. Lipoprotein metabolism in the macrophage: Implications for cholesterol deposition in atherosclerosis. Ann Rev Biochem 1983;52;223-261.

16.   Kurihara Y, Matsumoto A, Itakura H, Kodama T. Macrophage scavenger receptors. Curr Opin Lipidol 1991;2;295-300.

17.   Brown MS, Ho YK, Goldstein JL. The cholesteryl ester cycle in macrophage from cells: Continual hydrolysis and re-esterification of cytoplasmic cholesteryl esters. J Biol Chem 1980;255;9344-9352.

18.   Bernini F, Paoletti R. Effects of calcium antagonists on lipids and atherosclerosis. Am J Cardiol 1989;64;129 I-133 I.

19.   Schmitz G, Hankovitz J, Kovacs EM. Cellular processes in atherogenesis: Potential targets of calcium channel blockers. Atherosclerosis 1991;88;109-132.

20.   Raiteri M, Corsini A, Soma MR, et al. Antiatherosclerotic drugs: A critical assessment. In: Catapano AL, Gotto AM, Jr., Smith LC, Paoletti R, editors. Drugs affecting lipid metabolism. Dordrecht, The Netherlands: Kluwer Academic Publishers, 1993;317-331.

21.   Corsini A, Raiteri M, Soma M, Fumagalli R, Paoletti R. Simvastatin but not pravastatin inhibits the proliferation of rat aorta myocytes. Pharmacol Res 1991;23:173-180.

22.   Corsini A, Mazzotti M, Raiteri M,et al. Relationship between mevalonate pathway and arterial myocyte proliferation: "In vitro" studies with inhibitors of HMG-CoA reductase. Atherosclerosis 1993,10:117-125.

23.   Bernini F, Didoni G, Bonfadini G, Bellosta S, Fumagalli R. Requirement for mevalonate in acetylated LDL induction of cholesterol esterification in macrophages. Atherosclerosis 1993;104:19-26.

24.   Stein O, Leitersdorf E, Stein Y. Verapamil enhances receptor-mediated endocytosis of low density lipoproteins by aortic cells in culture. Arteriosclerosis 1985;5;35-44.

25.   Bernini F, Fantoni M, Corsini A, Fumagalli R. "In vitro" inhibition of arterial myocyte growth and stimulation of low density lipoprotein metabolism by SIM 6080, a new calcium antagonist. Pharmacol Res 1990;22:27-35.

26. Maggi FM, Bernini F, Barberi L., Fantoni M, Catapano AL. SIM 6080, a new calcium antagonist, reduces aortic atherosclerosis in cholesterol-fed rabbits. Pharmacol Res 1993;28:219-227.

27. Paoletti R, Bernini F, Fumagalli R, Allorio M, Corsini A. Calcium antagonists and LDL receptors. Ann NY Acad Sci 1988;522;390-398.

28. Daugherty A, Rateri DL, Schonfeld SB. Inhibition of cholesteryl ester deposition in macrophages by calcium entry blockers:An effect dissociable from calcium entry blockade. Br J Pharmacol 1987;91;113-118.

29. Schmitz G, Robenek H, Beuck M, Krause R, Schurek A, Niemann R. Ca++ antagonists and ACAT inhibitors promote cholesterol efflux from macrophages by different mechanisms. Arteriosclerosis 1988;8;46-56.

30. Etinjin OR, Hajjar DP. Nifedipine increases cholesteryl ester hydrolitic activity in lipid-laden rabbit arterial smooth muscle cells. A possible mechanism for its antiatherogenic effect. J Clin Invest 1985;75;1554-1558.

31. Bernini F, Bellosta S, Didoni G, Fumagalli R. Calcium antagonists and cholesteryl ester metabolism in macrophages. J Cardiovasc Pharmacol 1991;18(Suppl. 10);S42-S45.

32. Brown MS, Dana SE, Goldstein JL. Cholesterol ester formation in cultured human fibroblasts. J Biol Chem 1975;250;4025-4027.

33. Stein O, Stein Y. Effect of verapamil on cholesteryl ester hydrolysis and reesterification in macrophages. Arteriosclerosis 1987;7;578-584.

34. Gaviraghi G, Godfraind T. New insights into the vascular properties of lacidipine. In: Godfraind T, et al, editors. Calcium Antagonists. Dordrecht, The Netherlands: Kluwer Academic Publishers and Fondazione G. Lorenzini, 1993;65-69.

35. Micheli D, Ratti E, Toson G, Gaviraghi G. Pharmacology of lacidipine, a vascular-selective calcium antagonist. J Cardiovasc Pharmacol 1991;17(Suppl. 4);S1-S8.

CLINICAL TRIAL DESIGN AND NONINVASIVE ATHEROSCLEROSIS END-POINTS FOR STUDYING LIPOPHILIC DIHYDROPYRIDINES

M. Gene Bond, Michele Mercuri, Renate Arens, and Fabrizio Gianfrate, for the ELSA Collaborative Research Group

Introduction

Atherosclerosis has been, and continues to be an important cause of cardiovascular morbidity and mortality in industrialized countries. This disease process is known to begin early-on in life, but does not become clinically manifest until plaques result in high-grade lumen stenosis, or until these lesions produce thromboembolism. As a result, considerable effort and resources are spent on evaluation and treatment of end-stage arterial disease which has already resulted in tissue ischemia and/or necrosis. Unfortunately, however, a considerable percentage of patients who develop clinical sequelae of atherosclerosis, die suddenly and unexpectedly. For those patients who do survive the effect of tissue ischemia and infarct, and are then surgically intervened upon, there is a substantial decreased life span and quality of life when compared to the general population. Within the last decade there has been increased emphasis on identifying subjects who are at risk for the eventual development of cardiovascular disease before clinical sequelae occur and treating these subjects medically to reduce the effect of risk factors on prevalent acute events. There is suggestive evidence in controlled clinical trials that treatment of risk factors in asymptomatic subjects, e.g. elevated LDL cholesterol concentrations, does reduce cardiovascular morbidity and mortality. Clearly however, these studies also document that a substantial percentage of patients who have been able to effectively reduce risk, go on to develop atherosclerosis-related ischemic events.

A relatively new class of compounds, the calcium antagonists, especially those of the dihydropyridine group, are currently used to reduce blood pressure in hypertensive patients. Although initially developed as antihypertensive agents, *in vitro* and *in vivo* studies using animal models, suggest that this class of compounds may have the potential to inhibit atherogenesis or atherosclerosis progression [1-4]. These studies have also demonstrated that the beneficial effects on atherosclerosis in animal studies are independent from blood pressure lowering. The *in vitro* studies suggest that calcium antagonists may also decrease vascular cell proliferation, alter the metabolism of smooth muscle and endothelial cells by regulating intracellular calcium levels, increase cellular uptake and degradation of liproproteins, and increase arterial cholesterol ester hydrolysis [1,4,5].

A.M. Gotto et al. (eds.), Multiple Risk Factors in Cardiovascular Disease, 117-124.

Information from these basic studies has stimulated the interest to perform clinical trials in high risk patients to determine whether these compounds are effective in the treatment of atherosclerosis. The Montreal Heart Institute Study was a double-blind, randomized, placebo-controlled study of 383 patients with known coronary artery disease. Patients were randomized into 2 groups to be treated either with the calcium antagonist nicardipine, or placebo. Coronary artery atherosclerosis was quantitated on the basis of coronary arteriography which was performed at baseline and again after 24 months of either treatment. The results when comparing angiograms showed no statistically significant differences in the extent and severity of coronary artery atherosclerosis analyzed on a per-lesion or per-patient basis. However, retrospective analysis aimed at determining whether calcium antagonist treatment had an effect on progression of early "minimal" lesions demonstrated that the number of patients with early disease progression was significantly less in the nicardipine-treated group when compared to the placebo. Although not definitive, because of the retrospective nature of the analysis and differences in risk factors between the two treatment groups, this information suggested that calcium antagonists may have a preferential effect on early stages of atherosclerosis progression [6,7]. The International Nifedipine Trial on Antiatherosclerotic Therapy (INTACT) also addressed the question of whether a calcium channel antagonist would beneficially effect coronary artery atherosclerosis. This was a randomized, placebo-controlled, double-blind study which compared the effects of nifedipine and placebo over a period of 36 months. Patients eligible for enrollment had clinically significant coronary artery atherosclerosis [8] that was assessed with quantitative coronary arteriography [9] performed at entrance into the study and after 3 years. Similar to the Montreal Heart Institute Study, INTACT found no significant differences between treatment groups when examining either the progression or regression of preexisting lesions, nor in the number of affected patients. However, according to a prospective protocol hypothesis, a comparison of coronary segments from similar arteriographic projection angles studied at entrance and at 36 months demonstrated that the rate of new lesion formation per patient was significantly lower in the group treated with nifedipine than in the placebo-treated group [10]. These 2 studies focused on patients, all of whom had significant coronary artery disease, late or end-stage, which had produced clinical sequelae severe enough to justify invasive arteriographic procedures.

A very different type of clinical trial was begun in 1988 to test the effect of treatment with a new calcium antagonist of the dihydropyridine group, isradipine, when compared to a diuretic on the evolution of asymptomatic carotid artery atherosclerosis. The Multicenter Isradipine Diuretic Atherosclerosis Study (MIDAS) was a double-blind, randomized, actively controlled study of 883 hypertensive patients, all of whom had preexisting asymptomatic carotid atherosclerosis diagnosed by noninvasive B-mode ultrasonography [11,12,13]. The results of this study with a complete discussion of the results has not been published. However, it is noteworthy that MIDAS was unique from several perspectives including the following: all patients had asymptomatic carotid artery atherosclerosis; the experimental design and treatment with either drug, sought to insure that all risk factors at the time of randomization, and during the course of the study, were similar in both treatment groups; the B-mode ultrasonography methods were noninvasive; and up to seven B-mode sequential evaluations were performed on patients during this 3-year trial. Perhaps the most important difference between MIDAS and other previous clinical trials which have sought to evaluate atherosclerosis progression/regression was that the primary and the majority of secondary outcomes were based on measurements of the arterial wall rather than of lumen dimensions. Thus, MIDAS was instrumental in expanding the goals of clinical trials to determine when and how to treat atherosclerosis. Furthermore, it posed the question of whether calcium antagonists offer additional advantages in preventing hypertension-related end-organ injuries over the simple reduction of blood pressure obtained with traditionally effective drugs.

Another type of clinical trial has recently been implemented, which takes advantage of a new dihydropyridine calcium antagonist which has lipophilic properties. Lacidipine has been described previously in this symposium, and has unique pharmacokinetic properties which suggest that this compound remains integrated within cellular membranes for a longer period of time when compared to other calcium antagonists. Further, basic studies suggest that lacidipine may have a pronounced effect in inhibiting atherogenesis. The European Lacidipine Study on Atherosclerosis (ELSA) will compare the effect of two antihypertensive treatments, the dihydropyridine calcium antagonist lacidipine, and the beta blocker atenolol, on carotid artery intima-media thicknesses in hypertensive patients stratified on the basis of the presence of existing plaques, or wall thickening or normal carotid artery walls. The two treatment groups will also be compared at the end of the trial for fatal and morbid cardiovascular events. Also, 24-hour Ambulatory Blood Pressure Monitoring (ABPM) will be used routinely to better evaluate and characterized blood pressure profiles during treatment and to determine the association between circadian blood pressure variations and the morphology of carotid arteries, analyzed cross-sectionally and longitudinally during the active treatment period. Specifically, the primary objectives of this study will be to compare the effects of these two antihypertensive treatments on the progression of early extracranial carotid atherosclerotic plaques and on the progression/regression of carotid artery intima-media thicknesses. The secondary objectives are to compare the effects of an antihypertensive treatment with either lacidipine or atenolol on the appearance of new atherosclerotic plaques, on the rate of cardiovascular morbid and fatal events, to evaluate whether, and the extent to which, the treatments reduce office blood pressure, ambulatory blood pressure, and blood pressure variability. Furthermore, ELSA will determine the correlates between and among ambulatory blood pressure values, clinic blood pressure values, blood pressure variability, and carotid artery morphology, i.e. plaque and intima-media thickness at recruitment. Finally, it will determine whether reduction in ambulatory blood pressure values, clinic blood pressures, or blood pressure variability are among the predictors of the effect of treatments on carotid lesions, and on cardiovascular events.

Study Design

ELSA is a multinational, multicenter, randomized, double-blind, parallel group trial with a four-year active treatment period. A total of 3,708 patients, aged between 45 and 75 years, with diastolic blood pressures between 95-115mmHg and systolic pressures between 150-

210mmHg at the end of a single placebo run-in period will be recruited into the trial, and divided into three strata according to B-mode ultrasound characteristics of the extracranial carotid arteries as follows:

STRATUM 1:   patients with at least one carotid plaque (1,044 patients), defined as having at least one carotid artery wall whose intima-media thickness measures between 1.3-4.0mm

STRATUM 2:   patients with carotid intima-media thicknesses (1,620 patients) with at least one wall having a single maximum intima-media thickness between 1.0-1.3mm

STRATUM 3:   patients with no ultrasound evidence of carotid wall alteration (1,044 patients) in which maximum intima-media thickness is below 1.0mm.

During the active treatment phase major cardiovascular events will be documented. Patients allocated to strata 1 and 2 will have carotid ultrasound assessment at recruitment, and at yearly intervals to monitor change over 4 years. Statum 3 patients will have carotid assessment at recruitment, after 2 years, and at the end of the study in order to obtain comparative evidence of change in wall thickness of what initially are ultrasonographically normal carotid arteries. This same schedule will be followed for ambulatory blood pressure measurements. After a one month run-in phase with placebo, patients will be randomized to receive either lacidipine 4 mg/day, or atenolol 50 mg/day. Drug dosage will be increased to 6 mg (lacidipine) or 100 mg (atenolol) in nonresponder patients after 1 month and 3 months of treatment. For patients whose blood pressure does not respond adequately to treatment with study drugs, hydrochlorothiazide (12.5-25 mg/day) will be given on an open label basis.

Outcome Variables

The primary outcome variable is the change in the mean of maximum intima-media thicknesses on the far walls of the common carotid artery and carotid bifurcation, bilaterally. Secondary ultrasound outcome measures include the following:1) the change in the mean of maximum intima-media thicknesses recorded on up to 12 preselected segments of the carotid arteries, including near and far walls of the common carotid, carotid bifurcation, and internal carotid arteries; 2) the change in the largest maximum intima-media thickness among the 12 sites; 3) the change in the carotid segment which shows the greatest relative progression in maximum intima-media thickness during the active treatment period, calculated as the mean change of both segment walls.

Study Organization

Many clinical units at each Referral Center will recruit, screen, treat, and follow-up patients in this study. These clinical units will refer patients to 23 Referral Centers (see Table 1)

Table 1. ELSA Principal Investigators and Sonographers.

FRANCE

- University of Grenoble:
  PI: Prof. J.M. Mallion, M.D.
  Sonographers:
  Christophe Cimadomo, M.D.
  Dominique Ploin, M.D., Ph.D.
- University of Nancy:
  PI: Prof. Feiez Zannad, M.D.
  Sonographers:
  Emanuel Gasakure, M.D.
  Philippe Mizzon, M.D.
- University of Paris:
  PI: Prof. Stéphane Laurent, M.D.
  Sonographers:
  Roland Asmar, M.D.
  Brigitte Laloux

GREECE

- Athens University:
  PI: Prof. Pavlos Toutouzas, M.D.
  Sonographers:
  Dorothea Tsekoura, M.D.
  Asimakis Sideris, M.D.

GERMANY

- University of Berlin:
  PI: Prof. Jürgen Scholze, M.D.
  Sonographers:
  Christiane Ludwig, M.D.
  Gundula Sthur
- University of Frankfurt:
  PI: Prof. Hans-Joachim Gilfrich, M.D.
- University of Hamburg:
  PI: Prof. Christian Hamm, M.D.
  Sonographers:
  Britta Goldmann, M.D.
  Catarina Todd, M.D.
- Ludwig Maximilians University, München:
  PI: Prof. H.Holzgreve, M.D.
  Sonographers:
  Anja Meurer Mastellotto, M.D.
  Sybille Reder
- Westfälische Wilhems University, Münster:
  PI: Prof. C. Spicker, M.D.
  Sonographers:
  Barbara Suwelack, M.D.
  Jan Witta, M.D.

SPAIN

- University of Barcelona:
  PI: Prof. Alejandro Roca-Cusachs, M.D.
  Sonographers:
  Carlos Paytubí Garí, M.D.
  Eugenia Negredo, M.D.
- University of Madrid:
  PI: Prof. Luis Miguel Ruilope, M.D.
  Sonographers:
  Maria Cruz Casal
  Maria Luisa Fernandez

ITALY

- University of Ancona:
  PI: Prof. Alessandro Rappelli, M.D.
  Sonographers:
  Roberto Catalini, M.D.
  Oriana Zingaretti, M.D.
- University of Bologna:
  PI: Prof. Ettore Ambrosioni, M.D.
  Sonographers:
  Massimo Piccoli, M.D.
  Marcello Schiaratura, M.D.
- University of Brescia:
  PI: Prof. Enrico Agabiti Rosei, M.D.
  Sonographers:
  Giorgio Bettoni, M.D.
  M. Lorenza Muiesan, M.D.
- University of Milano:
  PI: Prof. Cesare Cuspidi, M.D.
  Sonographers:
  Roberta Paliotti, M.D.
  Antonio Lanfranchi, M.D.
- University of Napoli:
  PI: Prof. Bruno Trimarco, M.D.
  Sonographers:
  Nicola de Luca, M.D.
  Gianluigi Iovino, M.D.
- University of Padova:
  PI: Prof. Achille Pessina, M.D.
  Sonographers:
  Valeria Pagliari, M.D.
- Università di Pisa:
  PI: Prof. Antonio Salvetti, M.D.
  Sonographers:
  Michela Simi, M.D.
- Università di Roma:
  PI: Prof. Antonello Bucci, M.D.
  Sonographers:
  Modestini, M.D.
  Saverio Gioia, M.D.

SWEDEN

- University of Lund:
  PI: Prof. Thomas Thulin, M.D.
  Sonographers:
  Lena Arefalk
  Karin Falk
- University of Stockholm:
  PI: Prof. Ulf de Faire, M.D.
  Sonographers:
  Linda Nilson
  Ulla Hellmark-Augustsson

UNITED KINGDOM

- University of Glasgow:
  PI: Prof. John L. Reid, M.D.
  Sonographers:
  Ros Carter
  Margaret Greene
- University of Sheffield:
  PI: Prof. Ramsey, M.D.
  Sonographers:
  Andrew Bell

Table 2. ELSA Steering Committee Members.

ELSA Steering Committee Members

Prof. Alberto Zanchetti, M.D., Chairman
Università di Milano, Italy

Prof. M. Gene Bond, Ph.D. and
Michele Mercuri, M.D., Ph.D.
Bowman Gray School of Medicine, Winston-Salem, N.C, USA

Prof. Cesare Dal Palù, M.D.
Università di Padova, Italy

Volker Gladigau, M.D.
BOEHRINGER INGELHEIM GmbH, Germany

Prof. Lennart Hansson, M.D.
University of Uppsala, Sweden

Prof. Giuseppe Mancia, M.D.
Università di Milano, Italy

Prof. A. B. Neiss, Ph.D.
Institut für Medizinische Statistik
und Epidemiologie der TUM, Munich, Germany

Prof. H.K. Rahn, M.D.
Westfälische Wilhems Universität
Münster, Germany

Prof. John L. Reid, M.D.
University of Glasgow, Scotland

Oriana Zerbini, M.D.
GLAXO SpA, Verona, Italy

Prof. José Rodicio, M.D.
Hospital 12 de Octobre, Madrid, Spain

Prof. Michel Safar, M.D.
Hôpital Broussais, Paris, France

Ultrasound Center

Division of Vascular Ultrasound Research
Bowman Gray School of Medicine
Medical Center Boulevard
Winston-Salem, NC 27157-1025
USA

Co-Director: Prof. M. Gene Bond, Ph.D.

Co-Director: Michele Mercuri, M.D. Ph.D.

Research Associate: Rong Tang, M.D.

Ultrasound Coordinator: Anne Safrit, B.Sc.

Ultrasound Readers:
Sharon Alcorn
Donna Angel
Judy Batten
Jean Craig
Billie Holley
Patricia Miller
Daniel Pozo
Miriam Rodriguez
Theresa Wagner
Bo Xiao

Communication and Translation Coordinator:
Rita Pignatelli, D.Litt.

Admin. Secretary: Chiquita Wilson

Statistical and Analysis Center

Institut für Medizinische Statistik und
Epidemiologie der TUM
Ismaninger Straße 22
81675 München
Germany

Director: Prof. A. B. Neiss, Ph.D.

Coordinator: Michael Hennig

Data Manager: Barbara Thomas

ABPM Center

Center of Clinical Physiology and Hypertension
Ospedale Maggiore di Milano, Italy
Director: Prof G. Mancia
Co-Investigators:
Gianfranco Parati, M.D.
Stefano Omboni, M.D.
Antonella Ravogli, M.D.
Cinzia Santucciu, M.D.
Luisa Ulian, M.D.

which are responsible of the accumulation of data related to carotid ultrasonography and ambulatory blood pressure. The 23 Referral Centers, each administered by a single principal investigator, are in England, France, Germany, Greece, Italy, Scotland, Spain, and Sweden, and are coordinated by an International Steering Committee (see Table 2).

Quality Control

The ELSA protocol includes substantial quality assessment and quality control for the primary and secondary ultrasound endpoints. The ultrasound equipment, i.e. Biosound 2000 II s.a., was competitively selected among several commercially available models. All ultrasound instruments were pretested and matched as closely as possible for axial resolution, calibration factors, and interface quality. In addition each unit is periodically monitored during the course of the study. Sonographers and readers receive initial standardized training in scanning and reading protocols, respectively, and are initially certified based on scan quality. Ultrasound readers are certified based on efficiency and proficiency of measurements using standard scans. All operators are recertified on an annual basis. In addition, qualitative assessment is performed on each scan received by the centralized Ultrasound Center. Ultrasound Center equipment including hardware and software was selected on a competitive basis, pretested, and is monitored routinely.

Cross-sectional quality control for sonographers is accomplished by blinded replicate scans of all patients at baseline, after 2 years of treatment and again at the final visit. Cross-sectional quality control of readers is also performed on a routine basis by performing replications of randomly selected scans. Longitudinal quality control is assessed by monthly re-readings selected from a standard sample of 300 scans performed at baseline. Data provided by these replicate scans and readings allow assessment of quality by an independent Statistical Analysis Center (Table 2) which will provide data on absolute differences in replicate scans and readings. Intra- and intersonographer, and reader reproducibility are therefore monitored on a routine basis throughout the course of the trial.

ELSA is one of the first studies in the second generation of clinical trials that use non-invasive, high-resolution B-mode ultrasonography to establish primary and secondary outcome measures. It differs significantly in experimental design, anatomic entrance criteria at the level of the artery wall, in the use of a new generation of lipophilic dihydropyridine calcium antagonists, and in its prospective use of quality control protocols to monitor longitudinal change in instruments, sonographers, and readers.

References

1. Chobanian A. Effects of calcium channel antagonists and other antihypertensive drugs on atherogenesis. J Hypertens 1987;5(Suppl.4):S43-48.
2. Chobanian AV. How antihypertensive drugs may influence atherosclerosis. Primary Cardiology 1991;17:42-48.
3. Weinstein DB, Heider JG. Antiatherogenic properties of calcium antagonists. Am J Cardiol 1987;59:163B-172B.

4.   Weinstein DB, Heider JG. Protective action of calcium channel antagonists in atherogenesis and experimental vascular injury. Am J Hypertens 1989;2:205-12.

5.   Sowers JR, Zemel PC, Zemel MB, Kasim SE, Khoury S. Hypertension and atherosclerosis: Calcium antagonists as antiatherogenic agents. J Vasc Med Biol 1990;2:1-6.

6.   Waters D, Lespérance J, Francetich M, et al. A controlled clinical trial to assess the effect of a calcium channel blocker on the progression of coronary atherosclerosis. Circulation 1990;82:1940-53.

7.   Waters D, Freedman D, Lesperance J, et al. Design features of a controlled clinical trial to assess the effect of a calcium entry blocker upon the progression of coronary artery disease. Controlled Clin Trials 1987;8:216-42.

8.   Lichtlen PR, Hugenholtz PG, Rafflenbeul W, Hecker H, Jost S, Deckers JW, on behalf of the INTACT Group Investigators. Retardation of angiographic progression of coronary artery disease by nifedipine: Results of the International Nifedipine trial on Antiatherosclerotic Therapy (INTACT). Lancet 1990;335:1109-13.

9.   Reiber JHC, Serruys PW, Kooijman CJ, et al. Assessment of short-, medium-, and long-term variations in arterial dimensions from computer-assisted quantitation of coronary cineangiograms. Circulation 1985;71:280-88.

10.   Lichtlen PR, Nellessen U, Rafflenbeul W, Jost S, Hecker H. International nifedipine trial on antiatherosclerotic therapy (INTACT). Cardiovasc Drug Ther 1987;1:71-79.

11.   Bond MG, Wilmoth SK, Enevold G, Strickland HL. Detection and monitoring of asymptomatic atherosclerosis in clinical trials. AM J Med 1989;86(4A)(Suppl.):33-36.

12.   Borhani NO, Brugger SB, Byington RP, on behalf of the MIDAS Research Group. Multicenter study with isradipine and diuretics against atherosclerosis. J Cardiovasc Pharmacol 1990;15(Suppl.1):S23-29.

13.   Bond MG, Strickland HL, Wilmoth SK, Safrit A, Phillips R, Szostak L, for the MIDAS Research Group. Interventional clinical trials using noninvasive ultrasound end points: the Multicenter Isradipine/Diuretic Atherosclerosis Study. J Cardiovasc Pharmacol 1990;15(Suppl.1):S30-33.

THE BIOLOGICAL ROLES OF N-3 FATTY ACIDS: METABOLIC AND NUTRITIONAL ASPECTS

Claudio Galli
Institute of Pharmacological Sciences
University of Milan
ITALY

The interest in the biological roles of the long chain (LC) polyunsaturated fatty acids (PUFA) (LCP) of the n-3 series, especially EPA (eicosapentaenoic acid, 20:5 n-3) and DHA (docosahexaenoic acid, 22:6 n-3), available for human consumption especially as components of fish oils, is documented by the large volume of biomedical research devoted to these compounds that has been carried out in the last few years. The initial observations and studies were based mainly on dietary approaches, but preparations that are highly enriched with EPA and DHA, the most active components in fish oils, either as triglycerides or ethyl esters are now available for human studies.

EPA and especially DHA are constituents of complex lipids in certain tissues and organs (e.g. the retina, the brain grey matter, and the heart) of higher animals and are found in appreciable concentrations especially in fish fats and tissues. Although EPA and DHA can be formed from the 18 carbon precursor α linolenic acid (α LNA), which can be provided by various types of fats and oils in the diet, the rates of conversion of the precursor to the products are low and their availability in the diet is rather limited, thus providing a rationale for the use of pharmaceutical preparations enriched with the compounds.

This paper focuses on some recent advances in the biochemistry (biosynthesis and metabolism) of the 22 carbon n-3 fatty acids and on the biological and nutritional implications of these new findings.

Formation and Metabolism of EPA and DHA

The biosynthesis of the LCP in the n-6 and n-3 series has been considered until recently as a sequence of alternating desaturation and elongation steps of the 18 carbon precursors, taking place in the endoplasmic reticulum, the liver being the most active site of synthesis. The desaturation steps (6, 5, and 4 desaturases), respectively involved in the desaturation of the 18 carbon ($\Delta 6$), of the 20 carbon ($\Delta 5$) and of the 22 carbon ($\Delta 4$) members of the series, are considered as the regulatory steps in the overall process. *In vitro* studies on the 4 desaturation in the n-3 series, responsible for the conversion of 22:5 to 22:6, revealed that

125

A.M. Gotto et al. (eds.), Multiple Risk Factors in Cardiovascular Disease, 125-131.
© 1995 *Kluwer Academic Publishers and Fondazione Giovanni Lorenzini.*

this is not a single step process and that cooperation between two subcellular particles (endoplasmic reticulum and peroxisomes) takes place [1]. A similar sequence is proposed for the formation of 22:5 from 22:4 in the n-6 series (Figure 1). More specifically, while the formation of EPA from 18:3 follows the classical desaturation-elongation alternate sequence, EPA is subsequently further converted through two elongation steps to a 24 carbon member (24:5). This is then desaturated in position 6 producing 24:6, finally β oxidized to 22:6 (DHA) in peroxisomes. This sequence has several implications :

a) A 6 desaturation reaction takes place at two different steps, i.e. in the desaturation of the 18 carbon (18:3 > 18:4) and 24 carbon (24:5 > 24:6) members, and is present in both the n-6 and n-3 fatty acid series. This suggests that competition between substrates may occur at two steps in the same series, in addition to the well-known competition between substrates of the two series. As a consequence, nutritional (i.e. the balance between n-6 and n-3 fatty acids in the diet) as well as metabolic (i.e. competition between substrates in the same fatty acid series) factors are involved in the regulation of the overall formation of LCP. It is not clear, however, whether there is only one type of Δ 6 desaturase or different ones for the various substrates and a similar question can be posed for the elongases.

b) The presence of peroxisomal steps in the metabolic sequence, opens up an interesting area of research, due to the involvement of peroxisomes in various aspects of lipid metabolism in physiological and pathological conditions and to the well-known responsiveness of these particles to activating agents. In fact, peroxisomes are primarily responsible for the β oxidation of long chain fatty acids as well as for the synthesis of plasmalogenic phospholipids. Differing from mitochondria, the peroxisomal system is inducible by various agents including the long chain fatty acid substrates, i.e. peroxisomes proliferate to deal with the excess substrate to be oxidized. This may apply also to the biosynthetic pathway in the formation of 22 carbon n-6 PUFA; we have recently reported that the production of 24 carbon PUFA from exogenous arachidonic acid (20:4 n-6), in THP-1 cells, is activated at relatively high substrate concentration [2]. In addition to the natural long chain fatty acids, various types of synthetic compounds of fatty acid nature and endowed of lipid lowering activity, the "fibric acids" or "fibrates," appear to exert their effects through the proliferation of peroxisomes, by interacting with nuclear receptors, the "peroxisome proliferator activated receptor" (PPAR), a member of the steroid hormone receptor superfamily [3]. It is therefore possible that the biosynthesis of LCP may be affected by the administration of peroxisome proliferators. On the other side, some of the long-term activities exerted by LCP of the n-3 series may be mediated by activation of nuclear processes, possibly through interactions with the PPAR receptor [4]. Although there is little information on the role of the peroxisomal pathway for the synthesis of 22 carbon PUFA *in vivo*, there is some evidence that in severe peroxisomal disorders, such as the Zellweger syndrome, the accumulation of 22:6 in tissues is greatly reduced [5].

The complexity of the pathways for the synthesis of n-3 LCP from the short chain precursor, may be responsible for the relatively low rates of formation of DHA from α LNA. It is thus possible that the levels of EPA and DHA in tissues depend more upon the supply of preformed compounds in the diet, such as it occurs in omnivores, rather than upon the *in vivo* biosynthesis, as it must occur in herbivores.

Fatty Acid Series

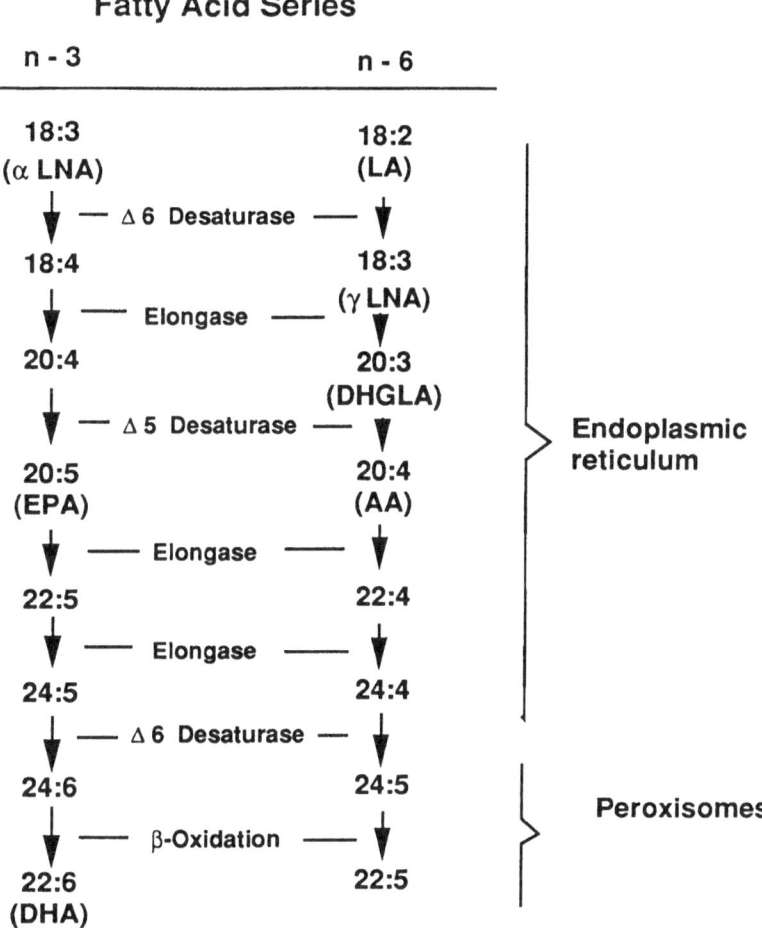

Figure 1. Metabolic conversion of 18 carbon to 22 carbon PUFA in the n-3 and n-6 series. AA, arachidonic acid; DHGLA, di-homo-gamma-linolenic acid. For other abbreviations, see text.

Another aspect of importance concerning the metabolism of the n-3 LCP is represented by the very low rates of their apparent turnover in plasma and cell lipids. This is indicated by the prolonged retention of elevated levels of EPA and DHA in plasma lipids and in lipids of circulating cells (platelets, leukocytes, and red blood cells), lasting for several months after cessation of treatment, in subjects receiving n-3 PUFA supplements [6]. While it is possible that the very low turnover is related to the turnover rates of the whole n-3 fatty acid-containing phospholipid molecule, the practical consequence is that trials with the use of these compounds cannot be carried out with a cross-over design.

Requirements and Availability of n-3 LCP

The known essentiality of DHA-containing phospholipids in the brain and the retina for neuronal functioning and visual acuity [7] and estimations of the convertibility of α-LNA to EPA and DHA has prompted some organization [8,9] to recommend minimal daily intakes for average populations, in grams per day, for n-3 PUFA. These recommendations include, in addition to dietary α-LNA, dietary EPA and DHA after considering the limited conversion of α-LNA to the above fatty acids and the antithrombotic potential of EPA plus DHA. Lowering the ratio of n-6 PUFA/n-3 PUFA to values between 4:1 and 10:1 was also advised in view of the competitive influence of high n-6 intakes on the synthesis of n-3 LCP. Although these values are just estimates and need to be confirmed by experimental data, they may be a starting point in the evaluation of the adequacy of the calculated average intakes in different population groups. The available estimated [10] and recommended [9] intakes for n-3 PUFA are presented in Table 1. It appears that the average intakes for EPA and DHA are only a small fraction of the recommendations, and this indicates a wide gap between the actual availability of these nutrients required for neuronal and visual functioning and for the prevention and management of chronic diseases, and the optimal intakes. It is also clear that the availability of preparations selectively enriched in EPA and DHA is very useful in order to provide adequate supply to individuals at risk for various chronic diseases who may need greater intakes.

Table 1. Estimated and Recommended Intakes for n-3 PUFA.

Fatty Acid	Estimated [10] g/day	Recommended [9] g/day
α-LNA	2.80	2.50
EPA + DHA	0.124	1.25

Cellular Basis for the Biological Effects of n-3 LCP

There is solid evidence that DHA is essential for visual function and for neuronal integrity [7]. A number of studies have also shown that various risk factors for cardiovascular disease are favorably affected by the administration of EPA and DHA (Table 2). The mechanisms responsible for the effects of n-3 LCP at the cellular level are certainly quite complex and diversified, since n-3 PUFA are ubiquitous constituents of structural lipids in cellular and subcellular membranes and also interact with various metabolic processes. A simplified representation of the possible sites of action (Figure 2) indicates an interplay among events taking place at the membrane level (generation of mediators and messengers in response to stimulation, ion transport processes, etc.), metabolic processes (fatty acid oxidation and peroxisomal activities) and events occurring at the nuclear level, where modulation of the

Table 2. Reported effects on risk factors for cardiovascular disease in human trials using pharmacological levels* of n-3 fatty acids (EPA + DHA).

Risk Factors	Effects
Plasma LDL-Cholesterol	Increase[†]
Plasma HDL, HDL_2	Increase
Plasma triglyceride	Decrease
Lipoprotein(a)	Decrease
Blood pressure	Decrease
Platelet function	
(adesion, aggregation, Tx A_2 synthesis)	Decrease
White cell count, leukocyte activation, LTB_4	
synthesis	Decrease
RBC filterability/deformability	Increase
Blood and plasma viscosity	Decrease
Plasma fibrinogen	Decrease

* Findings in human trials using EPA and DHA levels in the range of 1.4 to 6 g/day.
† Only in types of hyperlipemia (type IIb, type IV/V), in which LDL-cholesterol is normal or only marginally elevated.

expression of various types of proteins may be involved. Research in progress along these lines will provide more detailed clues on the biological roles of n-3 fatty acids in the near future.

Conclusions and Future Developments

The recent developments in our understanding of the biochemistry of the n-3 fatty acids (e.g. the involvement of the peroxisomal pathway, the interactions with the PPAR system) provide the basis for the appreciation of some of the unique physiological properties of these compounds, especially the long-term effects, possibly mediated by gene expression. The poor rates of endogenous synthesis of n-3 LCP from the precursor α-LNA supplied by the diet and their low availability in most foods, call for increments in the consumption of n-3 rich foods (fish) and, in some instances, the use of readily available highly enriched preparations for supplementation to subjects with enhanced requirement.

From a practical point of view, there is a need to define better the nutritional equivalency of the various n-3 fatty acids (? α-LNA = ? EPA = ? DHA) as well as their relative biological potencies. More specifically, the comparative potencies of EPA and DHA on some of the major effects (lipid/lipoproteins, membrane function, peroxisomes, nuclear events) are still largely unexplored.

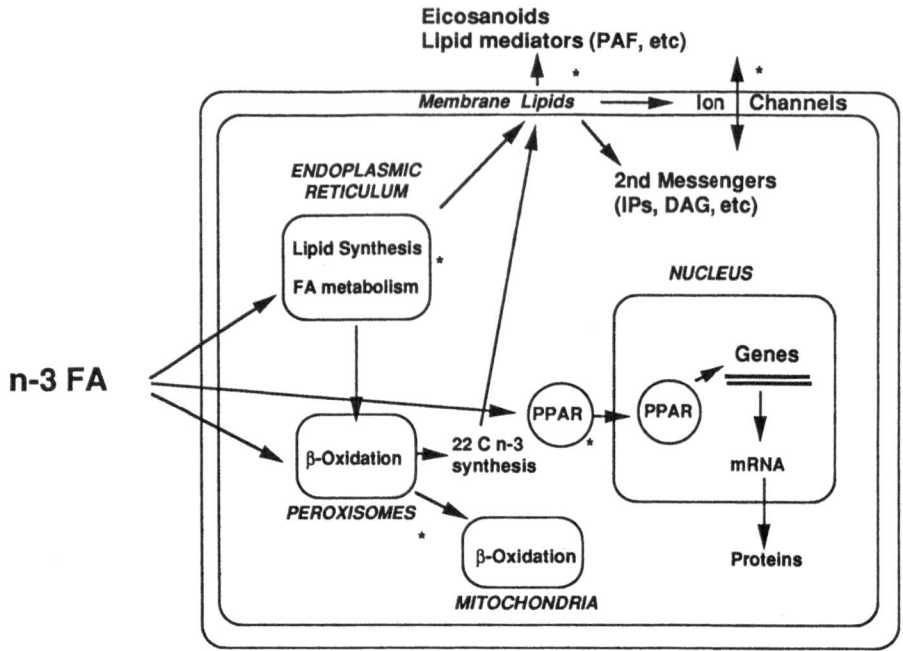

Figure 2. Possible sites of action of n-3 fatty acids at the cellular level (*):
-Lipid synthesis
-Membrane lipids and related processes (fluidity, eicosanoids, ion channels, 2nd messengers)
-Fatty acid oxidation (energy and 22 C PUFA synthesis)
-Peroxisomal proliferation, PPAR activation and nuclear processes

References

1.   Voss A, Reinhart M, Sankarappa S, Sprecher H. The metabolism of 7,10,13,16,19-docosahexaenoic acid in rat liver is independent of a 4-desaturase. J Biol Chem 1991;266:19995-20000.
2.   Caruso D, Risé P, Galella G, et al. Formation of 22 and 24 carbon 6-desaturated fatty acids from exogenous deuterated arachidonic acids is activated in THP-1 cells at high substrate concentrations. FEBS Letters 1994;343:195-199.
3.   Issemann I, Green S. Activation of a member of the steroid-hormone receptor superfamily by peroxisome proliferators. Nature 1990;347:645-650.
4.   Keller H, Dreyer C, Medin J, et al. Fatty acids and retinoids control lipid metabolism through activation of peroxisome proliferator activated receptor, retinoid - x receptor heterodimers. Proc Natl Acad Sci USA 1993;90:2160-2164.
5.   Martinez M. Abnormal profiles of polyunsaturated fatty acids in the brain, liver, kidney and retina of patients with peroxisomal disorders. Brain Res 1992;583:171-

182.

6.   Marangoni F, Angeli MT, Colli S, et al. Changes of n-3 and n-6 fatty acids in plasma
        and circulating cells of normal subjects, after prolonged washout. Biochim Biophys
        Acta 1993;1210:55-62.

7.   Neuringer M, Anderson GJ, Connor WE. The essentiality of n-3 fatty acids for the
        development and function of the retina and brain. Ann Rev Nutr 1988;8:517-41.

8.   Health and Welfare Canada: Nutrient Recommendations: The Report of the
        Scientific Review Committee. Ottawa: Supply and Services Canada, 1990

9.   British Nutrition Foundation: Unsaturated Fatty Acids:Nutritional and Physiological
        Significance. Andover, England: Chapman and Hall, 1992.

10.   Raper NR, Cronin JF, Exler J. Omega-3-fatty acids content of the United States
        food supply. J Am Coll Nutr 1992;11:304.

EFFECT OF SUPPLEMENTATION WITH MODERATE DOSES OF n-3 FATTY ACID ETHYL ESTERS TO HYPERTRIGLYCERIDEMIC PATIENTS ON LIPID AND HEMOSTATIC VARIABLES

Elena Tremoli, Susanna Colli, Paola Maderna, Sonia Eligini, Eduardo Stragliotto[1],
Patrizia Risé, Franco Pazzucconi, Cesare R. Sirtori, and Claudio Galli
Enrica Grossi Paoletti Center
Institute of Pharmacological Sciences
University of Milan
Via Balzaretti 9
20133 Milan
and
[1] Pharmacia Carlo Erba
Milan
ITALY

Introduction

The evidence of a reduced incidence of cardiovascular disease in the Eskimos, a population with a high dietary intake of n-3 fatty acids derived from fish, has suggested that dietary supplementation with n-3 fatty acids may be beneficial in the prevention of cardiovascular risk [1,2]. Recently, preparations of n-3 fatty acids as ethyl esters, enriched in eicosapentaenoic (EPA) and docosahexaenoic (DHA) acids, have become available. These preparations are well absorbed and can influence the plasma and cell compartments in a fashion comparable with that of n-3 fatty acids in other forms (triglycerides, fish or purified fatty acids) [3-5]. Initial studies indicate that n-3 fatty acid ethyl esters (n-3 FAs) administered at the dose of 3 g/day for 18 weeks to healthy subjects effectively influence plasma triglyceride levels and platelet function [6]. Moreover, the same treatment schedule was shown to inhibit the capacity of monocytes to generate thrombin, that is the expression of tissue factor activity by these cells [7]. In the study below described we demonstrate that n-3 FAs administered for 18 weeks at the dose of 3 g/day to hypertriglyceridemic patients consistently affect plasma triglycerides as well as the behavior of platelets and monocytes.

133

A.M. Gotto et al. (eds.), Multiple Risk Factors in Cardiovascular Disease, 133-140.
© 1995 *Kluwer Academic Publishers and Fondazione Giovanni Lorenzini.*

Materials and Methods

DESIGN OF THE STUDY

Thirty hypertriglyceridemic patients were selected at the E. Grossi Paoletti Center and randomly assigned, according to a double-blind placebo design, to receive either 3 g/day n-3 FAs or 3 g/day olive oil for 18 weeks. Patient selection was based on the diagnosis of type IV hyperlipoproteinemia according to WHO criteria [8]. None of the patients had clinical signs of atherosclerotic disease, nor were they hypertensive or diabetic. None of the patients was taking hormonal therapies or drugs known to interfere with lipid or coagulation parameters. Twenty-nine out of the 30 patients completed the study. One patient taking the active treatment dropped out because of gastrointestinal disturbances. Blood was drawn at time 0 (baseline) and 18 weeks after starting the treatments.

During the study period the patients were asked to continue their usual diet and to refrain from consuming foods rich in n-3 fatty acids, e.g. salmon, herring, and tuna. They were, from at least one month, on a low lipid-carbohydrate diet according to established guidelines in Italy: 40% from fats with a polyunsaturated-to-saturated fat ratio >1.8; 38-40% from carbohydrates; and 20% from proteins [9]. The project was approved by the Ethical Committee of the E. Grossi Paoletti Center. All the participants were carefully informed of the end points of the study. Informed consent was obtained from patients participating to this study.

PLASMA LIPIDS

Total cholesterol (TC) and triglyceride (TG) concentrations in plasma were measured by enzymatic methods [10,11]. High density lipoproteins (HDL) levels were determined as previously described [12]. Lipid determinations were standardized within the WHO Quality Control Program, the coefficient of variation for TC and TG being of 1.5% and 2.3%, respectively.

PLATELET AGGREGATION

Platelet-rich plasma (PRP) and platelet-poor plasma (PPP) were obtained from citrated anticoagulated blood by centrifugation at 150 and 600g for 18 min, respectively. Platelets were counted using a Coulter Counter (Coulter Electronics Ltd, Luton, England) and the platelet number adjusted to $3x10^{11}$/L using autologous PPP. Platelet aggregation was determined by the Born turbidimetric technique as previously described [13] in an Elvi 840 aggregometer (Elvi Logos, Milan, Italy), using collagen (Mascia Brunelli, Milan, Italy) as aggregating agent. For each subject, the concentration of collagen giving a 50% decrease in optical density (AC_{50}) was defined on the basis of a linear regression curve obtained by plotting the concentrations of collagen used to stimulate PRP versus the decrease in optical density determined 5 minutes after the addition of the agonist [14].

PLATELET THROMBOXANE B$_2$ FORMATION

Thromboxane B$_2$ (TXB$_2$) formation by platelets was determined in PRP samples incubated for 7.5 min at 37° C (stirring 1,000 rpm) with collagen (2.5 mg/L). The reaction was stopped by the addition of 2.5 mL methanol and TXB$_2$ levels were determined after solvent evaporation by a specific radioimmunoassay, using a commercially available kit (New England Nuclear, Boston, MA, USA).

MONOCYTE ISOLATION AND STIMULATION

All the procedures for monocyte isolation were performed under sterile conditions. Blood, anticoagulated with 3.8% sodium citrate (9:1, vol/vol), was centrifuged at 150g for 18 minutes to obtain PRP, that was discarded. The residue was processed for mononuclear cell isolation by adding an equal volume of phosphate-buffered saline (PBS) containing 0.5% bovine serum albumin and 0.1% glucose. Mononuclear cells were separated by centrifugation on Ficoll-Paque. Monocytes were isolated starting from the mononuclear cell fraction as previously described [15]. The purity of monocyte preparations was > 90%, as defined by cytochemical reactivity for alfa-naphthyl-acetate esterase [16]. Cell viability was determined by trypan blue dye exclusion. For fatty acid analyses adherent monocytes were gently scraped off, subjected to osmotic lysis with distilled water and the final pellets were stored at -80° C. For tissue factor activity (TFa) determination, adherent monocytes were incubated for 4 hours at 37° C in 5% CO$_2$ humid atmosphere in the absence and in the presence of 10 µg/mL bacterial lipopolysaccharide (LPS). At the end of the incubation period, cells were scraped off and subjected to three cycles of freezing and thawing.

ASSAY OF TISSUE FACTOR ACTIVITY (TFA)

Total cellular content of TFa was determined by a one-stage clotting assay on disrupted monocytes [17]. Assay mixture contained 0.1 mL of cell lysates, 0.1 mL citrated pooled normal plasma, and 0.1 mL of 25 mM CaCl$_2$. Clotting times were determined at 37° C and results were expressed in arbitrary units (U) by comparison with a standard curve of clotting times, which were obtained by serial dilutions of a preparation of human placental thromboplastin to which an arbitrary value of 2000 U was assigned. Assays performed with plasma from donors who were congenitally deficient in factor VII, consistently demonstrated no TFa. TFa was expressed as U/µg of protein.

FATTY ACID ANALYSES

For measurement of plasma fatty acids, blood was collected in EDTA (1 mg/mL of blood) and centrifuged for 20 minutes at 800 g. Lipids were extracted from plasma by stepwise addition to 1 volume of plasma of 2 volumes of distilled water, 4 mL of methanol, and 8 mL of chloroform containing 5 g/L of the antioxidant butylated hydroxytoluene (BHT). After phase separation at low temperature, the aqueous phase was collected and, after solvent evaporation, redissolved in chloroform/methanol 2:1 vol/vol. [18,19]. The contents of the extracts were determined by microgravimetry on aliquots of the extracts after solvent evaporation. The fatty acid methyl esters were prepared from total lipid extracts by transmethylation using methanolic HCl. The methyl esters were separated by gas liquid chromatography on capillary columns (Supelcowax 10, Fused silica 30μ, 0.32 ID, 0.25 mm film thickness) at a programmed temperature (140-210° C in 2.5/minute increments). Quantification of fatty acids was carried out by the use of the internal standard C 19:0 and calibration curves obtained with reference compounds.

Results

EFFECT OF TREATMENT WITH N-3 FAS ON PLASMA LIPIDS AND HEMOSTATIC VARIABLES

A significant accumulation of 20:5 n-3 and 22:6 n-3 levels in plasma was observed at 18 weeks of treatment with 3g/day n-3 FAs. As far as n-6 fatty acids are concerned, 20:4 n-6 levels decreased slightly in the hypertriglyceridemic patients who received n-3 fatty acids, whereas levels of 18:2 n-6 remained unchanged (Figure 1).

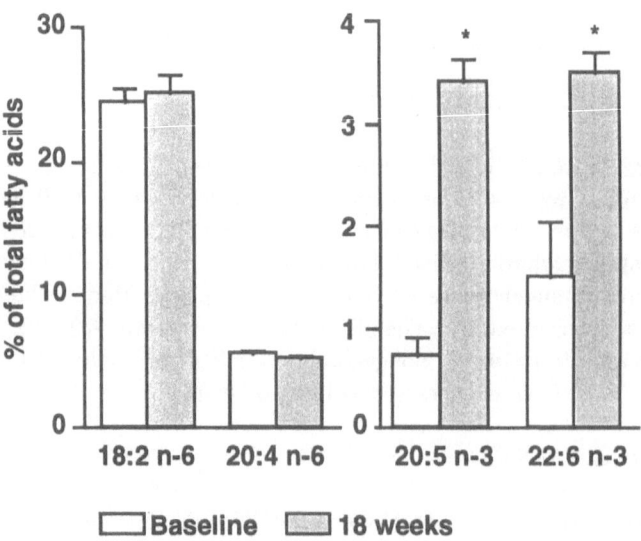

Figure 1. Fatty acid composition in plasma of hypertriglyceridemic patients at baseline and after 18 weeks treatment with n-3 FAs. Values are the means ± SEM. * p < 0.01 versus baseline.

Placebo treatment did not influence plasma lipids and platelet variables. In contrast, administration of 3 g/day n-3 FAs for 18 weeks significantly reduced plasma triglyceride levels (Table 1). The reduction of plasma triglyceride levels was accompanied by a slight increase in the HDL fraction confirming previous results obtained by our group in hypercholesterolemic patients [20].

Table 1. Effect of teatment with either 3 g/day n-3 FAs or olive oil for 18 weeks on plasma lipids and on platelet variables.

	n-3 FAs (n=14)		Olive Oil (n=15)	
	Baseline	18 weeks	Baseline	18 weeks
Total Cholesterol (mg/dl)	248 ± 10	252 ± 12	231 ± 10	232 ± 7
Triglycerides (mg/dl)	314 ± 38	200 ± 12*	371 ± 40	315 ± 37
HDL (mg.dl)	40.2 ± 2.1	41.9 ± 2.7	34.6 ± 1.7	37.6 ± 1.6
AC_{50} for Collagen (μg/ml)	0.61 ± 0.1	0.84 ± 0.1*	0.82 ± 0.1	0.85 ± 0.1
TXB_2 (ng/ml)	72.7 ± 4.8	47.7 ± 3.1**	74.9 ± 5.0	63.5 ± 6.0

Values are the average ± SEM; n=number of patients; *$p < 0.01$ and **$p < 0.001$ versus baseline

Concomitant with the beneficial effect of n-3 FAs on plasma lipids was the reduction in platelet reactivity. Indeed, in patients assigned to n-3 FAs treatment the concentration of collagen required to elicit 50% platelet aggregation was significantly increased (Table 1). A significant reduction in platelet TXB_2 formation was also observed following 18 weeks of n-3 FAs administration (Table 1).

EFFECT OF TREATMENT WITH N-3 FAS ON MONOCYTE TISSUE FACTOR ACTIVITY

Monocytes are known to generate thrombin through the expression of tissue factor (TF). TF is a transmembrane glycoprotein that mediates the initiation of the coagulation serine protease cascade. Monocytes, under basal condition do not express TF, but they do it following stimulation with a number of agonists [21]. In addition the adhesion process of monocytes to foreign surfaces induces per se the expression of relatively small amounts of TF. Cellular initiation of coagulation requires the formation of a binary complex between

TF and factor VII/VIIa. The complex TF-factorVII/VIIa leads to the activation of factor IX and X to IXa and Xa with consequent formation of thrombin [22].

As shown in Figure 2, treatment with n-3FAs for 18 weeks, significantly reduced TFa in unstimulated adherent monocytes and in monocytes exposed to 10 µg/mL LPS.

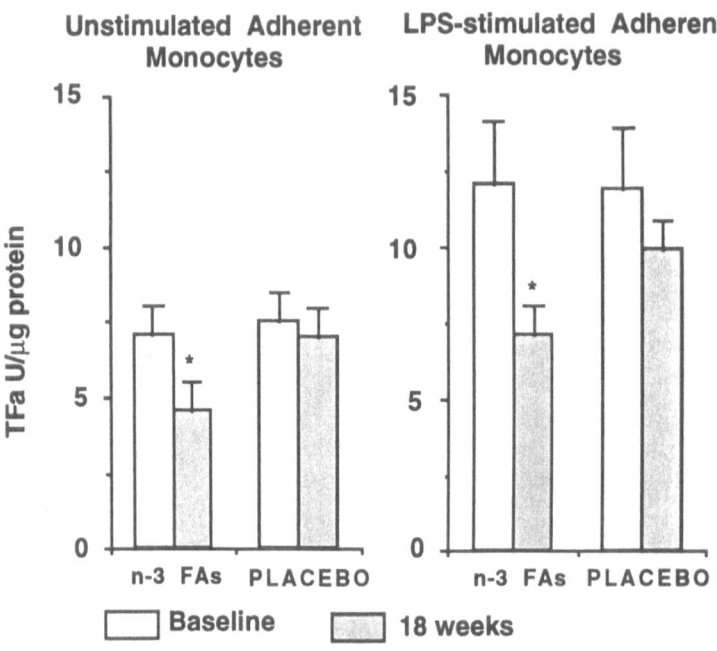

Figure 2. Tissue factor activity (TFa) in monocytes isolated from hypertriglyceridemic patients at baseline and after 18 weeks of treatment with n-3 FAs or with olive oil. Values are the means ± SEM. * p < 0.05 versus baseline.

Conclusions

The results described above indicate that a relatively prolonged administration of n-3 fatty acids, under the form of ethyl esters, improves the plasma lipid profile and the platelet reactivity in hypertriglyceridemic patients. Moreover the same treatment schedule reduces the capacity of monocytes to express TF activity, thus attenuating the prothrombotic potential of these cells.

This latter finding appears to be relevant in consideration of the observation that in hypertriglyceridemia a procoagulant state exists, due to elevated amounts of the essential cofactor for TF activity, i.e. factor VII/VIIa [23]. Because the TF-VIIa complex is the initiator of the coagulation cascade, the reduction of TF activity following n-3 FAs administration, may be relevant to this pathological condition.

In conclusion, the effects of n-3 FAs here reported add further explanation to their antithrombotic activity.

References

1.   Kromhout D, Bosschieter EB, Coulander C. The inverse relation between fish consumption and 20-year mortality from coronary heart disease. N Engl J Med 1985;312:1205-9.

2.   Dyerberg J, Bang HO. Haemostatic function and platelet polyunsaturated fatty acids in Eskimos. Lancet 1979;2:433-5.

3.   Hamazaki T, Urakaze M, Makuta M, et al. Intake of different eicosapentaenoic acid-containing lipids and fatty acid pattern of plasma lipids in the rat. Lipids 1987;22:994-8.

4.   Nørdoy A, Barstad L, Connor WE, Hatcher L. Absorption of the n-3 eicosapentaenoic acids as ethyl esters and triglycerides in humans. Am J Clin Nutr 1991;53:1185-90.

5.   Terano T, Hirai A, Hamazaki T, et al. Effect of oral administration of highly purified eicosapentaenoic acid on platelet function, blood viscosity and red cell deformability in healthy human subjects. Atherosclerosis 1983;46:321-31.

6.   Tremoli E, Maderna P, Marangoni F, et al. Prolonged inhibition of platelet aggregation following n-3 fatty acid ethyl ester administration to healthy volunteers. Am J Clin Nutr, submitted.

7.   Tremoli E, Eligini S, Colli S, et al. n-3 fatty acid ethyl ester administration to healthy subjects and to hypertriglyceridemic patients reduces tissue factor activity in adherent monocytes. Arterioscler Thromb 1994, in publication.

8.   WHO Memorandum. Classification of hyperlipoproteinemias. Circulation 1972; 45:501-8.

9.   Sirtori CR, Franceschini G, Gianfranceschi G, et al. Effects of gemfibrozil on plasma lipoprotein-apolipoprotein distribution and platelet reactivity in patients with hypertriglyceridemia. J Lab Clin Med 1987;110:279-86.

10.   Roschlau P, Bernt E, Gruber W. Enzymatic determination of total cholesterol in man. Z Klin Chem Klin Biochem 1974;12:403-7 (in German).

11.   Bucolo G, David H. Quantitative determination of serum triglycerides by the use of enzymes. Clin Chem 1973;19:476-82.

12.   Warnick GR, Benderson J, Albers JJ. Dextran sulfate-Mg^{2+} precipitation for quantitation of high-density lipoprotein cholesterol. Clin Chem 1982;28:1379-88.

13.   Tremoli E, Maderna P, Colli S, Morazzoni G, Sirtori M, Sirtori CR. Increased platelet sensitivity and thromboxane B_2 formation in type II hyperlipoproteinaemic patients. Eur J Clin Invest 1984;14:329-33.

14.   Maderna P, Colli S, Sirtori CR, Di Minno G, Tremoli E. Trial of low doses of Iloprost and aspirin in normal volunteers: Aspirin-induced enhancement of platelet anti-aggregating potential of Iloprost. Thromb Haemorrh Dis 1990;1:17-22.

15.   Stragliotto E, Camera M, Di Minno G, Postiglione A, Sirtori M, Tremoli E. Functionally abnormal monocytes in hypercholesterolemia. Arterioscler Thromb

140 E. TREMOLI ET AL.

1993;13:944-50.

16. Li CY, Lam KW, Yam LT. Esterases in human leukocyte. J Histochem Cytochem 1973;21:1-12.

17. Colli S, Tremoli E. Multiple effects of dipyridamole on neutrophils and mononuclear leukocytes: Adenosine-dependent and adenosine independent mechanisms. J Lab Clin Med 1991;118:136-45.

18. Folch J, Lees M, Sloan-Stanley GH. A simple method for isolation of total lipids from animal tissues. J Biol Chem 1957;226:497-509.

19. Rouser G, Kritchevsky G, Yamamoto A, Simon G, Galli C, Bauman AJ. Diethylaminoethyl and triethylaminoethyl-cellulose column chromatographic procedures for phospholipids, glycolipids and pigments. In: Lowenstein JM, editor. Lipids, Methods in Enzymology. New York: Academic Press, 1969;14:272-317.

20. Sirtori CR, Gatti E, Tremoli E, et al. Olive oil, corn oil, and n-3 fatty acids differently affect lipids, lipoproteins, platelets and superoxide formation in type II hypercholesterolemia. Am J Clin Nutr 1992;56:113-22.

21. Edgington TS, Mackman N, Brand K, Ruf W. The structural biology of expression and function of tissue factor. Thromb Haemost 1991;66:67-79.

22. Osterud B, Rapaport SI. Activation of factor IX by the reaction product of tissue factor and factor VII: Additional pathway for initiating blood coagulation. Proc Natl Acad Sci USA 1977;74:5260-4.

23. Meade TW, Mellows WS, Brozovic M, et al. Haemostatic function and ischemic heart disease: principal results of the Northwick Park Heart Study. Lancet 1986;2:533-7.

LONG-LASTING INHIBITION OF PLATELET AGGREGATION FOLLOWING A RELATIVELY SHORT-COURSE ADMINISTRATION OF N-3 FATTY ACID ETHYL ESTERS

Anna Maria Cerbone, Tullio Cusano, Elena Tremoli[1], Claudio Galli[1], Ferdinando Cirillo, Antonio Coppola, Eduardo Stragliotto[2], Aldo Amoriello[3], Vincenzo Marottoli[3], Gennaro Vecchione[4], and Giovanni Di Minno
Institute of Internal Medicine and Metabolic Diseases
University of Naples
Naples
[1]Institute of Pharmacological Sciences
University of Milan
Milan
[2]Medical Department, Pharmacia Farmitalia-Carlo Erba
Milan
[3]Divisions of Hematology and ImmunoHematology
Cardarelli Hospital
Naples
and
[4]I.R.C.S.S. "Casa Sollievo della Sofferenza"
San Giovanni Rotondo
ITALY

Introduction

Over the last 10 years, several studies have investigated the mechanisms through which fish oils rich in n-3 fatty acids may exert their antithrombotic activity [1]. Concerning the effects on platelets, the majority of *ex vivo* studies [2-5] show that the supplementation of n-3 fatty acids results in prolonged bleeding time and changes in the ability of platelets to aggregate and to adhere to collagen or fibrinogen-coated surfaces. Pathophysiological and clinical data [6] suggest that the aggregation of platelets involves, to some extent, the synthesis of prostaglandins/thromboxane. On the other hand, recently Tremoli et al. [7] have shown that, following cessation of the administration of a prolonged regimen of n-3 fatty acids ethyl esters, a long-lasting inhibition of platelet aggregation takes place, that minimally involves the synthesis of prostaglandins and thromboxane. We reasoned that it would be clinically important to evaluate whether a long-lasting platelet inhibitory effect of n-3 fatty acids could

A.M. Gotto et al. (eds.), Multiple Risk Factors in Cardiovascular Disease, 141-145.

be detected after a relatively short-course supplementation. This approach would also help elucidate potential antiplatelet mechanisms n-3 fatty acids independent of the synthesis of prostaglandins and thromboxane.

Methods

The study was carried out in 10 healthy volunteers (8 males, 2 females; 24-30 years old), who were instructed to ingest twice daily, during the meals, 2.55 grams of n-3 fatty acids ethyl esters (EPA/DHA ratio: 1.4) for 4 weeks. Immediately before starting the supplementation (-30), 28 days later (i.e. on the day when it was withdrawn) (time 0), and monthly for 3 months after the cessation of the supplementation (+30, +60, and +90), the skin bleeding time was assessed, and blood platelets were tested for the following variables: cAMP formation; membrane glycoprotein content as evaluated by Fluorescence Activated Sorter (FACS) analysis; adhesion to glass; aggregation in response to collagen, arachidonic acid, and ADP; thromboxane B_2 formation; ATP secretion; and binding of radiolabelled fibrinogen in response to thrombin. The skin bleeding time; platelet adhesion to glass; platelet aggregation in response to threshold concentrations of ADP, collagen and arachidonic acid; fibrinogen purification, characterization and labelling; TXB_2 measurements; intraplatelet cAMP; platelet secretion of nucleotides and binding to platelets of radiolabelled fibrinogen were carried out as previously reported [6,8]. FACS analysis of membrane glycoproteins was carried out as recently reported for monocytes [9].

Results and Discussion

Table 1 shows that at the cessation of the supplementation, the bleeding time was slightly although not significantly prolonged, and that platelet adhesion to glass was unchanged. Both these measurements were unchanged in the 3 months that followed cessation of n-3 fatty acids supplementation. In contrast, aggregation in response to collagen was greatly affected. At the cessation of the supplementation, the amount of collagen needed to cause 50% aggregation within 3 minutes was almost twice as much as that required before starting the supplementation ($p < 0.01$). The effect on the aggregation of platelets was long-lasting, the significant differences reported above being detectable 1 and 2 months after withdrawing the supplementation. Similar results were found when ADP was the agonist employed. In contrast the response to arachidonic acid was unchanged throughout the study. Together, the data were taken to suggest that the inhibitory effect observed when collagen or ADP were the agonists, was, at least in part, independent of the synthesis of thromboxane.

On the other hand, platelet secretion of ATP was normal, as were intraplatelet levels of cAMP. Thus other directions were explored. The binding of fibrinogen to specific platelet receptors is a prerequisite for the aggregation of platelets [6]. Therefore we wondered whether the impaired aggregation of platelets that followed cessation of the n-3 fatty acids supplementation, could involve an abnormal binding of this protein to platelets, and the data obtained showed that this was not the case. On the other hand, FACS analysis (Table 2)

Table 1. Bleeding time and platelet aggregation and adhesion during and at different time intervals following 1-month supplementation of n-3 FA ethyl esthers (Mean ± 1 SD).

	time of sampling (d)				
	-30	0	+30	+60	+90
Bleeding Time	265	319	339	294	nd°
(sec)	±63	±107	±111	±78	
Aggregation					
ADP	1.04	1.17	1.64^	1.50^	1.42
AC_{50} (μM)	±0.5	±0.4	±0.5	±0.5	±0.5
Collagen	0.45	0.73^	0.69^	0.72^	0.65
AC_{50} (μg/ml)	±0.2	±0.3	±0.3	±0.2	±0.3
Arachidonic Acid	0.42	0.46	0.44	0.44	0.41
AC_{50} (mM)	±0.2	±0.1	±0.1	±0.1	±0.2
Adhesion to Glass	89	84	89	89	nd°
(%)	±6	±3	±4	±5	

° nd: not determined; ^p < 0.05

showed that the glycoproteins IIb-IIIa complex, the receptor for fibrinogen on the platelet surface, was normal in cells from these volunteers. Thus the long-lasting impaired platelet aggregation of subjects who had ingested n-3 fatty acids did not appear to involve thromboxane B_2 formation, nucleotide secretion, intraplatelet cAMP, or abnormalities of the glycoprotein IIb-IIIa. On the other hand, n-3 FA did not appear to affect the glycoprotein Ib, the glycoprotein Ib-IX complex, and the glycoprotein receptors for thrombospondin, PADGEM, and vLAß. Recent data from Tremoli et al. [7] suggest that the long-lasting impaired aggregation of platelets that follows the cessation of a prolonged n-3 fatty acids supplementation, is associated with changes in the platelet membrane lipid composition. The association between the two phenomena is now under intensive investigation in our lab, and is supported by *in vitro* studies [10], in which enrichment of platelets with eicosapentaenoic (EPA) and/or docosahexanoic acids (DHA) is associated with changes of aggregation comparable to those induced in our volunteers.

In conclusion, we have found that following cessation of a relatively short-course supplementation of n-3 fatty acids ethyl esters, a long-lasting inhibition of platelet aggregation occurs, that is independent on the binding of fibrinogen to its specific receptor.

Table 2. FACS analysis of some platelet surface glycoproteins during and at different time intervals following 1-month supplementation of n-3 FA (Means ± 1 SD)

Glycoprotein	time of sampling (d)			
(Gp)	-30	0	30	90
Flow cytometry (% subject/control ratio)*				
Gp IIb-IIIa (P2)	1.17	1.10	0.98	0.89
Gp IIb (SZ.22)	1.39	0.99	1.27	nd
Gp IIIa (Y2/51)	1.09	0.99	0.95	1.01
Gp Ib (SZ1)	1.10	1.18	1.15	1.06
Gp Ib/IX (SZ2)	1.26	1.06	1.16	1.24
TSP Rec	1.48	1.26	1.13	0.87
VLAß (K20)	1.07	1.00	0.96	0.92
PADGEM (CBL-thr/6)	1.15	1.08	nd	nd

nd: not determined

*The values reported are means ± 1 SD of three determinations, those for controls are composite data from 10 normal platelet suspensions evaluated in parallel studies. Except for the TSP receptor at time 90 ($p < 0.05$) all other comparisons are not statistically significant.

References

1.   Cirillo F, Coppola A, Piemontino U, et al. Platelet effects of w3 fatty acid ethyl esters. World Rev Nutr Diet, Basel Karger, 1994;75: in press.

2.   Thorngren M, Gustafson A. Effects of 11-week increase in dietary eicosapentaenoic acid on bleeding time, lipids and platelet aggregation. Lancet 1981;2:1190-1193.

3.   Hirai A, Terano T, Hamazaki T, et al. The effects of the oral administration of fish oil concentrate on the release and the metabolism of ^{14}C arachidonic acid and ^{14}C-eicosapentaenoic acid by human platelets. Thromb Res 1982;28:285-298.

4.   von Schacky C, Fisher S, Weber PC. Long-term effects of dietary marine n-3 fatty acids upon plasma and cellular lipids, platelet function, and eicosanoid formation in humans. J Clin Invest 1985;76:1626-1631.

5.   Li X, Steiner M. Fish oil: A potent inhibitor of platelet adhesiveness. Blood 1990;76:938-945.

6.   Di Minno G, Cerbone AM, Mattioli PL, et al. Functionally thrombasthenic state in normal platelets following the administration of ticlopidine. J Clin Invest 1985;75:328-338.

7.   Tremoli E, Maderna P, Marangoni F, et al. Prolonged inhibition of platelet

aggregation following n-3 fatty acid-ethyl ester administration in healthy volunteers. Am. J Clin Nutr, in press.

8.   Di Minno G, Silver MJ, de Gaetano G. Prostaglandins as inhibitors of human platelet aggregation. Br J Haematol 1979;43:637-647.
9.   Stragliotto E, Camera M, Postiglione A, et al. Functionally abnormal monocytes in hypercholesterolemia. Arterioscl Thrombos 1993;13:944-950.
10.   Croset M, Lagarde M. In vitro incorporation and metabolism of eicosapentaenoic and docosahexaenoic acids in human platelets. Effect on aggregation. Thromb Haemostas 1986;56:57-62.

INSULIN RESISTANCE AND CARDIOVASCULAR RISK FACTORS IN NON-INSULIN-DEPENDENT DIABETES MELLITUS

K. George M. M. Alberti
Department of Medicine
University of Newcastle
The Medical School
Framlington Place
Newcastle upon Tyne NE2 4HH
UNITED KINGDOM

Introduction

It has long been known that macrovascular disease is a major cause of morbidity and mortality in noninsulin-dependent diabetes mellitus (NIDDM). Ischemic heart disease, cerebrovascular disease, and peripheral vascular disease are two to five times commoner in NIDDM than in the nondiabetic population. This has emerged from a range of sources including the classical Framingham and MRFIT studies [1,2]. CVD is far the commonest cause of death in NIDDM. There has thus been considerable interest in CVD risk factors (CVDRF) in NIDDM. In general, apart from smoking, most of the commoner risk factors are indeed more common in NIDDM than in the general population. Table 1 shows cross-sectional data from our own clinic in Newcastle.

Table 1. Cardiovascular Disease Risk Factors in NIDDM.

	%
Overweight	71
Obesity	25
Hypertension	55
Raised Triglycerides	68
Low HDL-Cholesterol	29

We have also shown in a separate cohort study that 1 year after diagnosis of NIDDM, 75% had hypertension, 65% had raised triglycerides, and marked hyper-cholesterolemia (> 65 mM) was present in 35% [3]. Similar data have been shown elsewhere. The major known risk factors do not however account for the entire risk.

147

A.M. Gotto et al. (eds.), Multiple Risk Factors in Cardiovascular Disease, 147-154.
© *1995 Kluwer Academic Publishers and Fondazione Giovanni Lorenzini.*

NIDDM itself confers additional risk as shown in the Framingham study.

Syndrome X

The clustering of CVDRF in diabetes was first noted by Avogaro and Crepaldi in 1965 [4]. Recently this has been emphasized by Reaven who labelled the quartet of risk factors, abnormal glucose tolerance, hypertension, dyslipidemia (raised triglycerides and low HDL-cholesterol), and obesity, "Syndrome X" [5]. The most important part of this observation was that he pointed out that each component part of Syndrome X was associated with insulin resistance and/or hyperinsulinemia, which Reaven suggested could have an etiological role. This was particularly pertinent in that others had postulated that hyperinsulinemia could have a direct role in promoting atherogenesis.

   Since the publication of Reaven's hypothesis, a whole range of other confirmed and putative CVD risk factors have been added to Syndrome X, which itself has been variously relabelled: the "metabolic syndrome," the "plurimetabolic syndrome," and the "insulin resistance syndrome." The original name is probably the most satisfactory in that it carries no connotations of causality, which remain largely speculative. There is, none the less, some confusion with cardiologic Syndrome X.

   The most important of the new components of Syndrome X are central obesity, microalbuminuria, raised sodium-lithium countertransport activity, PAI-1, hyper-fibrinogenemia, and physical activity. All of these may be associated with NIDDM and are commoner in NIDDM than in those with normal glucose tolerance although there is considerable overlap.

   In the rest of this brief review the association of insulin-resistance with each of the major risk factors will be discussed with particular respect to NIDDM.

Insulin Resistance and Cardiovascular Disease Risk Factors

Insulin resistance as usually measured implies only that there is impaired clearance of glucose from the circulation in response to exogenous or endogenous insulin. The euglycemic hyperinsulinemic clamp, the glucose-insulin-somatostatin infusion, and the short IV insulin tolerance test rely on exogenous insulin while the Bergman minimal model IV glucose tolerance test and he HOMA (homeostatic model assessment) method depend on endogenous insulin (see [6] for review of methods).

   A much broader definition of insulin resistance is desirable. There is clear evidence, that, if sought, many other resistant metabolic pathways can be identified. Thus adipose tissue resistance is generally found when glucose clearance is decreased and may be of considerable pathological importance. A definition such as "impaired action of insulin on carbohydrate, lipid, and protein metabolism" may be preferable while realizing that most studies are restricted to carbohydrate metabolism alone. The combination of the "clamp" with isotopic turnover, indirect calorimetry, and lipid intermediates can, indeed, give considerably more information, particularly if low doses of insulin are used in the clamp.

NIDDM

The presence of insulin resistance in NIDDM has been known for more than 50 years. It is associated particularly with failure of glucose storage in muscle and impaired activation of muscle glycogen synthase activation, and failure to suppress hepatic glucose production. In our own hands there was a 70% decrease in so-called "M" value (the amount of glucose infused per unit time to maintain euglycemia in the clamp) in normal weight new NIDDM patients [7]. There was a small additional effect of obesity: 85% decrease in those with BMI > 30 kg/m². It is worth noting that there is overlap with the nondiabetic population due perhaps to physical inactivity in some of the latter. There is also a tendency for insulin resistance to cluster in families. NIDDM is probably a heterogenous collection of disorders and in some insulin resistance will be dominant while in others impaired insulin secretion is more important.

OBESITY

Total body obesity of itself is clearly associated with insulin resistance [8]. A close correlation has been shown with total body fat in several groups of patients e.g., Pima Indians and our own Europid subjects. Several defects in insulin action have been shown in the grossly obese at both receptor and postreceptor level including down-regulation of the receptor and impaired tyrosine kinase activity of the receptor.

The emphasis now, however, is much more in fat distribution than on total obesity. The importance of androgenous fat distribution i.e., central adiposity, was pointed out nearly 50 years ago by Vague [9] but has only come into prominence in the last decade. Central obesity is much more closely associated with insulin resistance than BMI at least in some studies [10]. In our studies in Mauritius we found an independent contribution of BMI and waist-hip ratio to both basal resistance and to the risk of developing NIDDM [11]. This relates particularly to intra-abdominal rather than subcutaneous fat.

It has been suggested that central obesity plays a key role in initiating the various components of Syndrome X, through induction of insulin resistance. This is discussed further below.

PHYSICAL INACTIVITY

Physical inactivity is closely associated with NIDDM and the other lifestyle disorders. Whether this is merely an association or causally related remains to be established. Certainly there is a close correlation between fitness as assessed by V_{02} max and insulin sensitivity. We found in multivariate analysis that fitness was a more significant determinant than either total body fat or central obesity. Physical inactivity also adds significantly to the risks of developing NIDDM, presumably through increasing insulin resistance. Inactivity is also associated with higher triglyceride and lower HDL-cholesterol levels. Several large studies have shown a protective effect of physical exercise against subsequent development of ischemic heart disease. In that the NIDDM population is likely to be less fit than the nondiabetic population, physical inactivity must be a significant CVDRF in NIDDM.

DYSLIPIDEMIA

The occurrence of dyslipidemia in NIDDM is clearly established. This relates particularly to raised triglycerides and lowered HDL-cholesterol concentrations both of which are likely to be significant CVDRF in NIDDM subjects. The raised triglycerides are strongly associated with a shift in the LDL profile towards small dense particles which are themselves atherogenic [12].

Several studies have shown that raised triglycerides are associated with insulin resistance [13] while lowering levels improves insulin sensitivity. In general when triglyceride levels are raised, plasma nonesterified fatty acid (NEFA) levels are also elevated and vice versa. NEFA themselves can cause insulin insensitivity via the Randle cycle [14] and it is thus difficult to establish whether triglycerides themselves directly cause insulin resistance or act via NEFA, the levels of which are nearly always raised in NIDDM and impaired glucose tolerance (IGT). The increased NEFA delivery to the liver combined with hepatic insulin insensitivity could result in more triglyceride synthesis with the situation exacerbated by impaired triglyceride clearance.

HYPERTENSION

An association between raised insulin levels and hypertension was first pointed out by Welborn et al. [15]. Raised insulin levels with normal blood glucose concentrations imply insulin resistance. This was confirmed by clamp studies by Ferrannini et al. [16] and now by many others. Treatment of the hypertension does not alter the insulin resistance. Using the glucose-insulin infusion technique in African patients we have shown a 30% fall in insulin sensitivity in untreated nonobese hypertensives. NIDDM had a bigger effect but there was no additional effect of hypertension in NIDDM patients (Ramaiya, McLarty, Alberti, unpublished observations) suggesting that in NIDDM patients hypertension does not play a significant role in causing insulin resistance.

Although the results of these detailed studies are not in doubt, it has been more difficult to show a major association between insulin resistance and hypertension in populations. We found at best weak independent associations of insulin sensitivity assessed by the HOMA method in Europids in Newcastle and in Mauritius and no association in a recent study of elderly rural Nigerians. Others have made similar observations. This does not affect the clear association of hypertension with NIDDM and IGT [17], and other components of Syndrome X, but casts doubt perhaps on the centrality of insulin resistance. On the other hand, animal models of spontaneous hypertension lend stronger support to the association. A more powerful argument comes from the studies of Haffner et al. [18] in the San Antonio Heart Study. They showed a relative risk of 2.0 for development of hypertension over an 8-year period in those in the upper quantile of fasting insulin concentration compared with those in the lowest quantile. This was, however, weaker than the risk of developing hypertriglyceridemia (3.5) or NIDDM (5.6).

Various suggestions have been made as to how insulin resistance may cause hypertension. These have been reviewed in [19]. They include alterations in muscle blood flow, elevated sympathetic nervous system activity secondary to an imbalance between catecholamine and insulin activity. There may also be a direct action of insulin to increase sympathetic activity. A further hypothesis relates to the antinatriuretic effects of insulin. It is uncertain whether this will be of importance chronically. Finally altered transmembrane cation transport may be the link between hypertension and insulin resistance. This is discussed further below.

OTHER CVD RISK FACTORS

Several other CVDRF, such as fibrinogen and PAI-1, are elevated in NIDDM. PAI-1 correlates strongly with fasting insulin levels and levels fall when measures are taken which decrease insulin resistance [20]. Other risk factors include microalbuminuria and sodium-lithium countertransport activity (SLC), both of which are also associated with impaired insulin action. Interestingly Doria et al. [21] showed that only hypertensive subjects with raised SLC were insulin resistant providing an interesting link.

Mechanisms

There is no doubt that there is clustering of many CVD risk factors, particularly in subjects with NIDDM. The major questions are first, whether this occurs by chance; and second, is this a common underlying mechanism? The answer to the first is that several studies have shown that the associations occur too often to be by chance alone [22]. The second is more difficult. Current wisdom suggests that insulin resistance/hyperinsulinemia underlies and connects the different parts of Syndrome X.

We have reviewed above the relation of the main CVDRFs which form Sydrome X to insulin resistance. In all cases there is positive evidence although the mechanisms are often obscure. A strong school views central adiposity as the main trigger [10]. This they suggest is related to androgen status which itself correlates with insulin insensitivity in some studies. It is postulated that in central obesity omental adipocytes release excess fatty acids directly into the portal system. These reach the liver and promote excess gluconeogenesis and hepatic glucose output, and triglyceride synthesis. Any excess fatty acids reaching the periphery will inhibit glucose utilization. Glucose levels will tend to rise releasing more insulin and a new steady state achieved. The increasing insulin levels, i.e. insulin resistance, will then promote higher triglyceride levels which will themselves worsen the insulin resistance. The other components of the syndrome then develop. This is an attractive hypothesis, but remains largely conjectural. In particular there is no clear evidence yet of excess NEFA entering the portal circulation in Syndrome X. A similar hypothesis has been developed involving excess glucocorticoid activity, but is also unproven.

There are other possible explanations (Table 2).

Table 2. Unifying Factors in Syndrome X.

Insulin Resistance
Hyperinsulinaemia
Central Obesity/Androgenization

Cation Transport Changes
Cell Membrane Defects

As stated above sodium-lithium countertransport activity correlates with insulin sensitivity independent of other risk factors, at least in IDDM [23]. SLC is also elevated in diabetes, hypertension, and hypertriglyceridemia. It is tempting to speculate therefore that there might be a causal association, or that they might all reflect a common antecedent mechanism. Microalbuminuria also enters the equation. This and SLC both reflect membrane functions. Other ion transporters are also abnormal in NIDDM. Thus elevated Na^+/H^+ antiport activity and altered Na^+/K^+ATPase has been noted. A less direct effect of insulin resistance would then not be surprising for some of the CVDRF as described above.

One may then propose the hypothesis that there is some fundamental change in cell membrane structure and formation which underlies all the changes of Syndrome X, and of insulin resistance. Some support is given to this by the observation that increased saturated fatty acids in muscle cell membrane phospholipids from NIDDM subjects correlates with insulin resistance. It is not difficult to imagine that dietary excess or "Westernization" could lead to similar changes. Perhaps we should talk of Syndrome M rather than Syndrome X.

Conclusions

NIDDM is associated with an excess of many cardiovascular risk factors, as well as conferring extra risk directly. The clustering of these risk factors has been termed Syndrome X. All components are related to a greater or lesser extent with insulin resistance/hyperinsulinemia, and it has been suggested that this is the causal link between the different components. The associations with insulin resistance are, however, of very variable strength and have not been found by some. This could reflect crude measurement methods, but we suggest that a different pathophysiological mechanism may be responsible involving a change in the structure and function of the cell membrane.

References

1.   Kannel WB, McGee DL. Diabetes and glucose tolerance as risk factors for cardiovascular disease: The Framingham Study. Diabetes Care 1979;2:120-126.
2.   MRFIT Research Group. Multiple Risk Factor Intervention Trial: Risk factor changes and mortality results. JAMA 1982;248:1465-1477.

3.   Marsiaj HI, Catalano C, Sum CF, Home PD, Alberti KGMM. Management of newly diagnosed non-insulin-dependent (type 2) diabetes mellitus: A retrospective audit. Diab Res Clin Pract 1991;12:129-136.
4.   Avogaro P, Crepaldi G. Essential hyperlipemia, obesity and diabetes. Diabetologia 1965;1:136-153.
5.   Reaven GM. Role of insulin resistance in human disese. Diabetes 1988;37:1595-1607.
6.   Fulcher GR, Walker M, Alberti KGMM. The assessment of insulin action *in vivo*. In: Alberti KGMM, DeFronzo RA, Keen H, Zimmet P, editors. International textbook of diabetes mellitus. Chichester: John Wiley, 1992:513-590.
7.   Johnson AB, Argyraki M, Thow JC, et al. Impaired activation of skeletal muscle glycogen synthase in non-insulin-dependent diabetes mellitus is unrelated to degree of obesity. Metabolism 1991;40:252-260.
8.   Kolterman OG, Insel J, Sackow JM, Olefsky JM. Mechanism of insulin resistance in human obesity. Evidence for receptor and post-receptor defects. J Clin Invest 1980;65:1272-1284.
9.   Vague J. La differentiation sexuelle. Facteur determinant des formes de l'obesité. Presse Med 1947;55:339-341.
10.   Bjorntorp P. Abdominal obesity and the development of non-insulin dependent diabetes mellitus. Diabetes Metab Rev 1988;4:615-622.
11.   Dowse GK, Qin H, Collins VR, et al. Determinants of estimated insulin resistance and β-cell function in Indian, Creole and Chinese Mauritians. Diab Res Clin Pract 1990;10:265-279.
12.   Stewart MW, Laker MF, Dyer RG, et al. Lipoprotein compositional abnormalities and insulin resistance in type II diabetic patients with mild hyperlipidaemia. Arterioscler Thromb 1993;13:1046-1052.
13.   Laws A, Reaven GM. Evidence for an independent relationship between insulin resistance and fasting plasma HDL-cholesterol, triglyceride and insulin concentrations. J Int Med 1992;231:25-30.
14.   Randle PJ, Gorland PB, Hales CN, Newsholme EA. The glucose fatty acid cycle. Its role in insulin sensitivity and the metabolic disturbances of diabetes mellitus. Lancet 1963;i:785-789.
15.   Welborn TA, Breckenridge A, Rubenstein AH, Dollery CT, Fraser TR. Serum insulin in essential hypertension and peripheral vascular disease. Lancet 1966;i:1336-1337.
16.   Ferrannini E, Buzzigoli G, Bonadonna R, et al. Insulin resistance in essential hypertension. New Engl J Med 1987;317:350-357.
17.   Jarrett RJ, Keen H, McCartney M, et al. Glucose tolerance and blood pressure in two population samples: Their relation to diabetes mellitus and hypertension. Int J Epidemiol 1978;7:15-24.
18.   Haffner SM, Valdez RA, Hazuda HP, Mitchell BD, Morales PA, Stern MP. Prospective analysis of the insulin resistance syndrome (Syndrome X). Diabetes 1992;41:715-722.

19.   Smith U. Insulin resistance in hypertension. In: Moller DE, editor. Insulin resistance. Chichester: John Wiley, 1993:327-354.
20.   Juhan-Vague I, Alessi MC, Vague P. Increased plasma plasminogen activator inhibitor 1 levels. A possible link between insulin resistance and atherothrombosis. Diabetologia 1991;34:457-462.
21.   Doria A, Fioretto P, Avogaro A, et al. Insulin resistance is associated with high sodium-lithium countertransport in essential hypertension. Am J Physiol 1991;261:E684-691.
22.   Zimmet PZ, Collins VR, Dowse GK, et al. Is hyperinsulinaemia a central characterisic of a chronic cardiovascular risk factor clustering symdrome? Mixed findings in Asian Indian, Creole and Chinese Mauritians. Diabetic Med 1994;11:388-396.
23.   Catalano C, Winocour PH, Thomas TH, et al. Erythrocyte sodium-lithium countertransport activity and total body insulin-mediated glucose disposal in normoalbuminuric normotensive type 1 (insulin-dependent) diabetic patients. Diabetologia 1993;36:52-56.

GLUCOSE AS A RISK FACTOR FOR ATHEROSCLEROSIS

Richard Bucala and Anthony Cerami
The Picower Institute for Medical Research
350 Community Drive
Manhasset, New York 11030
USA

Background

When compared to the general population, individuals with diabetes mellitus suffer a 3-4-fold increased risk for developing atherosclerosis and vascular insufficiency. Since diabetes afflicts at least 10 million individuals in the United States alone, the contribution of hyperglycemia and insulin resistance to the overall mortality of heart disease and stroke is considerable [1,2,3].

Among the pathological processes believed to be central in the development of atherosclerosis are biochemical modifications that affect the functional integrity of low-density lipoprotein (LDL) [4]. A dyslipidemia characterized by increased levels of LDL, VLDL, and IDL is common in diabetics and increases significantly the likelihood that these patients will suffer from the atherosclerotic complications of heart attack and stroke [5,6]. Lipoproteins isolated from diabetic plasma also have been shown to exhibit important qualitative abnormalities, such as an impaired capacity to be taken up by fibroblast or tissue LDL receptors [6,7,8,9]. The precise molecular basis for this uptake abnormality is unknown but is of considerable interest since persistent elevation of either LDL or its metabolic precursor, VLDL, has been shown repeatedly to be an important risk factor across different populations for the development of atherosclerosis [1,2,3,4,6,9].

Oxidative Modification

One type of chemical modification that has been proposed to render the LDL particle more atherogenic is "oxidative modification." LDL that has been oxidized *in vitro* by exposure to transition metals exhibits diminished recognition by cellular LDL receptors and preferential uptake by macrophage "scavenger" receptors. It has been proposed that as a result of this process, vascular wall macrophages become transformed into lipid-laden "foam" cells, leading to the development of fatty streaks and the complex, proliferative lesions that characterize atherosclerotic plaque [4].

A.M. Gotto et al. (eds.), Multiple Risk Factors in Cardiovascular Disease, 155-163.

Over the years it has been established that unsaturated fatty acids (i.e. fatty acids bearing one or more double bonds in their carbon backbone) readily undergo peroxidative degradation. Lipid peroxidation occurs when an unspecified oxidant abstracts the relatively labile allylic hydrogen atom from the fatty acid side chain. In the case of polyunsaturated fatty acids, diene conjugation occurs, producing a resonance-stabilized pentadienyl radical. The addition of molecular oxygen then generates a lipid peroxyl radical (R-OO'). This serves to propagate oxidative degradation by initiating hydrogen atom abstraction at additional unsaturated bonds. Fatty acid peroxidation and breakdown then ensues, producing a variety of shorter chain, α,β-unsaturated aldehydes such as the hydroxy-alkenals. These species in turn can react with nucleophilic sites on proteins to form Michael addition products and resonance-stabilized Schiff bases [10,11,12]. Although transition metal-catalyzed lipid peroxidation occurs readily *in vitro* and continues to be studied as a model for the "propagative" phase of oxidative degradation, it should be noted that the identity of the oxidant(s) responsible for initiating lipid peroxidation *in vivo* has never been established. This situation has led to certain conceptual difficulties in assessing the prevalence and the pathological significance of lipid peroxidation, particularly with respect to atherogenesis [11].

Transition metals catalyze oxidative chemistry by lowering the energy barrier for electron transfer between two substrates. In effect, the unoccupied, outer *d* orbitals of transition metals act as molecular "wires" to facilitate the transfer of electrons between lipids and molecular oxygen which, in the absence of metals, is insufficiently reactive toward carbon-carbon double bonds. Although oxygen is frequently invoked as the molecule responsible for producing oxidative damage *in vivo*, it is in fact a poor oxidant. The electronic structure of triplet (ground state) oxygen has two unpaired electrons at the π anti-bonding level ($^3\Sigma g$), making the reaction between oxygen and molecules of singlet multiplicity such as unsaturated fatty acids spin forbidden. Significant amounts (0.1 - 1.0 μM) of the superoxide anion (O_2^-) do form *in vivo*, however superoxide also is incapable of abstracting *bis*-allylic hydrogens from unsaturated aliphatic residues. Under acidic conditions, superoxide may initiate oxidative modification by forming perhydroxyl radicals (HOO'), or by reacting with transition metals to form reactive hydroxyl radicals (HO') [12,13,14]. Nevertheless, low trace metal concentrations, the high availability of ligands that form tight coordination complexes with metals, and the abundant anti-oxidant capacity of plasma provide overwhelming evidence against the possibility that metal-catalyzed oxidation plays a significant role in mediating lipid peroxidation *in vivo* [15,16,17].

Advanced Glycosylation

In diabetes, persistent hyperglycemia leads to an increase in the level of nonenzymatically glycosylated or "glycated" protein amino groups [18,19]. This post-translational modification process is initiated by the attachment of glucose residues to primary amino groups and proceeds from freely reversible Schiff bases to more stable, slowly reversible Amadori rearrangement products (Figure 1). Amadori products were considered several years ago to be one potential source of apolipoprotein modification that might alter LDL metabolism *in vivo*. These adducts form on a number of plasma proteins and increased amounts of Amadori products have been found to be present in LDL isolated from diabetic patients than in LDL from nondiabetic patients [20]. Early glycosylation products such as the Schiff base or the Amadori product are slowly reversible however, and these adducts do not affect LDL clearance unless the ketoamine linkage has been first stabilized [20]. Although this can be achieved experimentally by chemical reduction with borohydride, reactions of this type do not occur *in vivo*. Instead, Amadori products either dissociate to yield free glucose, or else slowly undergo additional rearrangement reactions to produce a class of late-forming, irreversibly bound moieties termed advanced glycosylation endproducts (AGEs) [18,19].

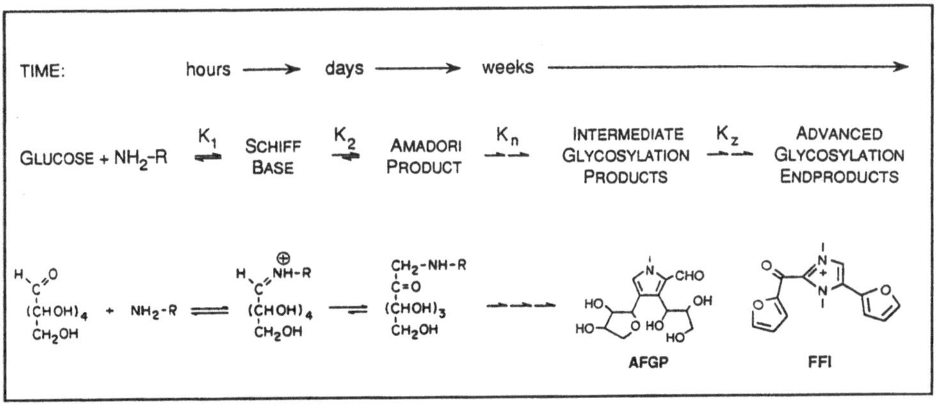

Figure 1.   Pathway for the formation of advanced glycosylation endproducts (AGEs).

AGEs have been shown to form through a succession of reactive intermediates which have the capacity to rapidly crosslink nearby lysine and arginine residues. These reactive AGEs circulate in blood and arise in large part from the entry into the plasma compartment of AGE-peptides produced by the normal catabolism of AGE-modified tissue proteins [21]. High concentrations of circulating AGE-peptides therefore occur even under non-hyperglycemic conditions if plasma filtration is impaired by renal failure. The reactive nature of AGE-peptides together with their inefficient removal by standard hemodialysis regimens has in turn led to the concept that circulating AGE-peptides comprise an important component of the so-called uremic toxins or "middle molecules" which accumulate during renal insufficiency and contribute to the morbidity and mortality of chronic renal failure [21,22]. Dyslipidemia and severe atherosclerotic vascular disease occurs in patients with renal insufficiency irrespective of diabetes. Diabetic patients with end-stage renal disease (ESRD) for example, suffer from a particularly poor long-term prognosis. Their two-year survival rate is ≤ 50% and cardiovascular complications account for the single most common cause of premature death [23,24].

Lipid Advanced Glycosylation and Oxidative Modification

Investigation into the advanced glycosylation of lipids and lipoproteins began several years ago after considering the possibility that phospholipids which contain primary amino groups could react with glucose to form AGEs in much the same way that polypeptide amines form AGEs [25]. In model studies, buffered suspensions of phosphatidylethanolamine (PE) or phosphatidylcholine (PC) were incubated with glucose and the metal chelator EDTA at 37°. PE but not PC (which contains a blocked, quaternary amine) was observed to react with glucose to form products with the same absorbance, fluorescence, and immunoreactive properties as the AGEs that form on proteins [25].

We hypothesized that intramolecular oxidation-reduction reactions, which are known to occur during advanced glycosylation [19,26], might act within the hydrophobic microenvironment of phospholipids to initiate fatty acid oxidation [25]. This oxidative pathway thus would proceed independently of added transition metals or exogenous, free-radical generating systems and might serve as an important mechanism for initiating lipid oxidation *in vivo*. As analyzed by thiobarbituric acid reactivity, lipid oxidation was observed to occur at a rate that was parallel to the rate of AGE formation. It is noteworthy that these products formed in the presence of metal chelators and in the absence of exogenously added transition metals, which frequently are used to catalyze lipid oxidation in model systems [4,10,11]. Control studies showed that lipid oxidation did not occur when glucose was incubated with PC, indicating that the reaction between glucose and the phospholipid amine was essential for initiating oxidative modification. The inclusion of free lysine to mixtures of glucose and PC also did not initiate oxidative modification, showing that AGEs must form directly within the hydrophobic microenvironment of the phospholipid to induce oxidation. In further studies, the addition of the advanced glycosylation inhibitor aminoguanidine prevented the formation of both lipid-AGEs and lipid oxidation products, verifying the essential role of advanced glycosylation in the initiation of lipid oxidation [25].

The contribution of advanced glycosylation to the oxidative modification of LDL was examined in a similar fashion *in vitro*. Purified human LDL was incubated with glucose (in the presence of metal chelators) and analyzed for both advanced glycosylation and oxidative modification. Incubation of LDL with 200 mM glucose for 3 days resulted in the formation of readily measurable levels of AGEs on both lipid and apoprotein. These studies also indicated that lipid-linked AGEs formed more rapidly than ApoB-AGEs, reaching a specific activity 100-fold greater than the ApoB-linked AGEs. These results were consistent with previously described increases in the rate of advanced glycosylation in the lipid, versus the polar, apoprotein phases. Measurements of oxidative modification further showed that LDL was oxidized concomitantly with the formation of AGEs [25].

Although thiobarbituric acid is widely used to test for lipid oxidation, the thiobarbituric acid reaction is relatively nonspecific and can produce chromophores after reaction with a number of possible aldehydes [27]. In more recent studies, gas chromatography-electron impact mass spectrometry analyses of AGE-modified LDL have identified specific oxidation products which form during either phospholipid- or LDL-advanced glycosylation. One product produced mass ions which were consistent with 4-

hydroxyhexenal, a previously characterized unsaturated fatty acid oxidation which forms by the oxidative decomposition of docosahexaenoic acid, the most prevalent fatty acid of the n-3 series [28]. These data provide further structural support for the concept that lipid-advanced glycosylation reactions can act directly to oxidize unsaturated fatty acids.

The recent identification of the AGE-reactive intermediate that is trapped by reaction with the advanced glycosylation inhibitor aminoguanidine has provided an important conceptual framework for considering how lipid-linked AGEs might act to initiate the oxidation of fatty acid side chains. Two years ago, an aminoguanidine-derived triazine was isolated from a solution of aminoguanidine and a propylamino-substituted Amadori product which were incubated under physiological conditions (Figure 2) [29]. The formation of the triazine was shown to proceed by the reaction of aminoguanidine with the reactive intermediate: 1-propylamino-1,4-dideoxyosone. The amine-substituted dideoxyosone is an interesting compound from the viewpoint that it may lead to pro-oxidant effects during advanced glycosylation reactions. Once attached to phospholipid head groups, dideoxyosones and related rearrangement products may interact with fatty acid side chains to initiate red-ox cycling directly within the hydrophobic, lipid microenvironment.

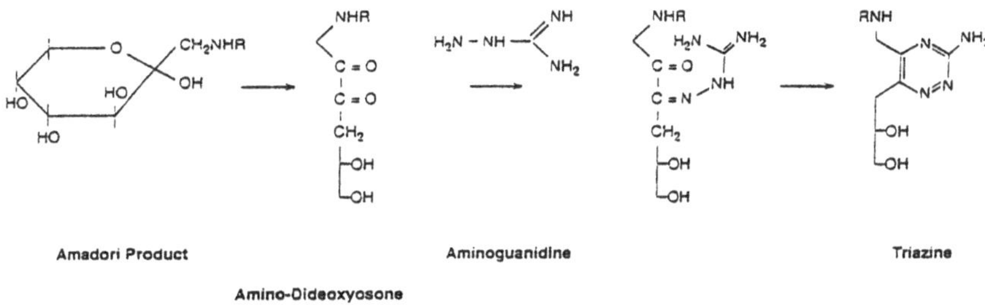

Figure 2. The formation of an aminoguanidine-derived triazine by the reaction of aminoguanidine with the reactive intermediate 1-propyl-amino-1,4-dideoxyosone (from [29]).

Lipoprotein Advanced Glycosylation

To better define the relationship between advanced glycosylation and LDL oxidation *in vivo*, we analyzed LDL from both nondiabetic and diabetic individuals by AGE-specific ELISA for the presence of phospholipid-AGEs, ApoB-AGEs, and oxidative modification [25,30]. LDL-advanced glycosylation also was examined in patients with diabetes and renal insufficiency. As discussed earlier, it had been determined that reactive AGEs circulate in high concentrations during renal insufficiency and that these AGEs can attach readily to plasma components such as LDL [21,22]. There was a significant elevation in the levels of ApoB-AGE and lipid-AGE in LDL when each of the patient groups was compared to the control (nondiabetic/normal renal function) group. The highest levels of AGE-modification were observed in patients with renal insufficiency, pointing to the important role of circulating, reactive AGE-peptides in producing AGE-modified LDL. LDL from diabetic or renal insufficient individuals also showed significantly greater oxidative modification than the LDL from control, nondiabetic individuals. These data support prior studies which have suggested that there is an increase in the thiobarbituric acid reactivity of LDL isolated from diabetic plasma [31,32]. It remains uncertain whether these measurements of LDL oxidation reflect an actual increase in lipid oxidation *in vivo*, or simply an increase in the susceptibility of LDL to oxidation once LDL is removed from the plasma for biochemical analysis. Nevertheless, linear regression analysis of these data revealed that there was a significant correlation between the level of AGE modification and LDL oxidation [25].

Chemical modification of basic residues within the LDL-receptor binding domain of ApoB has been shown to interfere with the ability of LDL to undergo receptor-mediated uptake and degradation [33,34]. Advanced glycosylation similarly modifies the lysine and arginine residues of proteins [18,19], and it was reasoned that LDL modified by AGEs might exhibit markedly delayed clearance kinetics *in vivo*. When the plasma clearance of AGE-LDL (modified *in vitro*) was examined in transgenic mice expressing the human LDL-receptor, markedly delayed clearance kinetics were observed when AGE-LDL was compared to control, native LDL [30]. Of note, the level of AGE-modification utilized in these studies was comparable to that observed in diabetic/ESRD patients *in vivo* (≈ 80 U AGE/mg ApoB). Overall, there was a significant relationship between the extent of ApoB-advanced glycosylation and impaired plasma clearance of LDL *in vivo* [30].

Lowering of Plasma LDL in Human Subjects By Aminoguanidine

To begin to assess the contribution of advanced glycosylation to altered LDL clearance kinetics in human subjects, we recently had the opportunity to study the lipoprotein profiles of diabetic patients who were enrolled in a 28-day, double-bind placebo-controlled trial of aminoguanidine [30]. Eighteen patients received aminoguanidine at an average daily dose of 1200 mg and 8 patients received placebo. Blood samples were obtained at the initiation and at the termination of treatment and analyzed for total cholesterol, triglycerides, VLDL-cholesterol, LDL-cholesterol, HDL-cholesterol, Hb-AGE, and HbA_{1c} (Table 1). The efficacy of aminoguanidine as an inhibitor of advanced glycosylation in these subjects was verified by the observation that circulating Hb-AGE levels decreased by almost 28% in the aminoguanidine-treated group [35]. Of significance, aminoguanidine therapy also was associated with a 19% decrease in total cholesterol, a 19% decrease in triglycerides, and a 28% decrease in LDL-cholesterol. There was a trend toward a decrease in VLDL-cholesterol as well, but this difference did not reach statistical significance.

Table 1. Biochemical analysis of blood specimens obtained from diabetic patients who received aminoguanidine (n=18) or placebo control (n=8) for 28 days. Values are expressed as percent (mean ± SE) of baseline value for each patient group (Day 28 value/Day 0 value x 100). P values are by paired Student's T-test. NS: not significant (from [30]).

Treatment	Cholesterol	Triglyceride	VLDL	LDL	HDL	HbAGE	HbA$_{1c}$
Aminoguanidine	81.3 ± 7.2	81.0 ± 6.2	68.5 ± 28.7	71.9 ± 9.9	104.7 ± 10.9	72.7 ± 7.5	89.7 ± 4.2
P value	< 0.04	< 0.02	NS	< 0.05	NS	< 0.025	NS
Placebo	97.4 ± 5.4	89.8 ± 5.8	96.4 ± 7.1	100.7 ± 11.2	96.7 ± 16.4	90.8 ± 6.7	100.0 ± 4.5
P value	NS	NS	NS	NS	NS	NS	NS

Conclusions

The elevated circulating level of AGE-modified LDL in diabetic patients together with the impaired plasma clearance kinetics of AGE-LDL in human LDL-receptor transgenic mice point to the important, contributory role of LDL-advanced glycosylation in diabetic atherogenesis. Impairment in the normal, receptor-mediated clearance of LDL is likely to act in concert with abnormalities in lipoprotein production, increases in lipoprotein oxidation and vascular wall lipoprotein trapping, and alterations in endothelial cell function to produce the rapidly progressive vasculopathy of diabetes or renal insufficiency. Lower levels of AGE-modified LDL occur in nondiabetic/nonrenally impaired individuals and it is worthwhile to consider that over a time period of many years, advanced glycosylation also may contribute to the age-related development of atherosclerosis in the general population.

References

1.   Kannel WB, McGee DL.   Diabetes and cardiovascular disease.   JAMA 1979;241:2035-2038.
2.   Ruderman NB, Haudenschild C. Diabetes as an atherogenic factor. Progress in Cardiovascular Diseases 1984;26:373-412.
3.   WHO Study Group. Diabetes mellitus. WHO Technical Report Series 1985;727:1-113.
4.   Steinberg D, Parthasarathy S, Carew TE, Khoo JC, Witzum JL. Modifications of low-density lipoprotein that increases its atherogenicity. Mechanisms of Disease 1989;320:915-924.
5.   Jensen T, Stender S, Deckert T.   Abnormalities in plasma concentrations of lipoproteins and fibrinogen in type I diabetic patients with increased urinary albumin excretion. Diabetologia 1988;31:142-145.
6.   Brown WV. Lipoprotein disorders in diabetes mellitus. Med Clin N Amer 1994; 78:143-161.
7.   Lopes-Virella MF, Sherer GK, Lees AM, et al. Surface binding, internalization and

degradation by cultured human fibroblasts of low density lipoproteins isolated from type I (insulin-dependent) diabetic patients: Changes with metabolic control. Diabetologia 1982;22:430-436

8.   Hiramatsu K, Bierman EL, Chait A. Metabolism of low-density lipoprotein from patients with diabetic hypertriglyceridemia by cultured human skin fibroblasts. Diabetes 1985;34:8-14.

9.   Goldstein JL, Brown MS. The low-density lipoprotein pathway and its relation to atherosclerosis. Annu Rev Biochem 1977;46:897-930.

10. Kanner J, German JB, Kinsella JE. Initiation of lipid peroxidation in biological systems. Crit Rev Food Sci Nutr 1987;25:317-365.

11. Dix TA, Aikens J. Mechanisms and biological relevance of lipid peroxidation initiation. Chem Res Toxicol 1992;6:2-18.

12. Esterbauer H, Schaur RJ, Zollner H. Chemistry and biochemistry of 4-hydroxynonenal, malonaldehyde and related aldehydes. Free Radical Biology and Medicine 1991;11:81-128.

13. Halliwell BM, Gutteridge JMC. Free radicals in biology and medicine. Oxford: Clarendon Press, 1989.

14. Bielski BHJ, Cabelli DE. Highlights of current research involving superoxide and perhydroxyl radicals in aqueous solutions. Int J Radiat Biol 1991;59:291-319.

15. Klaasen CD. In: Gillman AG, Goodman LS, Rall TW, Murad F, editors. The pharmacological basis of therapeutics. New York: Macmillian, 1985:1605-1627.

16. Frei B, Yamamoto Y, Niclas D, Ames BN. Evaluation of an isoluminol chemiluminescence assay for the detection of hydroperoxide in human blood plasma. Anal Biochem 1988;175:120-130.

17. Frei B, Stocker R, Ames BN. Antioxidant defenses and lipid peroxidation in human blood plasma. Proc Natl Acad Sci USA 1988;85:9748-9752.

18. Njoroge FG, Monnier VM. The chemistry of the maillard reaction under physiological conditions: A review. Prog Clin Biol Res 1989;304:85-107.

19. Bucala R, Cerami A. Advanced glycosylation: Chemistry, biology, and implications for diabetes and aging. Adv Pharmacol 1992;23:1-34.

20. Witztum JL, Mahoney EM, Branks MJ, Fisher M, Elam R, Steinberg D. Nonenzymatic glycosylation of low-density lipoprotein alters its biologic activity. Diabetes 1982;31:283-291.

21. Makita Z, Radoff S, Rayfield E, et al. Advanced glycosylation endproducts in patients with diabetic nephropathy. N Engl J Med 1991;325:836-842.

22. Makita Z, Bucala R, Rayfield EJ, et al. Diabetic-uremic serum advanced glycosylation endproducts are chemically reactive and resistant to dialysis therapy. Lancet 1994;343:1519-1522.

23. United States Renal Data System: USRDS 1992 Annual Data Report. The National Institutes of Health, National Institute of Diabetes and Digestive and Kidney Disease. Bethesda, MD.

24. Friedman EA. Treatment options for diabetic nephropathy. Diabetes Spectrum 1992;5:6-16.

25. Bucala R, Makita Z, Koschinsky T, Cerami A, Vlassara H. Lipid advanced glycosylation: Pathway for lipid oxidation *in vivo*. Proc Natl Acad Sci USA 1993;90:6434-6438.
26. Namiki M, Hayashi T. Formation of novel free radical products in an early stage of maillard reaction. Prog Ed Nutr Sci 1981;5:81-91.
27. Kikugawa K, Kato T, Iwata A. Determination of malonaldehyde in oxidized lipids by the Hantzsch fluorometric method. Anal Biochem 1988;174:512-521.
28. van Kuijk FJ, Thomas DW, Stephens RJ, Dratz EA. Occurrence of 4-hydroxy-alkenals in rat tissues determined as pentafluorobenzyl oxime derivative by gas chromatography--mass spectrometry. Biochemical and Biophysical Research Communications 1986;139:144-149.
29. Chen HJC, Cerami A. Mechanism of inhibition of advanced glycosylation by aminoguanidine *in vitro*. J Carbohydrate Chemistry 1993;12:731-742.
30. Bucala R, Makita Z, Vega G, et al. Modification of LDL by advanced glycosylation endproducts contributes to the dyslipidemia of diabetes and renal insufficiency. Proc Natl Acad Sci USA 1994;91:9441-9445.
31. Nishigaki I, Hagihara M, Tsunekawa H, Maseki M, Yagi K. Lipid peroxide levels of serum lipoprotein fractions of diabetic patients. Biochem Med 1981;25:373-378.
32. Morel DW, Chisolm G. Antioxidant treatment of diabetic rats inhibits lipoprotein oxidation and cytotoxicity. J Lipid Res 1989;30:1827-1834.
33. Mahley RW, Innerarity TL, Pitas RE, Weisgraber KH, Brown JH, Gross E. Inhibition of lipoprotein binding to cell surface receptors of fibroblasts following selective modification of arginyl residues in arginine-rich and B apoproteins. J Biol Chem 1977;252:7279-7287.
34. Mahley RW, Innerarity TL, Weisgraber KH, Oh SY. Altered metabolism (*in vivo* and *in vitro*) of plasma lipoproteins after selective chemical modification. J Clin Invest 1979;64:743-750.
35. Makita Z, Vlassara H, Rayfield E, et al. Hemoglobin--AGE: A circulating marker of advanced glycosylation. Science 1992;258:651-653.

DYSLIPIDEMIA IN NIDDM: NEW INSIGHTS

Marja-Riitta Taskinen, Mikko Syvänne*, and Sanni Lahdenperä
*First Department of Medicine
Third Department of Medicine
University of Helsinki
Helsinki
FINLAND

Introduction

The lipoprotein pattern in noninsulin-dependent diabetes mellitus (NIDDM) and insulin resistance syndrome (IRS) is characterized by elevation of serum and very low density lipoprotein (VLDL) triglycerides and lowering of high density lipoprotein (HDL) cholesterol whereas the concentrations of serum total and LDL cholesterol are commonly normal or only slightly increased. These lipid abnormalities are most frequent in poorly controlled NIDDM patients. Substantial evidence indicate that high triglycerides/low HDL cholesterol are strong risk factors for coronary heart disease (CHD) in NIDDM cohorts. The power of triglycerides as a CHD risk factor in NIDDM populations was clearly demonstrated in the Paris Prospective Study [1]. More recently Laakso et al. [2] reported that low HDL cholesterol was the most important single predictor of future CHD events in NIDDM patients followed over 7 years. In addition high triglycerides were associated with an increased risk of CHD events. Recently it has been questioned whether hypertriglyceridemia is directly atherogenic or if it is just a marker of underlying metabolic abnormalities like lowering of HDL cholesterol, insulin resistance, and hyperinsulinemia.

Metabolic Consequences of Hypertriglyceridemia

The recognition of the fact that hypertriglyceridemia is associated with multiple metabolic consequences (Table 1) which are potentially atherogenic may be a key link to explain the excess risk of CHD in NIDDM. Of note is that any of these abnormalities separately or in concert may raise the risk for CHD in a hypertri-glyceridemia individual. Importantly mild or moderate hypertriglyceridemia and low HDL cholesterol is very common in NIDDM patients, being present about in 20% of the patients.

A.M. Gotto et al. (eds.), Multiple Risk Factors in Cardiovascular Disease, 165-172.
© 1995 Kluwer Academic Publishers and Fondazione Giovanni Lorenzini.

POSTPRANDIAL LIPEMIA IN NIDDM

The concept that atherosclerosis is a postprandial phenomenon was introduced by Zilversmit fifteen years ago [3]. Substantial evidence have accumulated to indicate that chylomicron remnants indeed are strong risk factors for CAD [4,5]. The magnitude of

Table 1. Metabolic consequences of hypertriglyceridemia.

•   Excessive postprandial lipemia
•   Lowering of HDL and compositional changes of HDL
•   Preponderance of small, dense LDL
•   Enhancement of thrombogenesis

postprandial triglyceride response is closely related to the fasting concentration of serum triglycerides. This association may be due to a competition between endogenous and exogenous triglyceride-rich particles for the common removal pathways [6]. Accordingly postprandial lipemia is enhanced in patients with mild hypertriglyceridemia and low HDL [7]. As stated above, the constellation of high triglycerides and low HDL is frequent in NIDDM and therefore it would be anticipated to find enhanced postprandial lipemia in NIDDM. Recently substantial evidence has accumulated to confirm that indeed postprandial lipemia is increased in NIDDM patients [8-10]. The majority of remnant particles derived from the hydrolysis of chylomicrons resides within Sf 60-400, which also includes large VLDL particles.

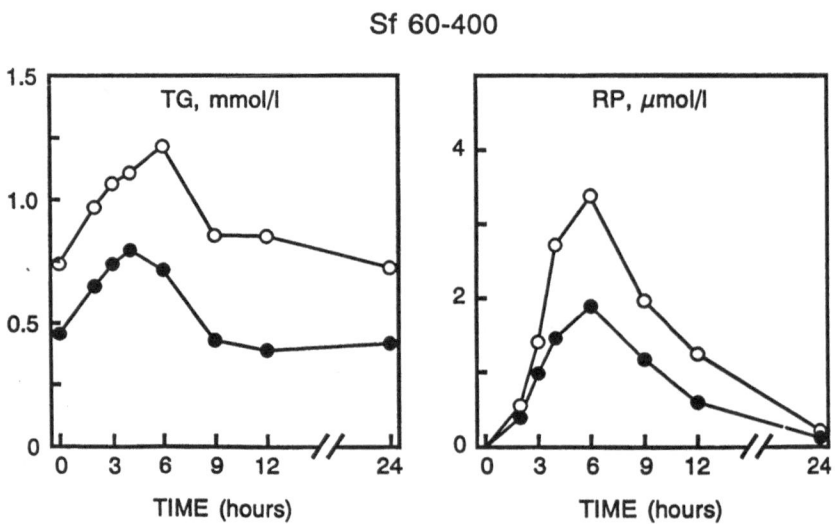

Figure 1. Responses of triglyceride (left panel) and retinylpalmitate (right panel) to oral fat load in VLDL$_1$ (Sf 60-400) fraction in Type 2 diabetic men (○) and in nondiabetic men (●).

Figure 1 shows the responses of triglyceride and retinylpalmitate used as a marker of chylomicron remnant particles in Sf 60-400 fraction during oral fat load in NIDDM as compared to nondiabetic men matched for age and BMI [10]. The postprandial responses of both triglycerides and retinylpalmitate are significantly larger in NIDDM men than in nondiabetic men. When we also followed the responses of triglycerides and retinylpalmitate in different fractions of triglyceride-rich particles (Sf > 400, Sf 20-60, and Sf 12-20 representing chylomicrons, small VLDL and IDL particles respectively) it was obvious that the most pronounced changes were observed in Sf 60-400 fraction. We conclude that NIDDM patients have defective removal of chylomicron remnants which have a long residence time in the circulation. We also reported a negative interrelationship between postheparin plasma LPL activity and postprandial increment of plasma triglycerides in nondiabetic men. However, we found no correlation between these parameters in NIDDM men indicating a defect in the hydrolysis of triglyceride-rich particles during alimentary lipemia. Thus dual defects characterizes exacerbation of postprandial lipemia in NIDDM. Although recent studies have consistently found that the magnitude of postprandial triglyceridemia is an independent predictor of coronary artery disease (CAD) in nondiabetic men [4,5] the responses of either postprandial triglycerides or retinylpalmitate did not distinguish for CAD in our NIDDM cohorts [10]. Interestingly Ginsberg et al. [11] have recently reported that postprandial lipemia does not predict the presence of CAD in nondiabetic women. Since excess of postprandial remnants are potentially atherogenic it remains appropriate to reduce postrandial lipemia in a high risk group like NIDDM patients.

HDL ABNORMALITIES IN NIDDM

Lowering of HDL cholesterol constitutes one of the characteristic lipoprotein abnormalities in NIDDM and insulin resistance syndrome. The recognition that HDL is heterogenous with respect to density and apolipoprotein content has focused the interest on the determinants of HDL subclasses. Traditionally HDL has been subfractionated into HDL_2 and HDL_3 according to the flotation rate. In most studies the concentration of HDL_3 is reduced more than that of HDL_2 in NIDDM patients [12]. Recently HDL particles have been separated into five subpopulations, which have different mean diameters of the particles, by gradient gel electrophoresis [13]. On the other hand the apolipoprotein composition of HDL can also be used to separate HDL subpopulations into particles which contain only apo A-I (LpA-I) and those containing both apo A-I and A-II (LpA-I:A-II)[14,15]. Recent data indicate that alterations of HDL subpopulations occur in patients with CAD and low HDL cholesterol [16-18]. However, so far little is known about HDL subpopulations in diabetic patients. To find out if diabetes induces specific alterations in the HDL subpopulations we measured the concentrations of LpA-I and LpA-I:A-II in 50 NIDDM men and in 30 non-diabetic men with similar age and BMI distribution [19]. The concentrations of both apo A-I and A-II were 7.1% lower in NIDDM men than in nondiabetic men. Interestingly we observed that NIDDM men had significantly lower concentrations of Lp A-I:A-II particles than nondiabetic men whereas the concentrations of Lp A-I particles were virtually similar in the two groups. Why Lp A-I:A-II particles are reduced in NIDDM and does this change interfere with mechanisms by which HDL protects against CAD remains to be established.

Recently we have also analyzed subpopulations of HDL particles by gradient gel electrophoresis (GGE) in NIDDM and nondiabetic men. Our preliminary data indicate that no consistent differences were observed in the distribution of HDL_{2B}, HDL_{2A}, HDL_{3A}, HDL_{3B}, and HDL_{3C} between the two groups. Likewise the mean diameter of particles sizes in each HDL subpopulations were closely similar. Interestingly the mean diameter of particles in each subclass seemed to decrease over the quintiles of fasting triglycerides. Chang LBF et al. [20] have reported that mean diameter of HDL subpopulations decreased when plasma triglycerides increased from 0.54 to 3.52 mmol/l. Altogether the data suggest that even mild hypertriglyceridemia is associated with a shift towards small HDL particles.

LDL SUBCLASSES IN NIDDM

Although the concentration of LDL in NIDDM patients is generally normal or slightly elevated the composition of LDL is altered (Figure 2). Our data shows that LDL (d 1.019 -

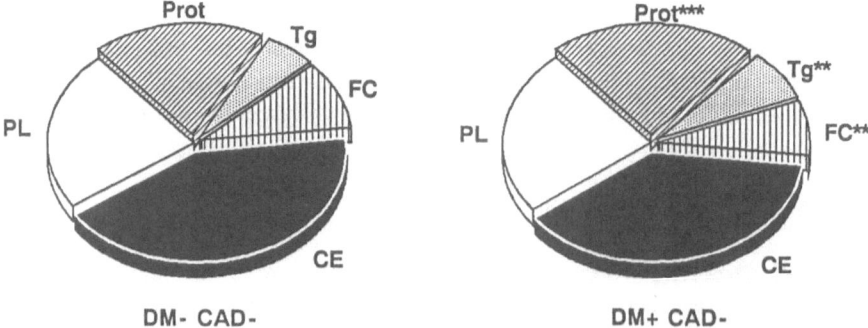

DM- CAD-   DM+ CAD-

Figure 2. Percentage composition of LDL (d 1.019-1.063) in Type 2 diabetic men and in nondiabetic men.

1.063) from Type 2 diabetic subjects is enriched in triglycerides but depleted in free cholesterol. In line other authors have reported that diabetic LDL is triglyceride rich although in the majority of previous studies IDL has not been separated from LDL [12]. LDL subclass comprises a heterogenous spectrum of particles that vary with respect to size, density and chemical composition [21]. Recent data indicate that LDL subclasses are functionally different and differ in their potential atherogeneity [22]. GGE is the most practical methodology to classify LDL subclasses [23]. Two characteristic patterns, designated as pattern A and B, can be distinguished. Pattern A consists of large more boyant LDL particles with the mean diameter of the major LDL peak being more than 255Å. In contrast pattern B comprises small dense LDL particles with the mean diameter of the major LDL peak less than 255Å. Substantial evidence indicate that preponderance of small dense LDL is associated with increased risk of CAD [24,25].

Although LDL subclass distribution seems to be under strong genetic influence [26], recent data indicate that much of the variation of LDL size can be explained by plasma triglycerides [27-29]. The constellation of high triglycerides, low HDL cholesterol and preponderance of small dense LDL is designated as the atherogenic lipoprotein phenotype [30]. Since raised plasma triglycerides and low HDL cholesterol are components of dyslipidemia in Type 2 diabetes it would be expected that small dense LDL also is a feature of dyslipidemia in Type 2 diabetes. Recent studies have confirmed that preponderance of small dense LDL, i.e. pattern B, is indeed a component of dyslipidemia in Type 2 diabetes [31-33]. Likewise Reaven et al. [34] reported that nondiabetic subjects with pattern B are more insulin resistant than subjects with pattern A. The question whether small dense LDL is an integral component of insulin resistance and Type 2 diabetes or due to raised triglycerides in these disorders is unresolved. In the majority of studies the peak LDL particle diameter is inversely correlated with plasma and VLDL triglycerides [33,35]. Our results are consistent with these findings (Figure 3). We have failed to confirm any relation between fasting insulin levels or insulin-mediated glucose disposal in Type 2 diabetic patients who have similar triglyceride values as nondiabetic control groups. We suggest that small dense LDL in Type 2 diabetes reflects the underlying pertubations of VLDL in this disorder.

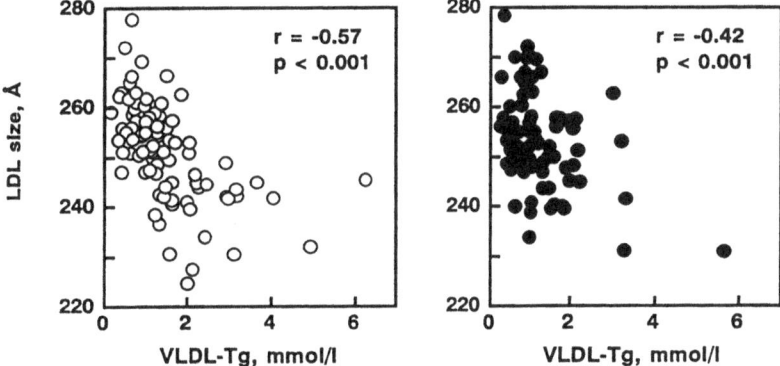

Figure 3. Correlations between the mean diameter of the major LDL peak and VLDL triglycerides in Type 2 diabetic men (left panel) and in nondiabetic men (right panel).

Summary

We conclude that in Type 2 diabetes hypertriglyceridemia has multiple detrimental effects on metabolism of remnant particles, LDL and HDL subclasses which are potentially atherogenic. The fact that plasma triglycerides influence the distribution of both LDL and HDL at a range of plasma triglyceride levels which represents upper normal range or mild hypertriglyceridemia suggests that steps should be taken to maintain plasma triglycerides as low as possible (< 1.5 mmol/l) in Type 2 diabetes.

References

1. Fontbonne A, Eschwége E, Cambien F, et al. Hypertriglyceridaemia as a risk factor of coronary heart disease mortality in subjects with impaired glucose tolerance or diabetes. Diabetologia 1989;32:300-4.

2. Laakso M, Lehto S, Penttilä I, Pyörälä K. Lipids and lipoproteins predicting coronary heart disease mortality and morbidity in patients with non-insulin-dependent diabetes. Circulation 1993;88:1421-30.

3. Zilversmit DM. Atherogenesis: A postprandial phenomenon. Circulation 1979;50:473-85.

4. Groot PHE, Stiphout WAHJ, Krauss XH, et al. Postprandial lipoprotein metabolism in normolipidemic men with and without coronary artery disease. Arterioscler Thromb 1991;11:653-62.

5. Patsch JR, Miesenbock G, Hoplerwieser T, et al. Relation of triglyceride metabolism and coronary artery disease. Arterioscler Thromb 1992;12:1336-45.

6. Schneeman BO, Kotite L, Todd KM, Havel RJ. Relationships between the response of triglyceride-rich lipoproteins in blood plasma containing apolipoproteins B-48 and B-100 to a fat-containing meal in normolipidemic humans. Proc Natl Acad Sci USA 1993;90:2069-73.

7. Ooi TC, Simo E, Yakichuk JA. Delayed clearance of postprandial chylomicrons and their remnants in the hypoalphalipopreinemia and mild hypertriglyceridemia syndrome. Arterioscler Thromb 1992;12:1184-90.

8. Lewis GF, O'Meara NM, Sollys PA. Fasting hypertriglyceridemia in non-insulin-dependent diabetes mellitus is an important predictor of postprandial lipid and lipoprotein abnormalities. J Clin Endocrinol Metab 1991;72:934-44.

9. Ida Chen Y-D, Swami S, Skowronski R, Coulston A, Reaven GM. Differences in postprandial lipemia between patients with normal glucose tolerance and non-insulin-dependent diabetes mellitus. J Clin Endocrinol Metab 1993;76:172-7.

10. Syvänne M, Hilden H, Taskinen M-R. Abnormal metabolism of postprandial lipoproteins in patients with non-insulin-dependent diabetes mellitus is not related to coronary artery disease. J Lipid Res 1994;35:15-26.

11. Ginsberg HN, Blaner W, Jones J, Thomas A, Sharrett AR, Begg M. Postprandial lipemia is a predictor of the presence of coronary heart disease in males but not females (abstract). Circulation 1993;88:I-363.

12. Taskinen M-R. Quantitative and qualitative lipoprotein abnormalities in diabetes mellitus. Diabetes 1992;41(Suppl.1):12-7.

13. Blanche PJ, Gong EL, Forte TM, Nichols AV. Characterization of human high-density lipoproteins by gradient gel electrophoresis. Biochim Biophys Acta 1981;665:408-19.

14. Cheung MC, Alberg JJ. Characterization of lipoprotein particles isolated by immunoaffinity chromatography: particles containing A-I and A-II and particles containing A-I but no A-II. J Biol Chem 1984;259:12201-9.

15. Fruchart J-C, Ailhaud G, Bard J-M. Heterogeneity of high density lipoprotein

particles. Circulation 1993;87(Suppl.III):III-22-III-27.

16. Puchois P, Kandoussi A, Fievet P, et al. Apolipoprotein A-I containing lipoproteins in coronary artery disease. Atherosclerosis 1987;68:35-40.

17. Parra HJ, Arveiler D, Evans AE, et al. A case-control study of lipoprotein particles in two populations at contrasting risk for coronary heart disease: The ECTIM Study. Arterioscler Thromb 1992;12:701-7.

18. Johansson J, Carlson LA, Landou C, Hamsten A. High density lipoproteins and coronary atherosclerosis. A strong inverse relation with the largest particles is confined to normotriglyceridemic patients. Arterioscler Thromb 1991;11:174-182.

19. Syvänne M, Kahri J, Taskinen M-R. Low levels of apo A-II containing particles are predictors of coronary artery disease in NIDDM and non-diabetic patients. 59th EAS Congress. Nice, May 17-21, 1992; Abstract..

20. Chang LBF, Hopkings GJ, Barter PJ. Particle size distribution of high density lipoproteins as a function of plasma triglyceride concentration in human subjects. Atherosclerosis 1985;56:61-70.

21. Krauss RM, Burke DJ. Identification of multiple subclasses of plasma low density lipoproteins in normal humans. J Lipid Res 1982;23:97-104.

22. Griffin BA, Packard CJ. Metabolism of VLDL and LDL subclasses. Curr Opinion Lipidol 1994;5:200-6.

23. Krauss RM, Blanche PJ. Detection and quantitation of LDL subfractions. Curr Opinion Lipidol 1992;3:377-83.

24. Austin MA, Breslow JL, Hennekens CH, Buring JE, Willett WC, Krauss RM. Low-density lipoprotein subclass patterns and risk of myocardial infarction. JAMA 1988;250:1917-21.

25. Musliner TA, Krauss RM. Lipoprotein subspecies and risk of coronary disease. Clin Chem 1988;34:B78-B83.

26. Austin MA. Genetics of low-density lipoprotein subclasses. Curr Opinion Lipidol 1993;2:125-32.

27. McNamara JR, Campos H, Ordovas JM, Peterson J, Wilson PWF, Schaefer EJ. Effect of gender, age, and lipid status on low density lipoprotein subfraction distribution. Arterioscler 1987;7:483-90.

28. Austin MA, Newman B, Selby JV, Edward K, Mayer EJ, Krauss RM. Genetics of LDL subclass phenotypes in women twins. Arterioscler Thromb 1993;13:687-95.

29. Griffin BA, Freeman DJ, Tait GW, et al. Role of plasma triglyceride in the regulation of plasma low density lipoprotein (LDL) subfractions: Relative contribution of small, dense LDL to coronary heart disease risk. Atherosclerosis 1994;106:241-53.

30. Austin MA, King M-C, Vranizan KM, Krauss RM. Atherogenic lipoprotein phenotype. A proposed genetic marker for coronary heart disease risk. Circulation 1990;82:495-506.

31. Barakat HA, Carpenter JW, McLandon VD, et al. Influence of obesity, impaired glucose tolerance, and NIDDM on LDL structure and composition. Diabetes 1990;39:1527-33.

32.   Feingold KR, Grunfeld C, Pang M, Doerrier W, Krauss RM. LDL subclass
      phenotypes and triglyceride metabolism in non-insulin-dependent diabetes.
      Arterioscler Thromb 1992;12:1496-502.
33.   Stewart MW, Laker MF, Dyer RG, et al. Lipoprotein compositional abnormalities
      and insulin resistance in type II diabetic patients with mild hyperlipidemia.
      Arterioscler Thromb 1993;13:1046-52.
34.   Reaven GM, Ida Chen Y-D, Jeppsen J, Maheux P, Krauss RM. Insulin resistance
      and hyperinsulinemia in individuals with small, dense, low density lipoprotein
      particles. J Clin Invest 1993;92:141-5.
35.   Selby JV, Austin MA, Newman B, et al. LDL subclass phenotypes and the insulin
      resistance and the insulin resistance syndrome in women. Circulation 1993;88:381-7.

DIABETES AND CARDIOVASCULAR RISK: EPIDEMIOLOGIC ASPECTS

Steven M. Haffner
Division of Clinical Epidemiology
Department of Medicine
University of Texas Health Science Center at San Antonio
7703 Floyd Curl Drive
San Antonio, Texas 78284-7873
USA

Introduction

Most studies of noninsulin dependent diabetes mellitus (NIDDM) suggest a two-fold increased risk of coronary heart disease (CHD) [1,2]. Women have a relatively greater excess risk of CHD risk with NIDDM than men with NIDDM in most [3-5], but not all studies [6,7]. The excess risk of CHD in NIDDM subjects is only partially explained by increases in traditional cardiovascular risk factors such as total cholesterol, smoking, and hypertension [3,8,9].

Hypertension

An excellent review of diabetes and hypertension has recently appeared [10]. Several studies have shown an increase in hypertension in NIDDM relative to normal subjects [11,12]. The relationship of duration of diabetes to hypertension is unclear with some studies showing a positive relationship [11] and other studies showing no association [12]. Impaired glucose tolerance is associated with an increased prevalence of hypertension [5,13]. Few prospective data are available on the relationship of blood pressure to the incidence of cardiovascular disease in diabetic subjects. However, hypertension is related to cardiovascular mortality in diabetes [8,14].

Hyperlipidemia

The characteristic pattern of dyslipidemia in NIDDM consists of hypertriglyceridemia and low HDL cholesterol [15-17]. Abnormalities of obesity and body fat distribution that occur in NIDDM do not totally account for dyslipidemia in NIDDM subjects relative to normoglycemic subjects [18,19]. Wilson et al. [15] have shown that the absolute

173

A.M. Gotto et al. (eds.), Multiple Risk Factors in Cardiovascular Disease, 173-184.
© 1995 *Kluwer Academic Publishers and Fondazione Giovanni Lorenzini.*

concentration of total and LDL cholesterol are similar in diabetic and nondiabetic subjects. Walden et al. [17] reported that the adverse effect of diabetes on dyslipidemia were more marked in women than in men and proposed that this phenomenon might explain why diabetes eliminates or attenuates a woman's protection against ischemic heart disease. Although similar findings (i.e., greater excess of dyslipidemia in women than in men with NIDDM) have been reported in other studies [9,19] this has not been reported in all studies [20,21].

In addition to quantitative changes, diabetic subjects may have qualitative changes in lipid and lipoprotein composition which may affect their atherogenicity. Biesbroeck et al. [22] have shown that HDL particles from NIDDM subjects are rich in triglyceride and poor in cholesterol, suggesting that the decrease in HDL cholesterol characteristically seen in diabetic patients is predominantly due to a reduction in the amount of cholesterol per particle rather than to a reduction in the number of particles. In addition, apolipoprotein (apo) A-I is decreased relative to apo A-II in type I diabetic subjects [22]. Because HDL_2 (the HDL subfraction thought to be protective against CHD) has relatively more A-I than A-II, the decrease in total HDL may underestimate the true atherogenic potential associated with the diabetic state [22]. Taskinen et al. [23] found that although intensive insulin therapy markedly decreased the concentration of VLDL, it had only a minor effect on total HDL. However, when these investigators examined the effects of insulin therapy on the principal subfractions of HDL, they observed that HDL_2 increased by 21%, whereas HDL_3 decreased by 13%. Thus the benefits of insulin therapy may be underestimated if only its effect on total HDL is monitored.

Elevations in the free cholesterol lecithin ratio have been described in diabetic subjects, a change that in nondiabetic subjects has been shown to be a strong predictor of CHD, comparable in effect to LDL cholesterol [24]. Several investigators [25,26] have shown in diabetic subjects that VLDL is enriched with free cholesterol and also that the free cholesterol lecithin ratio is increased in hypertriglyceridemic subjects. These changes were not reversed by improved metabolic control. Lane et al. [27] described a compositional change in normolipidemic diabetic subjects, an increase in the free cholesterol to lecithin ratio of the HDL_2 subfraction. The mechanisms whereby changes in the composition of surface and core lipids may enhance cardiovascular risk are unknown but could relate to the capacity of HDL to exchange cholestyl ester with other lipoproteins and to transport free cholesterol from cell membranes to circulating lipoproteins [28].

LDL composition may also be altered in type II diabetes. Polydispersion of LDL particle size has been reported associated with hypertriglyceridemia in both diabetic and nondiabetic subjects [29,30]. Recent data suggests that small dense LDL may be a risk factor for CHD [31,32]. Austin et al. found that most individuals can be assigned two LDL subclass patterns (A or B) [31]. Small dense LDL (type B) has been associated with increased triglyceride and decreased high density lipoprotein cholesterol, male gender, hyperinsulinemia, and insulin resistance [31,33-37]. LDL size has been reported to be lower in diabetic women [33,35,38] and diabetic men [38,39]. In one study, there was a stronger association between LDL size and diabetes in women than in men [38] which may also partially explain the greater relative risk of CHD observed in women with NIDDM observed in some studies. The increase in small dense LDL observed in diabetic subjects also occurs in normolipidemia NIDDM men [39] suggesting that association may be only partially dependent on the elevated triglyceride and decreased HDL common in NIDDM subjects. The composition of LDL has not been well explained in subjects with insulin dependent diabetes mellitus. No study has examined the association of small dense LDL to CHD risk in diabetic subjects.

Increased glycosylation of LDL is also characteristic of the diabetic state, although this modification of LDL has not been shown to increase coronary risk either in diabetic or in nondiabetic subjects [40]. Oxidized LDL, by contrast, may increase the risk of CHD because it is more atherogenic than native LDL [41]. Increased peroxidation of LDL, which may reflect increased oxidation has been described in diabetic subjects [42]. Although, it is apparent why glycosylated LDL would be elevated in diabetic subjects, it is less clear why oxidized LDL would also be elevated. A possible mechanism is suggested by the data of Steinbrecher and Witztum [43] which indicated that glycosylation of LDL may slow its removal via the LDL-apo B 100 receptor pathway.

Recent data suggests that in nondiabetic subjects, Lp(a) may be a strong risk factor for CHD [44]. The area of Lp(a) in diabetes has recently been reviewed [45]. In subjects with IDDM, Lp(a) concentrations are usually increased [46]. In addition Lp(a) levels usually decline with improved metabolic control [47,48]. Whether Lp(a) concentrations are elevated in NIDDM subjects is still controversial [45]. While early studies have indicated an increase in Lp(a) in NIDDM subjects [49], later studies [50,51] have seen no significant effect of NIDDM on Lp(a) concentrations. In one recent study, Lp(a) concentrations were lower in subjects with NIDDM than in nondiabetic subjects after control for apo(a) phenotype [52]. Improved glycemic control does not decrease Lp(a) levels [50,52]. Microalbuminuria has been reported with increased Lp(a) levels in IDDM [53] but whether there is an increase in Lp(a) with NIDDM is still controversial [54,55]. Little data is available on the relationship of Lp(a) to CHD in diabetic subjects. While Jenkins et al. [54] have found such a relationship in NIDDM subjects, other studies have not found a relation between Lp(a) and CHD in either IDDM [56,57] or NIDDM subjects [57,58]. One problem in the assessment of Lp(a) and CHD has been the lack of prospective studies. Only one study has examined this issue prospectively [57]. With cross-sectional studies, a survival bias could occur with subjects having both diabetes and elevated Lp(a) levels dying before being examined and thus a cross-sectional study might shown no relationship.

Diabetic Risk Factors: Glycemia and Duration of Diabetes

Many epidemiologic studies show that duration of diabetes and degree of hyperglycemia are the principal risk factors for the development of microvascular complications of diabetes [59-61]. In the DCCT trial, tight control of diabetes in IDDM was shown to reduce the risk of retinopathy, nephropathy, and neuropathy by about 50% in a large, randomized controlled trial [62]. These, however, are not the principal risk factors for the development of macrovascular disease. In the WHO Multinational Study [63], no relationship was found between either plasma glucose concentration on diabetes duration and major Q wave abnormalities.   Similarly in a population-based study of IDDM and NIDDM [64] in Denmark, Nielsen and Ditzel found no association between glycosylated hemoglobin levels and the prevalence of macrovascular complication, although they did confirm that diabetic control was correlated with diabetic retinopathy. These two studies just cited are cross-sectional, but prospective studies have also failed to uncover an association between duration of clinical diabetes (i.e., the duration of hyperglycemia and macrovascular hyperglycemia) and macrovascular complications [65,66]. Also, in the London cohort of the WHO Multinational Study, which was followed prospectively, no effect of diabetes duration on cardiovascular mortality was observed among NIDDM subjects [67]. However, in two recent prospective studies from Finland, a modest relationship between severity of glycemia and duration of NIDDM was observed [68,69].

Cardiovascular Risk Factors in Prediabetic Subjects

A possible explanation for the weak association between severity and duration of hyperglycemia and risk of macrovascular complications is that the latter are influenced by the metabolic derangements that precede diabetes - that is those that are present during the prediabetic phase. Prospective data from several epidemiologic studies [70-73] have suggested a prolonged period (perhaps decades) of hyperinsulinemia precedes the onset of clinical diabetes. This hyperinsulinemia is presumed to be a compensatory response to insulin resistance, which is also characteristic of the prediabetic state.   Moreover, prospective studies in both whites [74] and Pima Indians [75] have shown that insulin resistance can predict the later occurrence of NIDDM.

Hyperinsulinemia may be a cardiovascular risk factor both by its effects on established risk factors and also possibly by a direct atherogenic effect on the arterial wall [76].   Several earlier studies suggested that serum insulin levels were independent risk factors for further cardiovascular disease in nondiabetic men [77-79]. However, in more recent studies in elderly subjects [80,81] and in high-risk men for coronary heart disease (Multiple Risk Factor Intervention Trial) serum insulin levels did not predict the incidence of CHD. Insulin resistance has been shown to be associated with increased carotid wall thickness or plaque in nondiabetic subjects [82,83]. The balance of these findings, combined with the hyperinsulinemia and insulin resistance present in prediabetic subjects, suggest that prediabetic should have an atherogenic pattern of risk factors. This has been confirmed in prediabetic subjects identified retrospectively in epidemiological studies [73,84]. The risk of atherogenic risk factors in confirmed prediabetic subjects was observed even in subjects who had normal glucose tolerance and were not obese [84].

We have summarized the above concepts using the "ticking clock" metaphor, in the case of microvascular complications, for which the principal risk factors are degree and duration of hyperglycemia, "the clock starts ticking" at the onset of clinical diabetes (i.e., at the onset of hyperglycemia). In contrast, for macrovascular complications in which insulin resistance with its concomitant metabolic derangements, including compensatory hyperinsulinemia are important factors, "the clock starts ticking" years or even decades earlier in the prediabetic phase.

It should be emphasized that the above arguments do not imply that the use of insulin in intensive control in diabetic subjects is harmful. In IDDM subjects in the DCCT trial [62], intensive control was associated with a modest (but not statistically significant) decline in cardiovascular events. In the VA Cooperative Trial [85], preliminary data suggests in NIDDM subjects an increase in cardiovascular disease in subjects treated with intensive insulin therapy. In summary, no conclusive data show a harmful effect of insulin therapy on cardiovascular disease in diabetic subjects although the United Kingdom Prospective Study will provide additional data on NIDDM subjects in the near future.

Conclusion

CHD is increased in NIDDM. Risk factors in NIDDM include hypertension, increased triglyceride, and decreased HDL cholesterol. Additional qualitative differences in lipoproteins may also contribute to risk of CHD. Triglyceride levels may be more related to risk of CHD in diabetic subjects than in nondiabetic subjects. In addition, the increase in CHD is not related strongly to the duration of diabetes nor to the severity of glycemia, suggesting that the increased risk may be due in part to the hyperinsulinemia and/or insulin resistance in the prediabetic phase.

References

1. Pyörälä K, Laakso M, Uusitupa M. Diabetes and atherosclerosis: An epidemiological view. Diabetes Metab Rev 1987;3:463-524.
2. Haffner SM, Stern MP, Rewers M. In: B Draznin, RH Eckel, editors. Diabetes and atherosclerosis: Epidemiological considerations in diabetes and atheroslcerosis: Molecular basis and clinical aspects. New York: Elsevier, 1992:229-254.
3. Garcia MJ, McNamara PM, Gordon T, Kannel WB. Morbidity and mortality in diabetics in the Framingham population: Sixteen-year follow-up. Diabetes 1974;23:105-111.
4. Barrett-Connor E, Wingard DL. Sex difference in ischemic heart disease mortality in diabetics: A prospective population-based study. Am J Epidemiol 1983;118:489-496.
5. Jarrett RJ, McCarthy P, Keen H. The Bedford Study: Ten year mortality rates in newly diagnosed diabetics, borderline diabetics and normoglycemic controls and risk indices for coronary heart disease in borderline diabetics. Diabetologia 1982;22:79-84.
6. Head J, Fuller JH. International variation in mortality among diabetic patients: the WHO Multinational Study of Vascular Disease in Diabetics. Diabetologia 1990;33:477-481.
7. Kleinman JC, Donahue R, Harris M, Finucane FF, Modans JH, Brock DB. Mortality among diabetics in a national sample. Am J Epidemiol 1988;128:389-401.
8. Stamler J, Vaccaro O, Neaton JD, Wentworth D, for the Multiple Risk Factor Intervention Trial Research Group. Diabetes, other risk factors and 12-year

mortality for men screened in the Multiple Risk Factor Intervention Trial. Diabetes Care 1993;16:434-444.

9.   Assman G, Schulte H. The Prospective Cardiovascular Monster (PROCAM) Study: Prevalence of hyperlipidemia in persons with hypertension and/or diabetes mellitus and the relationship to coronary heart disease. Am Heart J 1988;116:1713-1724.

10.   Epstein M, Sowers JR. Diabetes and hypertension. Hypertension 1992;19:403-418.

11.   Uusitupa M, Siitonen O, Aro A, et al. Prevalence of coronary heart disease, left ventricular failure and hypertension in middle-aged, newly diagnosed type 2 (non-insulin-dependent) diabetic subjects. Diabetologia 1985;28:22-27.

12.   Jarrett RJ, Keen H, McCarthney M, et al. Glucose tolerance and blood pressure in two population samples: their relation to diabetes mellitus and hypertension. Int J Epidemiol 1978;63:54-64.

13.   Modan M, Halkin H, Almog S, et al. Hyperinsulinemia: A link between hypertension, obesity and glucose intolerance. J Clin Invest 1985;75:809-817.

14.   Kannel WB, McGee DL. Diabetes and cardiovascular disease: The Framingham study. JAMA 1979;2035-2038.

15.   Wilson PWF, Kannel WB, Anderson KM. Lipids, glucose intolerance and vascular disease: The Framingham Study. Monogr Atheroscler 1985;13:1-11.

16.   Hanefeld M, Schultze J, Fischer S, et al. The Diabetes Intervention Study (DIS): A cooperative multi-intervention trial with newly manifested type II diabetics: preliminary results. Monogr Atheroscler 1985;13:98-103.

17.   Walden CE, Knopp RH, Wahl PW, et al. Sex differences in the effect of diabetes on lipoprotein triglyceride and cholesterol concentrations. N Engl J Med 1984;311:953-959.

18.   Haffner SM, Stern MP, Hazuda HP, et al. Do upper body adiposity and centralized adiposity measure different aspects of regional body fat distribution? Relationship to non-insulin dependent diabetes mellitus, lipids and lipoproteins. Diabetes 1987;36:43-51.

19.   Laakso M, Barrett-Connor E. Asymptomatic hyperglycemic hyperglycemia is associated with lipid and lipoprotein changes favoring atherosclerosis. Arteriosclerosis 1989;9:665-672.

20.   Falko JM, Parr JH, Simpson RN, et al. Lipoprotein analyses in varying degrees of glucose intolerance: comparison between non-insulin dependent diabetic, impaired glucose tolerant and control populations. Am J Med 1987;83:641-647.

21.   Briones ER, Mao SJT, Palumbo PJ, et al. Analyses of plasma lipids and apolipoproteins in insulin dependent and non-insulin dependent diabetics. Metabolism 1984;33:42-49.

22.   Biesbroeck B, Albers JJ, Wahl PW, et al. Abnormal composition of high density lipoproteins in non-insulin dependent diabetics. Diabetes 1982;31:126-131.

23.   Taskinen MR, Kuusi T, Helve E, et al.. Insulin therapy induces atherogenic changes of serum lipoproteins in non-insulin dependent diabetes. Arterioscler 1988;8:168-177.

24.   Kuksis A, Myher JJ, Geher K, et al.. Decreased plasma phosphotidlcholine (free

cholesterol) ratio as an indicator of risk for ischemic vascular disease. Arteriosclerosis 1982;2:296-302.

25.   Fielding CJ, Reaven GM, Fielding P. Human non-insulin-dependent diabetes: Identification of a defect in plasma cholesterol transport normalized in vivo by insulin and in vitro by selective immunoabsorption of apolipoprotein. Proc Natl Acad Sci USA 1982;79:6365-6369.

26.   Bagdade JD, Buchanor WE, Kuusi T, et al.. Persistent abnormalities in lipoprotein composition in non-insulin dependent diabetes following intensive therapy. Arteriosclerosis 1990;10:232-239.

27.   Lane JGT, Subbiah PU, Otto ME, et al. Lipoprotein composition and HDL particle distributions in women with non-insulin dependent diabetes mellitus and the effects of probucol treatment. J Lab Clin Med 1991;118:552-560.

28.   Morton RE. Interaction of lipid transfer protein with plasma lipoproteins and cell membranes. Experentia 1992;46:552-560.

29.   Fisher WR. Heterogenity of plasma low density lipoproteins: Manifestations of the physiological phenomenon in man. Metabolism 1983;32:283-291.

30.   Vega GL, Grundy SM. Kinetic heterogenity of low density lipoproteins in primary hypertriglyceridemia. Arteriosclerosis 1986;6:395-406.

31.   Austin MA, Breslow JL, Hennekens CHD, Buring JE, Willett WC, Krauss RM. Low density lipoprotein subclass patterns and risk of myocardial infarction. JAMA 1988;260:1917-1921.

32.   Crouse JR, Parkes JS, Schey HM, Kahl FR. Studies of low density lipoprotein molecular weight in human beings with coronary artery disease. J Lipid Res 1985;26:566-574.

33.   Bakarat HA, Carpenter JW, McLendon VD, Klazarie P, Legget N, Health J, Marks R. Influence of obesity, impaired glucose tolerance and NIDDM on LDL structure and composition: Possible between hyperinsulinemia and atherosclerosis. Diabetes 1990;39:1527-1533.

34.   McNamara JR, Campos H, Ordovas JM, Peterson RM, Wilson PWF Schaefer EJ. Effect of gender, age and lipid status on low density subfraction distribution: Results of the Framingham Offspring Study. Arteriosclerosis 1987;7:483-490.

35.   Selby JV, Austin MA, Newman B, Zhang D, Quesenberry CP, Mayer EJ, Krauss RM. LDL subclass phenotypes and the insulin resistance syndrome in women. Circulation 1993;85:381-387.

36.   Reaven GM, Chen YDI, Jeppesen J, Maheux P, Krauss RM. Insulin resistance in individuals with small dense lipoproteins. J Clin Invest 1993;92:141-146.

37.   Haffner SM, Mykkänen L, Valdez R, Paidi M, Stern MP, Howard BV. LDL size and subclass pattern in a biethnic population. Arteriosclerosis 1993;3:1623-1634.

38.   Haffner SM, Mykkänen L, Stern MP, Paidi M, Howard BV. Greater effect of LDL size in women than in men. Diabetes Care, in press.

39.   Feingold KR, Grunfeld C, Doerrler W, Krauss RM. LDL subclass phenotypes and triglyceride metabolism in non-insulin dependent diabetes. Arteriosclerosis and Thrombosis 1992;12:1496-1502.

40.   Lyons TJ. Oxidized low density lipoproteins: a role in the pathogenesis of atherogenesis in diabetes? Diabetic Med 1991;8:411-419.

41.   Steinberg D, Parthasarthy S, Carew TE, et al.. Beyond cholesterol: modifications of low density lipoprotein that increase its atherogenicity. N Engl J Med 1989;320:913-924.

42.   Nishigaki I, Hagihara M, Tsunekawa H, et al. Lipid peroxide levels of serum lipoprotein fractions of diabetic patients. Biochem Med 1981;25:373-378.

43.   Steinbrecher WP, Witztum JML. Glucosylation of low density lipoproteins to an extent comparable to that seen in diabetes slows their catabolism. Diabetes 1984;33:130-134.

44.   Seed M, Hoppichler F, Reavley D, et al. Relationship of serum lipoprotein(a) concentration heart disease in patients with familial hypercholesterolemia. N Engl J Med 1990;322:1494-1499.

45.   Haffner SM. Lipoprotein(a) and Diabetes. An update. Diabetes Care 1992;16:835-840.

46.   Levitsky L, Scanu A, Gould SH. Lipoprotein(a) levels in black and white children and adolescents with IDDM. Diabetes Care 1991;14:283-287.

47.   Buckert E, Davidoff P, Grimaldi F, Truffert J, Giral P, Doumith R, Thervent F, DeGennes JL. Increased serum levels of lipoprotein(a) in diabetes mellitus and their reduction with glycemic control (Letter). JAMA 1990;263:35-36.

48.   Haffner SM, Tuttle KR, Rainwater DL. Decrease of lipoprotein(a) with improved metabolic control in IDDM subjects. Diabetes Care 1991;14:302-307.

49.   Ramirez LC, Arauz Pacheco C, Lackner C, Albright G, Adims BV, Raskin P. Lipoprotein(a) levels in diabetes mellitus: Relationship to metabolic control. Ann Intern Med 1992;117:42-47.

50.   Taskinen MR, Enholm C, Jaubianen M, Kaupinen-Makelin R, Yki-Jarvinen H, FINMIS group. The concentration of Lp(a) is not influenced by the degree of glycemic control in NIDDM (Abstract). Proceedings of 9th International Symposium on Atherosclerosis; 1991 Oct; Rosemont, IL:196.

51.   Haffner SM, Morales PA, Stern MP, Gruber MK. Lp(a) concentrations in NIDDM. Diabetes 1992;41:1267-1272.

52.   Rainwater DL, MacCleur JW, Stern MP, Vanderberg JL, Haffner SM. Effects on non-insulin dependent diabetes mellitus on Lp(a) concentrations and apolipoprotein(a) size. Diabetes, in press.

53.   Jenkins AJ, Steele JS, Jones ED, Best JP. Increased plasma apolipoprotein(a) levels in IDDM subjects with microalbuminuria. Diabetes 1991;40:787-790.

54.   Jenkins AJ, Steele JS, Jones ED, Santamaria JD, Best JD. Plasma apolipoprotein(a) is increased in type II (non-insulin dependent) diabetic patients with microalbuminuria. Diabetologia 1992;35:1055-1059.

55.   Haffner SM, Morales PA, Gruber MK, Hazuda HP, Stern MP. Lack of association of lipids, lipoproteins and Lp(a) with microalbuminuria in NIDDM. Arteriosclerosis 1993;13:205-210.

56.   Maser RE, Usher D, Becker DJ, Drash AL, Kuller LH, Orchard TJ. Lipoprotein(a)

concentration shows little relationship to IDDM complications in the Pittsburgh epidemiology of diabetes complications study cohort. Diabetes Care 1993;16:755-758.

57. Haffner SM, Klein BEK, Moss SE, Klein R. Lack of association between Lp(a) concentrations and coronary heart disease mortality in diabetes: the Wisconsin Epidemiologic Survey of Diabetic Retinopathy. Metabolism 1992;41:194-197.

58. Niskanen L, Mykkänen L, Karonen SL, Uusitupa M. Apoprotein(a) levels in relation to coronary heart disease and risk factors in type II (non-insulin dependent diabetes). Cardiovasc Risk Factors 1993;3:76-81.

59. Diabetes Drafting Group. Prevalence of small vessel and large vessel disease in diabetic patients from 14 centers: the World Health Organization Multinational Study of Vascular Disease in Diabetics. Diabetologia 1985;28:615-640.

60. Ballard DJ, Melton LJ, Dwyer MS, et al. Risk factors for diabetic retinopathy: A population-based study in Rochester, Minnesota. Diabetes Care 1986;9:334-342.

61. Klein R, Klein BEK, Moss SE, et al. Glycosylated hemoglobin predicts the incidence and progression of diabetic retinopathy. JAMA 1988;260:2864-2871.

62. The Diabetes Control and Complications Trial (DCCT) Research Group: The effect of intensive treatment of diabetes on the development and progression of long-term complications in insulin dependent diabetes mellitus. N Engl J Med 1993;329:977-986.

63. West KM, Ahuja MMS, Bennett PH, et al. The role of circulating glucose and triglyceride concentrations and their interactions with other "risk factors" as determinations of arterial disease in nine diabetic population samples from the WHO Multinational Study. Diabetes Care 1983;6:361-369.

64. Nielsen NV, Ditzel J. Prevalence of macro- and microvascular disease as related to glycosylated hemoglobin in type I and II diabetic subjects: An epidemiologic study in Denmark. Horm Metab Res 1985; (Suppl.15):19-23.

65. Fuller JH, Shipley MJ, Rose G, et al. Coronary heart risk and impaired glucose tolerance: the Whitehall Study. Lancet 1980;1:1373-1376.

66. Herman JB, Medalie JH, Goldbourt U. Differences in cardiovascular morbidity and mortality between previously known and newly diagnosed adult diabetics. Diabetologia 1977;13:229-234.

67. Morrish NJ, Stevens LK, Head J, et al. A prospective study of mortality among middle-aged diabetic patients (the London Cohort of the WHO Study of Vascular Disease in Diabetics). II Associated risk factors. Diabetologia 1990;33:542-548.

68. Kuusisto J, Mykkänen L, Pyörälä K, Laakso M. Non-insulin dependent diabetes and its metabolic control predict coronary heart disease in elderly subjects. Diabetes, in press.

69. Laakso M, Lehto S, Pentilä I, Pyörälä K. Lipids and lipoproteins predicting coronary heart disease mortality and morbidity in patients with non-insulin dependent diabetes mellitus. Circulation 1993;88:1421-1430.

70. Saad MF, Knowler WC, Pettit DJ, et al. The natural history of impaired glucose tolerance in Pima Indians. N Engl J Med 1988;319:1500-1506.

71.   Sicree RA, Zimmet PZ, King HOM, et al. Plasma insulin response among Nauruans: Prediction of deterioration of glucose tolerance over six years. Diabetes 1987;36:179-186.
72.   Haffner SM, Stern MP, Mitchell BD, et al. Incidence of type II diabetes in Mexican Americans predicted by fasting insulin and glucose levels, obesity and body fat distribution. 1990;39:283-288.
73.   Mykkänen L, Kuusisto J, Pyörälä K, Laakso M. Cardiovascular disease risk factors as predictors of type 2 (non-insulin-dependent) diabetes mellitus in elderly subjects. Diabetologia 1993;36:553-559.
74.   Warram JH, Martin BC, Krolewski AS, et al. Slow glucose removal rate and hyperinsulinemia precede the development of type II diabetes in the offspring of diabetic parents. Ann Intern Med 1990;113:909-915.
75.   Lillioja S, Mott DM, Spraul M, et al. Insulin resistance and insulin secretory dysfunction as precursors of non-insulin dependent diabetes mellitus. Prospective Studies of Pima Indians. N Engl J Med 1993;329:1988-1992.
76.   Stout RW. Insulin and atheroma: 20 yr. perspective. Diabetes Care 1990;13:631-654.
77.   Pyörälä K, Savalainen E, Kaukola S, Haapakoski J. Plasma insulin as coronary heart disease risk factor: Relationship to other risk factors and predictive value during 9 1/2 year follow-up of the Helsinki study population. Acta Med Scand 1985;(Suppl.) 701:38-52.
78.   Eschwege E, Ducimetiere P, Thibault N, Richard JL, Claude JR, Rosselin GE. Coronary heart disease mortality in relation with diabetes, blood glucose and plasma insulin levels. The Paris Prospective Study, ten years later. Horm Metab Res 1985;(Suppl. Series) 15:41-45.
79.   Welborn TA, Wearne K. Coronary heart disease incidence and cardiovascular mortality in Busselton with reference to glucose and insulin concentrations. Diabetes Care 1979;2:154-160.
80.   Welin L, Eriksson H, Larsson B, Ohlson LO, Svardsudd K, Tibblin G. Hyperinsulinemia is not a major coronary risk factor in men. The study of men born in 1913. Diabetologia 1992;35:766-770.
81.   Kuusisto J, Mykkänen L, Pyörälä K, Laakso M. Hyperinsulinemic microalbuminuria: A new risk factor for coronary heart disease. Circulation, in press.
82.   Orchard TJ, Kuller LK, Eichner J, Kuller LH, Becker DJ, McCollum LM, Grandits GH. Insulin as a predictor of coronary heart disease: Interaction with apolipoprotein E phenotype: A report from the Multiple Risk Factor Intervention Trial. Ann Epidemiol 1994;4:40-45.
83.   Howard G, O'Leary D, Ayad M, Wagenknecht L. Lower insulin sensitivity is related to atherosclerosis in nondiabetics: The Insulin Resistance Atherosclerosis Study (IRAS). Diabetes 1994;43:(Suppl.1):60A.
84.   Haffner SM, Stern MP, Hazuda HP, et al. Cardiovascular risk factors in confirmed prediabetes: Does the clock for coronary heart disease start ticking before the onset

of clinical diabetes? JAMA 1990;263:2893-2898.

85.   Abraira C, Johnson N, Colwell J and the VA CSDM Group. VA Cooperative Study on glycemic control and complications in type II diabetes (VA CSDM): Results of completed feasibilty trial. Diabetes 1994;43(Suppl.1):59A.

RATIONAL TREATMENT OF THE "PLURIMETABOLIC SYNDROME"

A. Tiengo, A. Avogaro, and S. Del Prato
Istituto di Medicina Clinica
Cattedra di Malattie del Ricambio
Universita' degli Studi di Padova
Padua
ITALY

Introduction

The "plurimetabolic syndrome," hypothisized by Padova group back in 1967 and subsequently defined by Reaven as "Syndrome X" [1] includes an array of metabolic and fibrinolytic alterations (impaired glucose tolerance, increased triglyceride levels, decreased HDL cholesterol, increased PAI-1 and fibrinogen levels, and hyperuricemia) which become phenotypically expressed in well-defined clinical syndromes (diabetes mellitus, type IV hyperlipedemia, hypertension, and gout). All these diseases are associated with a premature atherosclerotic involvement of the vascular tree. On the other hand it was clearly shown that the prevalence of these diseases is significantly higher in those patients affected by atherosclerotic cardiovascular disease [2] or that they were associated with hypertension [3]. The plurimetabolic syndrome could be considered clinically as the "New World Disease" since its prevalence and incidence has significantly increased among Western industrialized countries where negative environmental factors, such as overnourishment and sedentariness, unmask genetic traits otherwise quiescent during food deprivation. In this perspective, rapidly modernizing populations retain the so called "thrifty" genotype, a genotype which allows an efficient fat deposition and survival during famine but is able to facilitate obesity and glucose intolerance once these communities change from the traditional to the urban diet high in refined carbohydrates. A peculiar genetic predisposition, along with an inappropriate life style, may induce a prevalence of the plurimetabolic syndrome in as high as 40-50% of these individuals. In Italy the prevalence of the plurimetabolic syndrome is around 10-15% among adults. It must be stressed that the plurimetabolic syndrome has gained credit from a epidemiological point of view since its presence is significantly associated with the premature onset of atherosclerotic cardiovascular disease. Therefore, with this perspective in mind, the prevention of this syndrome must be rationally approached.

A.M. Gotto et al. (eds.), Multiple Risk Factors in Cardiovascular Disease, 185-196.
© 1995 *Kluwer Academic Publishers and Fondazione Giovanni Lorenzini.*

The Treatment of Insulin Resistance

As previously outlined, the vast array of metabolic, hemodynamic, and fibrinolytic alterations present in the plurimetabolic syndrome, originates from the presence of insulin resistance, i.e. higher plasma insulin in order to elicit a normal biological action. Several cross-sectional studies have confirmed the close correlation between hyperinsulinemia and the disturbances observed in the plurimetabolic syndrome [4-6]. Insulin resistance is a major risk factor in the development of noninsulin-dependent diabetes [7,8]. Recently Haffner et al. [9] examined the relationship of fasting insulin concentration (as an index of insulin resistance) and the incidence of multiple metabolic abnormalities in the 8-year follow-up of the cohort enrolled in the San Antonio Heart Study. Fasting insulin levels were related to the incidence of hypertension, decreased high-density lipoprotein cholesterol concentration, increased triglyceride concentration, and noninsulin-dependent diabetes mellitus. These results were not attributable to differences in baseline obesity and were similar in Mexican-Americans and non-Hispanic whites. Therefore it seems that elevation in insulin concentrations precede and predict a cluster of different metabolic disorders including dysplipidemia, hypertension and NIDDM. On the other hand, insulin-resistance and the consequent hyperinsulinemia, is involved in the pathogenesis and progression of coronary ischemic disease [10,11] and atherosclerotic events.

The rationale for a therapeutic strategy of the plurimetabolic syndrome therefore should be to correct: 1) the primary condition of insulin resistance and hyperinsulinemia and 2) the different metabolic abnormalities.

In the absence of known genetic defects and of a consequent genetic therapeutic approach, we should direct our aims at improving insulin action, i.e. reduce the fasting and postprandial plasma insulin concentration (Table 1). This will increase glucose uptake in target tissues and will also improve the other metabolic abnormalities of the plurimetabolic syndrome.

Table 1. Goals of the Treatment of the Plurimetabolic Syndrome.

· Relief of insulin resistance
· Reduction of hyperinsulinemia
· Improvement in glucose tolerance
· Amelioration of other metabolic and clinical abnormalities

Diet, physical activity, insulin-sensitizer drugs, and antihyperinsulinemic agents represent the useful tools of this strategic approach. Interventions such as diet and exercise to achieve weight reduction could improve all the metabolic disturbances of the syndrome

(Table 2).

Table 2. Rationale Treatment of the Plurimetabolic Syndrome.

Genetic defects	?
Insulin resistance	Diet, Exercise Insulin sensitizer drugs.
Hyperinsulinemia	Slowing carbohydrate absorption compounds.

NONPHARMACOLOGIC THERAPY

Weight loss improves glucose tolerance through a reduction of both fasting and postprandial insulin levels. An hypocaloric diet improves both peripheral glucose disposal and hepatic glucose production in obese-diabetic patients [12]. The normalization of the daily glucose profiles, along with a significant reduction of both systolic and diastolic blood pressure, insulin, triglyceride, cholesterol, and fibrinogen levels, has been observed after a significant weight loss. Weight loss can significantly decrease hyperinsulinemia and insulin resistance in obese patients with visceral obesity [13]. A high-carbohydrate diet increases both plasma insulin and triglyceride levels and can deteriorate blood glucose control in the postprandial period in patients with the plurimetabolic syndrome [14]. However, the adverse metabolic effects of the high-carbohydrate diet are neutralized when fiber and carbohydrates are increased simultaneously. A high-carboydrate/high-fiber diet significantly improves blood glucose control and does not increase plasma insulin and triglyceride concentrations.

However, the partial replacement of complex carbohydrates with monounsaturated fatty acids in the diet may improve glycemic control and the levels of plasma triglyceride, and reduce the postprandial insulin concentration [15].

Exercise is considered another first-line measure to reduce plasma lipids, improve glucose profile, and increase insulin sensitivity. Regular physical exercise (three times per week for 20-45 minutes at 50-70% of maximum capacity) can improve glucose and lipid metabolism in patients with impaired glucose tolerance, hypertriglyceridemia, and hypertension [16]. In humans, physical activity may reduce basal hepatic glucose production rather than improve insulin-stimulated glucose disposal [17] despite a significant increase in GLUT4 (glucose transporters) levels in skeletal muscle. The addition of moderate physical training to an appropriate diet improves insulin sensitivity by reducing plasma insulin concentration and increasing carbohydrate storage [18].

INSULIN-SENSITIZER DRUGS

Once diet and exercise fail to normalize the metabolic abnormalities, drug treatment should be considered. Theoretically, useful drugs for the treatment of the plurimetabolic syndrome should improve tissue insulin sensitivity without increasing β-cell secretion. These drugs may be defined as "insulin sparing" or "insulin sensitizers".

Only some of the drugs listed in Table 3 are currently available in clinical practice and their metabolic effects against insulin-resistance are limited. Several new drugs, have been tested only in animals and it is not known whether their use in humans is safe.

Table 3. Insulin-sensitizer Drugs.

Present	Future
Biguanides	Thiazolidinediones
Sulphonilureas	Fatty acid oxidation inhibitors
Acipimox	Dichloroacetate
Benfluorex	Insulin-like growth factors
ACE-inhibitors	Vanadate
Fibrates	β-adrenergic agonists

Among the insulin-sensitizer drugs currently available, we should mention sulfonylureas, even though these compounds exert their hypoglycemic effect principally by enhancing insulin secretion. On the other, hand several studies have shown an improved insulin sensitivity and insulin receptor binding during chronic sulfonylurea therapy [19]. The improvement in glucose levels during sulfonylurea treatment can also ameliorate triglyceride and HDL-colesterol levels [20]. Nevertheless their efficacy in overcoming the insulin-resistant state in the plurimetabolic syndrome is still debated. On the contrary, the glucose-lowering effect of biguanides occurs without increased insulin secretion since they principally act by stimulating glucose utilization by peripheral tissues. It has been shown convincingly that chronic metformin treatment improves glucose metabolism both in basal and insulin-stimulated state [21,22].

In baseline conditions, but not during euglycemic hyperinsulinemia, this improvement is associated with a parallel reduction in free fatty acid (FFA) oxidation and with an increase in glucose oxidation. During insulin-stimulated condition, the significant increase in non-oxidative glucose metabolism is secondary to an improvement in glucose disposal. On the other hand, it seems that the primary antihyperglycemic effect of metformin in NIDDM patients after acute treatment is due to the suppression of hepatic glucose production in the absence of an increase in peripheral and portal plasma insulin concentrations. The suppression of FFA oxidation and FFA plasma concentration induced by metformin seems to be the principal mechanism through which this drug improves both hepatic and whole body glucose metabolism. A positive correlation between the rate of hepatic glucose production and of lipid oxidation has been demonstrated by Perriello et al. [23] in NIDDM patients after placebo or metformin administration, before and during hyperinsulinemic-isoglycemic clamp. Parenthetically it must be emphasized that prolonged metformin administration does not interfere with protein and aminoacid metabolism [24]. The positive effects of metformin on lipoprotein profile and the recent observations of its favorable action on PAI-1 activity and on arterial blood pressure [25,26] indicate that this drug not only improves glycemic control and lowers insulin resistance, but also corrects other risk factors for atherosclerotic cardiovascular disease. For all these reasons metformin could be considered positively in the treatment of the plurimetabolic syndrome.

The use of antilipolytic drugs could be considered for treatment of the plurimetabolic syndrome. These patients do have increased plasma FFA, and FFA turnover rate; furthermore, an inverse correlation between FFA oxidation and glucose utilization at the muscle level has been demonstrated. It has also been shown that FFA specifically decreases glucose uptake and oxidation in obese and NIDDM subjects [27]. Acipimox (a nicotinic analogue) inhibits lipolysis and depresses FFA levels thus improving insulin and noninsulin-mediated glucose utilization in both normals and NIDDM patients [28]. Although these encouraging results were observed during acute studies, long-term studies have been disappointing.

Benfluorex (a derivative of fenfluramine), another drug utilized in some European countries, may decrease hyperglycemia after short-term administration. It was shown that it improves insulin sensitivity at liver, muscle, and adipose tissue sites [29-30]. These effects are qualitatively similar to those elicited by biguanides. Long-term studies with benfluorex are needed to establish the real antihyperglycemic potency of this drug and its possible use in the insulin-resistance syndrome. Fenfluramine itself exerts a positive effect on body weight, glucose homeostasis, and serum lipoproteins in NIDDM patients [31]

Recently, in contrast to other antihypertensive drugs such as diuretics and beta-blockers which may have a negative effect on insulin action, ACE-inhibitors, and particularly captopril, may improve insulin sensitivity in type II diabetes and hypertension, at least on a short-term basis [32]. According to the hemodynamic hypothesis, ACE-inhibition would enhance insulin action through arterial vasodilatation and increased blood flow. A similar mechanism has been observed after prazosin treatment [33].

The treatment of hypertriglyceridemia, which represents a constant feature of the plurimetabolic syndrome, could positively affect the insulin-resistance state. An inverse correlation between serum triglycerides and total glucose metabolism has been demonstrated in hypertriglyceridemic diabetic patients [34]. Lipid disturbances could not only be the consequence of insulin resistance but they also tend to aggravate insulin resistance. Therefore hypolipidemic treatment could interfere positively on insulin action [35].

An improvement in glucose tolerance in NIDDM after a secondary fall in plasma FFA clofibrate and bezafibrate treatment [36] has been reported. We [37] recently observed that the normalization of plasma VLDL-TG levels obtained by gemfibrozil therapy is associated with a significant improvement in glucose metabolism not only in nondiabetic but particularly in diabetic-hypertriglyceridemic patients.

FUTURE DRUGS

In the past decade a new class of antidiabetic agents with a specific efficacy for insulin-resistant states have been extensively studied. Many studies on the use of these agents have been carried out in insulin-resistant animal models, and the use of one or more of these agents in human phase I and II studies is being pursued actively.

Thiazolidinedione Derivatives

The thiazolidinedians are the only new class of agents that have been shown to increase insulin sensitivity in insulin-resistant animals [38] but few of these drugs have been evaluated clinically. The earliest member of this class of drugs and the most extensively studied are ciglitazone, followed by eglitone, pioglitazone, and troglitazone.

In animal models of insulin resistance and human diabetes, ciglitazone improves glucose tolerance and lowers plasma insulin levels. In the hyperglycemic, hyperinsulinemic fa/fa rat, a ciglitazone derivative enhances insulin inhibition of hepatic glucose production and increases insulin-stimulated glucose disposal [39].

The oral administration of thiazolidinediones induces a sensitization of adipose tissue, skeletal muscle, and liver to insulin action. The potentiation of insulin action on target tissues is mediated by the effects of these drugs on intracellular insulin action subsequent to past insulin-receptor binding. Increased glucose oxidation by adipose tissue and muscle, and increased glycogen and lipid synthesis from glucose and decreased glycogenolysis have been shown after thiazolidinedione treatment.

Troglitazone, the last compound of this class, is being tested as a new oral antidiabetic agent. Evidence exists from animal studies and clinical trials with noninsulin-dependent diabetes mellitus patients that troglitazone might reduce insulin resistance. It could antagonize the glucose induced inhibition of the insulin receptor kinase. In NIDDM patients troglitazone improves significantly insulin resistance, reduces insulinemia, lowers hepatic glucose production, and improves both fasting and postprandial plasma glucose [40]. Using a new agent (BRL 49653), Oakes et al. [41] showed that thiazolidinediones may act through an altered lipid availability.

Fatty Acid Oxidation Inhibitors

Inhibitors of fatty acid oxidation have potential beneficial effects in reducing plasma glucose. They reduce substrate availability for gluconeogenesis and hepatic glucose production. On the other hand, increased fatty acid oxidation curbs glucose oxidation through the inhibition of pyruvate dehydrogenase. This inhibition may occur at levels of long-chain acyl-CoA-carnitine acytransferase I (LCAT I) or of long-chain acylcarnitine translocase or of pyruvate carboxylase. A fatty acid oxidation inhibitor, as well as methyl-2-tetradecyl-glicidate, leads, in hyperglycemic man, to a greater decrease in blood glucose and β-hydroxybutyrate without any significant modification of insulin levels [42]. Clomoxir and etomoxir, inhibitors of carnitine palmitoyltransferase I, seem to lower both hepatic glucose production and plasma lipid levels in a dose-dependent manner, but at the expense of increases in free fatty acid level.

Dichloracetate

The agent, dichloracetate, is able to reduce both blood glucose and lipid concentrations without stimulating insulin secretion. Dichloroacetate inhibits hepatic glucose production and increases glucose clearance by stimulating pyruvate dehydrogenase (PDH), the rate-limiting enzyme of aerobic glucose oxidation. In patients with NIDDM it simultaneously reduces insulin requirement, plasma glucose, and serum triglycerides. Several derivatives of dichloroacetate have been synthesized and found to have some biological activity in animals. However, it seems premature to consider dichloroacetate an important part of the chronic treatment of plurimetabolic syndrome.

Insulin-Like Growth Factors

IGF-I is an insulin analogue with direct effects on glucose uptake; it acts through its binding to a specific receptor. IGF-I seems to decrease plasma glucose with a kinetic pattern similar to that of insulin but with lower potency. Studies in animals demonstrate that IGF-I is less potent than insulin in inhibiting hepatic glucose output as compared to its ability to stimulate glucose uptake in peripheral tissues [43].

Intravenous infusion of IGF-I lowers insulin and C-peptide levels while it is able to maintain normal glucose tolerance during either an oral glucose tolerance test or a mixed meal, in humans. On the other hand, euglycemic clamp studies in normal volunteers have demonstrated that IGF-I has a potency in stimulating glucose disposal approximately 7% that of insulin. In addition IGF-I is able to reduce plasma triglucerides and LDL cholesterol and to raise HDL cholesterol. Therefore IGF-I might appear useful in reducing hyperinsulinemia and some alteration of metabolic syndrome [44].

Other Agents

The oxidized form of the trace element vanadium, vanadate, was reported to have an insulin-like effect. Vanadate normalizes basal hepatic glucose production and restores glucose utilization through mechanisms distal to the insulin receptor kinase [45]. In genetically obese hyperinsulinemic insulin-resistant rats, vanadate improves glucose metabolism in skeletal muscle without altering the number or the expression of the glucose transporter GLUT4. Unfortunately the positive effect on glucose metabolism is overcome by several negative side effects which preclude, at the moment, its use in clinical trials. A β-adrenoceptor agonist, recently developed, is able to stimulate thermogenesis; chronic treatment with this drug leads to weight loss and to improvement in glucose tolerance, insulin sensitivity, and hyperlipidemia in obese hyperinsulinemic diabetic rodents [46].

In the last months a new oral agent, derived from lipid lowering substances and named 515261, has been developed for the treatment of the so-colled "insulin resistance syndrome" [47]. It induces a marked decrease in plasma insulin and triglyceride levels and an increase in glucose disposal rate in rats.

ANTIHYPERINSULINEMIC AGENTS

An alternative way of reducing hyperinsulinemia is to modulate or at least to slow down carbohydrate absorption from gut. This will eventually lead to a reduction of both post-prandial hyperglycemia and hyperinsulinemia.

This goal is partially achieved by the use of fiber. Natural fiber improves glucose tolerance and reduces insulin response. The extractive-soluble fiber may be associated to carbohydrates inducing the same improvement in glucose tolerance and in insulin levels. High-fiber diet improves insulin sensitivity [48] and prevents the elevation of triglyceride level. The introduction of the α-glucosidase inhibitors allows a reduced rate of absorption of simple sugars by inhibiting brush-border enzymes that cleave oligo- and disaccharides into monosaccharides. Three of these compounds, acarbose, miglitol, and emiglicate, lower postprandial hyperglycemia and hypertriglyceridemia in patients with NIDDM. Fasting C-peptide and insulin concentrations remain unchanged during therapy, but a decrease in postprandial insulin concentration has been reported [49].

The delayed glucose absorption from complex carbohydrates and disaccharides leads to a diminished stimulation of the β-cells of the pancreas. Therefore, a long-lasting reduction of postprandial hyperinsulinemia by more than 30% has been observed in controlled studies with acarbose. For NIDDM, this is beneficial for the following reasons: it protects the β-cell secretory capacity and it reduces the harmful effect of hyperinsulinemia on hypertriglyceridemia. Consistent data indicate a reduced increment in postprandial hypertri-glyceridemia [50] secondary to a decrease in VLDL synthesis and a decrease in total cholesterol. The positive effects on hyperinsulinemia suggests that the chronic use of α-glucosidase inhibitors may be useful in the treatment of the plurimetabolic syndrome.

Conclusions

Insulin-resistance plays a key role in the development of the different abnormalities of the plurimetabolic syndrome. The increased insulin concentration predicts a cluster of metabolic disorders. Therefore, it seems rationale to normalize this fundamental defect. The lifestyle changes characterized by increased physical activity, hypocaloric and low-fat diet and consequent weight loss improve insulin-sensitivity. In this way the plurimetabolic abnormalities of urbanized Australian aborigines (type II diabetes, obesity, hypertri-glyceridemia, hypertension) improved or are completely abolished by a relatively short reversal from the urbanized to the traditional life-style [51].

Other than diet and physical activity, very few drugs are available to be used against insulin-resistance of the plurimetabolic syndrome. Nevertheless we must use them, when appropriate, when nonpharmacological treatment has failed, to increase the tissue sensitivity to insulin, to ameliorate glucose profile, lipid levels, etc., and to reduce above all hyperinsulinemia, the central feature of the plurimetabolic syndrome. In the near future, the thiazolidinedione derivatives and the fatty acid inhibitors should allow achievement of this goal. As we wait for a more effective specific treatment of insulin resistance, we cannot reject the multifactorial therapy which is, at least, able to improve the different metabolic abnormalities of the plurimetabolic syndrome.

References

1. Reaven GM. Role of insulin resistance in human disease. Diabetes 1988;37:1595-1607.
2. Castelli WP, Garrison RJ, Wilson WF, Abbot RD, Kalonsdian S, Kannel WB. Lipoprotein cholesterol: Incidence of coronary hearth disease and lipoprotein cholesterol levels. JAMA 1986;256:2835-2838.
3. Williams RR, Hunt SC, Hopkins PN, et al. Familiar dysplipidemic hypertension. JAMA 1988; 59:3579-3586.
4. Zavaroni I, Bonora E, Pagliara M, et al. Risk factors for coronary artery disease in healthy persons with hyperinsulinemia and normal glucose tolerance. N Eng J Med 1989;320:702-706.
5. Orchard TJ, Becker DJ, Bates M, Kuller LH, Drash AL. Plasma insulin and lipoprotein concentrations: An atherogenic association? Am J Epidemiol 1983;118:326-337.
6. Haffner SM, Fong D, Hazuda HP, Pugh JA, Patterson JK. Hyperinsulinemia, upper body adiposity and cardiovascular risk in non-diabetics. Metabolism 1988;37:338-345.
7. Lillioja S, Matt DM, Spraul M, et al. Insulin resistance and insulin secretory dysfunction as precursors of non-insulin-dependent diabetes mellitus. N Engl J Med 1993;329:1988-1992.
8. Haffner SM, Stern MP, Mitchell BD, Hazuda HP, Patterson JK. Incidence of type II diabetes mellitus in Mexican-Americans predicted by fasting insulin and glucose levels, obesity and body fat distribution. Diabetes 1990;39:283-289.
9. Haffner PA, Valdez RA, Hazuda H, Mitchell DD, Morales PA, Stern M. Prospective analysis of the insulin-resistance syndrome. Diabetes 1992;41:715-722.
10. Pyorala K. Relationship of glucose tolerance and plasma insulin to the incidence of coronary heart disease: Results from two population studies in Finland. Diabetes Care 1979;2:131-141.
11. Fontbonne A, Charles A, Thiebult N, et al. Hyperinsulinemia as predictor of coronary heart disease mortality in a healthy population: The Paris Prospective Study, 15-year follow-up. Diabetologia 1991;34:356-361.
12. Henry RR, Wiest-Kent TA, Scheaffer L, Koltermann OG, Olefsky JM. Metabolic consequences of very-low-calorie diet therapy in obese non-insulin-dependent diabetic and non diabetic subjects. Diabetes 1986;35:155-164.
13. Busetto L, Digito M, Inelmen EM, Carraro R, Enzi G. Modifications of metabolic

abnormalities after massive weight loss. In: Crepaldi G, Tiengo A, Manzato E, editors. Diabetes, obesity and hyperlipidemias V. The plurimetabolic syndrome. Excerpta Medica. Int Congr Ser 1039, 1993:255-270.

14. Riccardi G, Rivellese A. Effects of dietary fiber and carbohydrate on glucose and lipoprotein metabolism in diabetic patients. Diabetes Care 1991;14:115-125.

15. Garg A, Bonanome A, Grundy SM, Zhang ZJ, Unger RH. Comparison of a high-carbohydrate diet with a high-monounsatured-fat diet in patients with non-insulin-dependent diabetes mellitus. N Engl J Med 1988;319:829-834.

16. Holloszy JD, Schultz J, Kusnierkiewicz J, Hagberg JM, Ehsani AA. Effects of exercise on glucose tolerance and insulin resistance: Brief review and some preliminary results. Acta Med Scand Suppl 1986;711:55-65.

17. Segal KR, Edamo A, Abalos A, Blando L, Tomas MB, Pin-Sunyer FX. Effect of exercise training on insulin sensitivity and glucose metabolism in learn, obese and diabetic men. J Appl Physiol 1991;71:2402-2411.

18. Bogardus C, Ravussin E, Robbins DC, Wolfe RR, Horton ES, Sims EA. Effect of physical training and diet theraphy on carbohydrate metabolism in patients with glucose intolerance and non-insulin-dependent diabetes mellitus. Diabetes 1984;33:311-318.

19. Groop LC. Sulphonylureas in NIDDM. Diabetes Care 1992;15:737,754.

20. Taskinen MR, Beltz WF, Harger I. Effects on NIDDM on VLDL-lipoprotein triglyceride and apolipoprotein B metabolism. Studies before and after sulfonylurea therapy. Diabetes 1986;35:1268-1277.

21. Nosadini R, Avogaro A, Trevisan R, et al. Effect of metformin on insulin-stimulated glucose turnover and insulin binding to receptors in type II diabetes. Diabetes Care 1987;10:62-67.

22. Riccio A, Del Prato 5, De Kreutzenberg S, Tiengo A. Glucose and lipid metabolism in non-insulin-dependent diabetes: Effect of metformin. Diabete Metabol 1991;17: 180-184.

23. Perriello G, Misericordia P, Volpi E, et al. Acute antihyperglycemic mechanisms of metformin in NIDDM. Diabetes 1994;43:920-928.

24. Tessari P, Biolo G, Bruttomesso D, et al. Effects of metformin treatment on whole-body and splanchnic amino-acid turnover in mild type 2 diabetes. J Clin Endocrinol Metab 1994, in press.

25. Nagi D, Yudkin JS Effects of metformin on insulin resistance, risk factors for cardiovascular disease and plasminogen activator inhibitor in NIDDM subjects. Diabetes Care 1993;16:621-629.

26. Giugliano D, De Rosa N, Di Maro G, et al. Metformin improves glucose, lipid metabolism and reduces blood pressure in hypertensive, obese women. Diabetes Care 1993;16:1387-1393.

27. Bevilacqua S, Buzzigoli G, Bonadonna R, Ferrannini E. Operation of Randle's cycle in patients with non-insulin-dependent diabetes. Diabetes 1990;39:383-391.

28. Piatti PM, Monti LD, Pacchioni M, Pontiroli AE, Pozza G. Forearm insulin- and non-insulin mediated glucose uptake and muscle metabolism in man: Role of free

fatty acids and blood glucose levels. Metab Clin Exp 1991;40:926-933.

29. De Feo P, Lavielle R, De Gregoris P, Bolli GB. Antihyperglycemic mechanisms of Benfluorex in type II diabetes mellitus. Diab Metab Rev 1993;9(Suppl.1):35-42.

30. Riccio A, Vigili de Kreutzenberg S, Dorella M, et al. Mechanism(s) of the blood glucose lowering action of benfluorex. Diab Metab Rev 1993; 9(Suppl.1):19-28.

31. Salmela PI, Sotaniemi EA, Viikari J, Solakivi-Jaakkala T, Jarvensivu P. Fenfluramine therapy in non-insulin-dependent diabetic patients: Effects on body weight, glucose homeostasis, serum lipoproteins, and antipyrine metabolism. Diabetes Care 1981;4:535-540.

32. Torlone E, Rambotti AM, Perriello G, et al. ACE-inhibition increases hepatic and extrahepatic sensitivity to insulin in patients with type 2 diabetes mellitus and arterial hypertension. Diabetologia 1991;34:119-125.

33. Pollare T, Lithell H, Selinus I, Berne C. Application of prazosin is associated with an increase of insulin-sensitivity in obese patients with hypertension. Diabetologia 1988;31:415-420.

34. Widen E, Ekstrand A, Saloranta C, et al. Insulin-resistance in type 2 (noninsulin-dependent) diabetic patients with hypertriglyceridemia. Diabetologia 1992;35:1140-1145.

35. Steiner G. Altering triglyceride concentrations changes insulin-glucose relationships in hypertriglyceridemic patients. Double-blind study with gemfibrozil with implications for atherosclerosis. Diabetes Care 1991;14:1077-1082.

36. Jones IR, Swai A, Taylor R, Miller M, Laker M, Alberti KGMM. Lowering of plasma glucose concentrations with bezafibrate in patients with moderately controlled NIDDM. Diabetes Care 1990;13:855-863.

37. Avogaro A, Beltramello P, Marin R, et al. Insulin action and glucose metabolism are improved by gemfibrozil treatment in hypertriglyceridemic patients. Atherosclerosis, in press.

38. Bressler R, Johnson D. New pharmacological approaches to therapy of NIDDM. Diabetes Care 1992;15:792-805.

39. Bowen L, Stein PP, Stevenson R, Shulman GI. The effect of CP 68722, a thiazolidinedione derivate, on insulin sensitivity in lean and obese Zucker rats. Metabolism 1991;40:1025-1030.

40. Suter S, Nolan JJ, Wallace P, Gumbiner B, Olefsky J. Metabolic effects of new oral hypoglycemic agent CS-045 in NIDDM subjects. Diabetes Care 1992;15:193-203.

41. Oakes ND, Kennedy CJ, Jenkins AB, Laybutt DR, Chisholm DJ, Kraegen EW. A new antidiabetic agent, BRL 49653, reduces lipid availability and improves insulin action and glucoregulation in the rat. Diabetes 1994;43:1203-1210.

42. Tutwiler GF, Kirsch T, Mohnbacher R, Ho W. Pharmacologic profile of methyl-2-tetradecylglucidate, an orally effective hypoglycemic agent. Metabolism 1978;37:1539-1555.

43. Zenobi PD, Graf S, Ursprung H, Froesch R. Effects of insulin-like growth-I on glucose tolerance, insulin levels, and insulin secretion. J Clin Invest 1992;89:1908-1913.

44.   Moses AC, Abrahamson MJ. Therapeutic approaches to insulin resistance. In: Moller DE, editor. Insulin Resistance. New York: J. Wiley and Sons Ltd., 1993: 385-410.

45.   Blondel O, Simon J, Chevalier B, Portha B. Impaired insulin action but normal insulin receptor activity in diabetic rat liver: Effect of vanadate. Am J Physiol 1990; 258:E459-467.

46.   Cawthorne MA, Sennitt MV, Jonathan RSA, Smith SA. BRL 35135, a potent and selective atypical 13-adrenoreceptor agonist. Am J Clin Nutr 1992;85:1525-1575.

47.   Duhault J, Lacour F, Boulanger M, et al. 515261, a new compound for the treatment of the insulin resistance. Diabetologia 1994;10:959-968.

48.   Fugowa NK, Anderson JW, Hagernon G, Young VR, Minakers KL. High carbohydrate, high fiber diets increase peripheral insulin sensitivity in healthy young and old adults. Am J Clin Nutr 1990;52:524-528.

49.   Hanefeld M, Fisher S, Schulze J, et al. Therapeutic potentials of acarbose as first-line drug in NIDDM insufficiently treated with diet alone. Diabetes Care 1991;14:732-737.

50.   Zavaroni I, Reaven GM. Inhibition of carbohydrate-induced hypertriglyceridemia by a disaccharidose inhibitor. Metabolism 1981;30:417-420.

51.   O'Dea K. Marked improvement in carbohydrate and lipid metabolism in diabetic australian aborigenes after temporary reversion to traditional lifestyle. Diabetes 1984;33:596-603.

KIDNEY PROTECTION IN DIABETES MELLITUS

Karl Heinz Rahn, Michael Barenbrock, Barbara Suwelack, Helge Hohage
Department of Medicine D
University of Münster
D-48149 Münster
GERMANY

Diabetes mellitus may cause several types of kidney disease, the most important of which is diabetic nephropathy. Besides chronic glomerulonephritis, diabetic nephropathy is now the most frequent disorder causing end-stage renal failure in Germany.

Clinical diabetic nephropathy is currently defined by the presence of a persistently positive urinary dipstick test for protein in a patient with diabetes mellitus when other renal disease is absent. A positive urinary dipstick test for protein means that protein excretion rate exceeds 300 mg/day. Clinical diabetic nephropathy as defined in this way is a relatively late manifestation of diabetic renal disease and is frequently accompanied by hypertension and impaired renal function. Diabetic renal disease can be divided into 5 stages, the final ones being clinical diabetic nephropathy and end-stage renal failure [1].

Stage 1 begins immediately with the onset of diabetes mellitus and is characterized by glomerular hypertrophy. The ensuing functional abnormality is an increase of glomerular filtration rate. Apparently in all patients with stage 1, progression to stage 2 follows which is characterized by increased thickness of the capillary basement membranes. In 35-40% of patients with stage 2, stage 3 develops. This stage is characterized by glomerulosclerosis and albuminuria exeeding 30 mg/day. Stage 4 may follow 10-30 years after onset of diabetes mellitus. The typical structural abnormality of this stage 4, the clinical diabetic nephropathy, is widespread glomerulosclerosis. In a high percentage of patients, clinical diabetic nephropathy progresses to end-stage renal disease requiring dialysis or renal transplantation. The sequence of stages described most clearly applies for patients with insulin-dependent diabetes mellitus. It is less clear whether this scheme is also typical for noninsulin-dependent diabetes mellitus.

Concomitantly with the alterations of kidney structure and function as described above, there are changes of the large and medium-sized arteries in diabetic patients. These can now be detected noninvasively by ultrasound techniques. Using high resolution ultrasound, the intima-media thickness of the carotid artery and other arteries of similiar size can be determined. In our studies, the maximum intima-media thickness is measured at 9-12 points in 3 defined segments of the common and the internal carotid arteries close to the

197

A.M. Gotto et al. (eds.), Multiple Risk Factors in Cardiovascular Disease, 197-200.
© 1995 *Kluwer Academic Publishers and Fondazione Giovanni Lorenzini.*

bifurcation.

We have determined the intima-media thickness in 4 normal subjects with an average age of 26 years and in 4 age-matched patients with insulin-dependent diabetes mellitus. The diabetic patients had no signs of incipient or clinical diabetic nephropathy. Their diabetes was known for periods ranging from 5-21 years. The mean of the intima-media thickness in the control subjects was 0.68 mm, a value which is normal for this age group. The intima-media thickness of the patients with diabetes mellitus was not different. Certainly, it was not increased as compared with the normal subjects. The picture is totally different in diabetic patients whose nephropathy has progressed to end-stage renal failure. In such patients, the intima-media thickness of the carotid artery is considerably increased.

The use of ultrasound techniques also allows us to study noninvasively the distensibility of large- and medium-sized arteries. We performed a number of studies in which the distensibility of the common carotid artery was determined. The method is based upon the processing of low frequency Doppler signals originating from the sample volumes coinciding with the anterior and posterior vessel walls [2]. From the degree of outward movement of the vessel walls and the concomitantly measured blood pressure, the distensibility coefficient and the cross-sectional compliance of the carotid artery can be determined.

We have measured these parameters in 10 normal subjects with an average age of 30 years and in age-matched patients with insulin dependent diabetes mellitus. The diabetic patients had no signs of incipient or clinical diabetic nephropathy. There was no difference between the two groups of subjects studied in the distensibility coefficient and the cross-sectional compliance. Again, the picture is totally different when normal subjects are compared with diabetic patients in whom diabetic nephropathy has progressed to end-stage renal failure. In such patients, the distensibility coefficient and the cross-sectional compliance of the carotid artery are significantly reduced as compared with age-matched control subjects. This indicates increased stiffness of the vessel wall.

Apparently, the most relevant alterations of the large- and medium-sized arteries occur in diabetic patients once diabetic nephropathy or end-stage renal failure have developed. It is, therefore, understandable that efforts have been made to slow the progression of organ damage particularly in diabetic patients whose renal disease has progressed to diabetic nephropathy. For a number of years, it has been known that treatment of elevated blood pressure inhibits the progression of diabetic nephropathy [3]. Recently, it has been demonstrated that in this respect ACE-inhibitors are superior to other antihypertensive drugs.

Björck et al. [4] compared the effects of the ACE-inhibitor enalapril and of the beta-blocker metoprolol in 40 patients with insulin-dependent diabetes mellitus and diabetic nephropathy. The target blood pressure during therapy was a mean arterial pressure between 90 and 110 mmHg in supine position. Furosemide and hydralazine or nifedipine were added if the target blood pressure was not obtained with the ACE-inhibitor or the beta-blocker. During the observation period of 3 years, glomerular filtration rate declined by an average of 16 ml/min in the patients treated with metoprolol. The decline was significantly less in the patients treated with enalapril.

This study has been criticized because at entrance supine diastolic blood pressure was 5 mmHg higher in the enalapril group than in the metoprolol group, the difference being statistically not significant. During treatment, the supine diastolic blood pressure averaged to 85 mmHg in the enalapril group and to 90 mmHg in the metoprolol group. This difference is statistically significant. However, mean arterial blood pressure was almost identical during treatment (102 mmHg in the enalapril group and 103 mmHg in the metoprolol group).

Considerably more patients were recruited for a study on the effect of the ACE-inhibitor captopril in patients with diabetic nephropathy [5]. Two hundred and two patients with diabetic nephropathy were treated with placebo, 207 with captopril. Presence of hypertension was not an inclusion criterium. However, 75% of the patients in the captopril group and 76% in the placebo group had systolic blood pressure levels above 140 mmHg or diastolic blood pressures above 90 mmHg at entrance into the study. The study was double-blind. If the target blood pressure of 140/90 mmHg was not obtained during the observation period, antihypertensive agents other than ACE-inhibitors and calcium antagon-tists were added. During the study, the difference in median diastolic blood pressure was consistently less than 4 mmHg between the two groups. During an observation period of 3.5 years, 23% of the patients in the placebo group died or required dialysis or renal transplantation. This percentage was considerably less in the captopril group. The difference was statistically significant.

The studies by Björck et al. [4] and by Lewis et al. [5] demonstrate that treatment with an ACE-inhibitor has a more pronounced renal protective effect than treatment with other antihypertensive agents in patients with diabetic nephropathy.

Summary

Long-standing diabetes mellitus causes serious alterations of the structure and function of large- and medium-sized arteries and of kidney function. The most severe diabetic complication of the kidneys is diabetic nephropathy which often progresses to end-stage renal failure. Recent studies have demonstrated that ACE-inhibitors are superior to other antihypertensive drugs in inhibiting the progression of diabetic nephropathy.

References

1.   Selby JV, FitzSimmons SC, Newman JM, Katz PP, Sepe S, Showstack J. The natural history and epidemiology of diabetic nephropathy. JAMA 1990;263:1954-1960.

2.   Barenbrock M, Spieker C, Laske V, Heidenreich S, Hohage H, Bachmann J, Hoeks APG, Rahn KH. Studies of the vessel wall properties in hemodialysis patients. Kidney International 1994;45:1397-1400.

3.   Mogensen CE. Long-term antihypertensive treatment inhibiting progression of diabetic nephropathy. BMJ 1982;285:685-688.

4.   Björck S, Mulec H, Johnsen SA, Norden G, Aurell M. Renal protective effect of

enalapril in diabetic nephropathy. BMJ 1992;304:339-343.
5.   Lewis EJ, Hunsicker LG, Bain RP, Rohde RD. The effect of angiotensin-converting-
         enzyme inhibition on diabetic nephropathy. N Engl J Med 1993;329:1456-1462.

ASSOCIATION OF SERUM URIC ACID WITH TRIGLYCERIDE LEVELS IN FEMALE PATIENTS WITH NIDDM

Wolfgang Rathmann, Hans Hauner, Burghard Haastert, Katrin Kirchner, and F. Arnold Gries
Diabetes Research Institute at the Heinrich-Heine-University
Düsseldorf
GERMANY

Introduction

There is increasing evidence that elevated serum uric acid (SUA) seems to be part of a cluster of abnormalities related to insulin resistance that include hypertension, impaired glucose tolerance, hyperinsulinemia, and dyslipidemia, characterized by low HDL-cholesterol concentrations and high triglyceride levels [1]. Hyperuricemia was reported to be closely associated with hypertension [2] as well as with elevated triglyceride levels [3] and resistance to insulin-mediated glucose uptake [1]. Insulin resistance appears to increase SUA levels by decreasing renal uric acid clearance [4]. This relation to major cardiovascular risk factors may explain why in some studies an association of elevated uric acid with coronary heart disease (CHD) was found in univariate analysis which disappeared in multivariate analysis after taking other risk factors into account [2,5]. However, prospective studies have reported an independent association of hyperuricemia with CHD and cardiovascular mortality in women [6,7]. Recently, we have shown a correlation of hyperuricemia with CHD in women with insulin-dependent diabetes mellitus (IDDM) and noninsulin-dependent diabetes mellitus (NIDDM) that was independent of hypertension, nephropathy, and obesity [8]. However, there are conflicting results on SUA levels in diabetic patients. Hyperuricemia has been reported to be more prevalent in subjects with impaired glucose tolerance [1] while mean SUA levels tended to be lower in diabetic patients compared with the nondiabetic population [9]. The aim of this study was to assess SUA levels in patients with NIDDM with poor metabolic control and to analyze possible sex-differences in the influence of several metabolic factors that are known to be related with SUA. We found that prevalence of hyperuricemia was low in both male and female patients with long-standing poorly controlled NIDDM (men 6%, women 8%, n.s.). There was a correlation of triglyceride levels with SUA in women but not in men that may partially explain the association of SUA with CHD in female diabetic patients.

A.M. Gotto et al. (eds.), Multiple Risk Factors in Cardiovascular Disease, 201-209.
© 1995 *Kluwer Academic Publishers and Fondazione Giovanni Lorenzini.*

Patients

Clinical data of 196 NIDDM patients (88 male, 108 female) with poor metabolic control (HbA1 > 9.5%) who were consecutively referred to the Diabetes Research Institute in 1993 were retrospectively analyzed. Exclusion criteria for the study were use of diuretic drugs or current medical treatment of serum lipid disorders or hyperuricemia. Furthermore, patients with previous disease that might influence SUA like myeloproliferative disorders or neoplasms were also excluded. All patients had been treated with oral antidiabetic drugs. The clinical variables considered for the statistical analyses are shown in Table 1.

Methods

Fasting blood samples for laboratory measurements were collected before an improvement of diabetic control by hypocaloric diet or insulin therapy. Serum uric acid levels were measured using an enzymatic method (Boehringer Mannheim, Germany). Hyperuricemia was defined as SUA levels above 7.0 mg/dl in men and 6.6 mg/dl in women. Plasma glucose levels were measured after an overnight period (fasting) and 2 hours after breakfast (postprandial). Glycosylated hemoglobin (HbA1) was measured using ion-exchange chromatography (Isolab Inc.,USA). The normal range of HbA1 in this laboratory is below 7.7%. Urinary protein excretion was determined by 24-hour samples collected at the ward and urine albumin was determined by an immunoprecipitation method. Urinary albumin excretion rate (μg/min) and systolic and diastolic blood pressure were given as means of triplicate measurements in every patient. Total cholesterol was determined by enzymatic test (Boehringer Mannheim, Germany). HDL- and LDL-concentrations were only measured in patients with elevated total cholesterol and data are not shown. Fasting insulin and insulin concentrations (IRI) 6 minutes after intravenous application of 1mg glucagon were assessed by an immunofluorometric method (IRI, Abbott Comp, England). Coronary heart disease was considered to be present if ECG-abnormalities characteristic for ischemia or clinical symptoms (angina) were present or patients were treated for CHD. This definition included patients with history of prior myocardial infarction.

Statistics

The data are given as arithmetic means with standard deviation or geometric means with standard deviation factor in log normally distributed parameters (triglycerides, creatinine, albuminuria, insulin). All analyses were performed separately for male and female patients. Means and prevalence rates were compared with t-test, chi-square, or Fisher's exact test, respectively. An univariate regression analysis was used to study the relationship between SUA and the variables under investigation (Table 1). Furthermore, a multivariate linear regression analysis concerning the effect of all independent parameters listed in Table 1 on SUA was performed. In addition, stepwise and backward selection procedures using the multivariate model were analyzed. The final model was formed by selecting significant influence factors on serum uric acid. Furthermore, some multivariate models with fixed sets of variables were analyzed. Statistical analysis was performed using the SAS program (Version 6.09 for UNIX; SAS Institute, Cary, USA).

Table 1. Descriptive data of serum uric acid levels (dependent variable) and several biomedical characteristics (independent variable) considered for regression analyses in 196 NIDDM separated for sex.

Parameter	Men (n=88)	Women (n=108)	p-Value*
serum uric acid (mg/dl)	5.14±1.23	4.70±1.28	<0.05
age (years)	59.58±10.81	63.67±11.27	<0.05
duration of diabetes (years)	10.78±7.63	9.25±6.96	n.s.
body mass index (kg/m²)	26.84±4.35	27.86±5.77	n.s.
fasting plasma glucose (mg/dl)	245.24±58.93	255.50±57.28	n.s.
pp plasma glucose (mg/dl)	300.76±58.73	325.03±66.77	<0.05
triglycerides (mg/dl)	$179.08 \cdot 2.30^{\pm 1}$	$185.49 \cdot 1.78^{\pm 1}$	n.s.
total cholesterol (mg/dl)	234.27±67.00	250.75±53.70	n.s.
creatinine (mg/dl)	$0.83 \cdot 1.20^{\pm 1}$	$0.67 \cdot 1.41^{\pm 1}$	<0.05
albuminuria (µU/min)	$16.57 \cdot 4.72^{\pm 1}$	$13.29 \cdot 3.99^{\pm 1}$	n.s.
fasting insulin (µU/ml)	$4.60 \cdot 2.17^{\pm 1}$	$5.36 \cdot 2.31^{\pm 1}$	n.s.
stim. insulin (µU/ml)	$12.06 \cdot 2.57^{\pm 1}$	$13.81 \cdot 2.82^{\pm 1}$	n.s.
systolic blood pressure (mm Hg)	144.86±24.86	$155.00 \cdot 28.15^{\pm 1}$	n.s.
diastolic blood pressure (mm Hg)	82.70±12.39	84.82±14.33	<0.05
alcohol consumption (n/%):			
no	37 (42%)	86 (80%)	
seldom or regularly	51 (58%)	22 (20%)	<0.05

Male and female patients were compared using t- or chi-square tests. *
Data is given as arithmetric means with standard deviation or geometric means comparing logarithms.

Results

The descriptive data for the variables considered for univariate and multivariate regression analyses are given in Table 1. Serum uric acid levels were higher in the male than in the female diabetic patients. The prevalence of hyperuricemia, defined as SUA levels above 7.0 mg/dl in men and above 6.6 mg/dl in women, was low both in male (6%) and female patients (8%, n.s.). There were no sex-differences for the quality of diabetic control (HbA1: men $11.8 \pm 1.4\%$ versus women $12.2 \pm 1.7\%$) except for higher postprandial blood glucose levels in the female patients. Sex-differences were found for age and diastolic blood pressure which were higher in women. In contrast, creatinine levels were higher in the male compared with the female patients. No difference was found for the prevalence of microalbuminuria (men 33% versus women 31%, n.s.). Prevalence of coronary heart disease (men 40% versus women 44%, n.s.) and history of myocardial infarction (men 10% versus women 9%, n.s.) was comparable in both gender (not shown). Alcohol consumption, which is also known to influence SUA levels, was more frequent in male diabetic patients. Fifty-eight percent of the male diabetic patients reported a seldom or regularly daily alcohol intake compared with 20% of the female patients (Table 1).

The results of the univariate regression analyses are shown in Table 2. In both genders, BMI, triglycerides, and serum creatinine were positively correlated with SUA. The R^2 value of triglycerides, in the female patients indicated a closer association with SUA than in the male patients (33% versus 9.6%). In male diabetic patients, there was a trend for an inverse correlation of SUA with postprandial blood glucose. In contrast, no association with blood glucose levels was found in women. In female diabetic patients, fasting insulin and insulin concentrations, after stimulation with glucagon, and total cholesterol showed a significant correlation with SUA (Table 2).

Table 3 demonstrates the results of the multivariate linear regression analysis. In the male diabetic patients, age, BMI, and creatinine were significant factors influencing SUA levels. The three parameters alone explained 33% of the variance of SUA. Serum uric acid levels increased with BMI (0.12 mg/dl increase per 1 kg/m²) and creatinine (2.78 mg/dl increase per 1 mg/dl of (log) creatinine). There was also a small decrease of SUA of 0.03 mg/dl per each year of age in men. Using the backward selection procedure, triglycerides, cholesterol, and fasting blood glucose turned out to be significant factors in male patients, too. However, performing another regression analysis with these three parameters as independent factors and BMI as dependent variable, the effect of serum lipids and blood glucose was closely related to the influence of BMI in men (data not shown). In the female diabetic patients, BMI, creatinine, and triglycerides alone explained 43% of the variance of SUA. An increase of each of these parameters corresponded with an increase of SUA as indicated in Table 3.

This relationship remained stable during further stepwise and backward selection procedures (data not shown). Concerning alcohol consumption, increased alcohol intake turned out to have significant influence on SUA only in female patients. However, this effect disappeared in a fixed model including BMI, triglycerides, creatinine, and alcohol (data not shown).

Table 2. Univariate linear regression analyses of the association of serum uric acid (mg/dl) with some biomedical parameters in 196 patients with NIDDM separated for sex.

Parameter	Men (n=88)		Women (n=108)	
	Estim. Parameter (Standard Error)	R^2-value (%)	Estim. Parameter (Standard Error)	R^2-value (%)
age (years)	-0.0118 (0.0140)	1.0	0.0012 (0.0125)	0.1
duration of diabetes (years)	0.0118 (0.0193)	0.1	0.0221 (0.0207)	1.3
body mass index (kg/m²)	0.1386 (0.0340)**	19.5	0.1162 (0.0222)**	24.4
fasting plasma glucose (mg/dl)	0.0018 (0.0023)	0.9	0.0000 (0.0023)	0.1
pp plasma glucose (mg/dl)	-0.0046 (0.0024)	5.1	0.0017 (0.0020)	0.8
triglycerides (mg/dl)	0.4306 (0.1589)*	9.6	1.2335 (0.1902)**	33.1
total cholesterol (mg/dl)	0.0025 (0.0020)	2.2	0.0063 (0.0027)*	6.3
creatinine (mg/dl)	2.3579 (0.7670)*	12.1	1.0584 (0.3721)*	8.7
albuminuria (µg/min)	0.0414 (0.0967)	0.3	0.1094 (0.1000)	1.4
fasting insulin (µU/ml)	0.1467 (0.2104)	0.8	0.4386 (0.1630)*	8.8
stim. insulin (µU/ml)	0.1505 (0.1719)	1.3	0.3186 (0.1361)*	6.8
systolic blood pressure (mm Hg)	0.0032 (0.0063)	0.4	-0.006 (0.0049)	0.1
diastolic blood pressure (mm Hg)	0.0072 (0.0122)	0.5	-0.006 (0.0096)	0.1

* <0.05
** <0.001

Discussion

Cross-sectional and two major prospective studies indicate that hyperuricemia is associated with CHD and cardiovascular mortality in women [6,7,8,10,11]. However, there is no evidence from experimental studies that elevated SUA can directly promote arteriosclerosis [12] but hyperuricemia is related to various major cardiovascular risk factors such as hypertension, dyslipidemia, obesity and insulin resistance [1,3,4]. Thus, the association between SUA and CHD in women might be dependent on the correlation with some of these risk factors. In the present study with NIDDM, SUA was positively correlated with trigly-

Table 3. Multivariate linear regression analyses of variables* associated with serum uric acid (mg/dl) in 196 NIDDM separated for sex.

Parameter	Men (n=88)	
	Estimated Parameter (Stand Error)	p-Value
age (years)	-0.0270 (0.0130)	0.043
body mass index (kg/m²)	0.1184 (0.0320)	<0.001
creatinine (mg/dl)	2.7818 (0.7576)	<0.001
	Women (n=108)	
	Estimated Parameter (Stand.Error)	p-Value
body mass index (kg/m²)	0.0582 (0.0232)	0.014
triglycerides (mg/dl)	0.8919 (0.2123)	<0.001
creatinine (mg/dl)	0.8040 (0.3003)	<0.001

Proportion of variance explained by the prognostic factors:

men: $R^2 = 33.2\%$ women: $R^2 = 42.8\%$

*   Other variables included in the model were duration of diabetes, fasting and pp plasma glucose, total cholesterol, albuminuria, fasting and stimulated insulin, systolic and diastolic blood pressure, and alcohol consumption.

ceride levels but not with total cholesterol and hypertension. In multiple linear regression analysis, an association of triglycerides with SUA was found only in female but not in male patients.

In a previous study, we showed that hyperuricemia is associated with the presence of coronary heart disease in women with IDDM and NIDDM [8]. Diabetes is well known to impose a greater risk of CHD in female than in male patients. The excess risk for ischemic heart disease and cardiovascular mortality among diabetic women might be largely explained by the high prevalence of elevated triglyceride levels and reduced concentrations of HDL-cholesterol among these women [13]. Diabetic dyslipidemia is more frequent and more pronounced in female patients than in diabetic men, even after adjustment for diabetes treatment, age, and BMI [14]. The metabolic base for this sex difference of lipoprotein disturbances is not clear. One clue for understanding this difference is the role of insulin resistance for the development of lipid abnormalities. Insulin resistance has been shown to be positively correlated with triglyceride levels and negatively with HDL-cholesterol [15,16]. Thus, insulin resistance might explain the excess risk for CHD in diabetic women, although there is no evidence that women are more insulin-resistant than men in general [17].

Another factor that might contribute to the sex difference of lipoprotein disturbances is the influence of sex hormones on insulin resistance. The majority of female patients with NIDDM are in the postmenopausal state [18] which seems to be accompanied by a worsening of insulin action. The loss of ovarian function during menopause might be involved in insulin resistance and this might be responsible for the increased risk of ischemic heart disease in women [19]. Hormone replacement therapy with estrogen and progestin in postmenopausal women leads to lower fasting glucose and insulin levels [20].

In postmenopausal women with angiographically defined coronary heart disease, SUA, and triglycerides levels are both associated with the severity of cardiovascular stenosis. In contrast, such correlations were not seen in male patients with CHD, matched for age and BMI [21]. The results of a major prospective study on the association of SUA with cardiovascular mortality supports that view that hyperuricemia is associated with an increased risk for CHD particularly in postmenopausal women. An increased mortality risk for cardiovascular events in conjunction with hyperuricemia was observed mainly in women in the age group of 55-64 years [7].

The aim of the present study was to assess a possible sex difference association of SUA with cardiovascular risk factors in patients with NIDDM. Although the conclusions from our data may be limited due to the fact that we studied only poorly controlled patients, the main results are in agreement with a previous study that had been performed in a large sample of patients with NIDDM [22]. Ishihara et al. reported the same sex-specific correlation between SUA and triglyceride levels whereas an important influence of BMI and serum creatinine on SUA was also found for both sexes. In contrast to our results, postprandial plasma glucose was inversely correlated with SUA [22]. Several studies have indicated that hyperglycemia may have a uricosuric activity which lowers serum uric acid in diabetic patients [9,24]. In the present study, the range of glucose levels was probably too small to allow the detection of a correlation with SUA. The uricosuric effect of hyperglycemia might explain the observation, that prevalence of hyperuricemia in diabetic patients is lower than in the nondiabetic population [9,23]. In conclusion, the major finding of this study was that SUA levels are correlated with triglyceride levels in female but not in male patients with NIDDM. These results suggest that both hyperuricemia and high triglyceride levels may be markers for an unfavorable cardiovascular risk factor profile in female diabetic patients. In addition, there was a positive association between serum uric acid and both fasting and stimulated insulin concentrations in the univariate regression analysis in diabetic women. Recent data suggest that SUA and elevated levels of triglycerides are both supposed to be a marker for insulin resistance [1,3,24]. Further studies including intervention studies are required to investigate the role of serum uric acid in the relationships among insulin resistance, NIDDM, and atherosclerosis.

References

1.   Modan M, Halkin, H, Karasik A, Lusky A. Elevated serum uric acid - a facet of hyperinsulinaemia. Diabetologia 1987;30:713-18.

2.   Brand FN, McGee DL, Kannel WB, Stokes III J, Castelli WP. Hyperuricaemia as a risk factor of coronary heart disease: The Framingham Study. Am J Epidemiol 1985;121:11-18.

3.   Vuorinen-Markkola H, Yki-Järvinen H. Hyperuricaemia and insulin resistance. J Clin Endocrinol Metab 1994;78:25-29.

4.   Facchini F, Jda Chen YD, Hollenbeck CB, Reaven GM. Relationship between resistance to insulin-mediated glucose uptake, urinary uric acid clearance, and plasma uric acid concentration. JAMA 1991;266:3008-11.

5.   Yano K, Rhoads GG, Kagan A. Epidemiology of serum uric acid among 8000 Japanese-American men in Hawaii. J Chron Dis 1977;30:171-84.

6.   Reunanen A, Takkunen H, Knekt P, Aromaa A. Hyperuricaemia as a risk factor for cardiovascular mortality. Acta Med Scand 1982;668(Suppl.):49-59.

7.   Levine W, Dyer AR, Shekelle RB, Schoenberger JA, Stamler J. Serum uric acid and 11.5-year mortality of middle-aged women: Findings of the Chicago Heart Association Detection Project in Industry. J Clin Epidemiol 1989;42:257-67.

8.   Rathmann W, Hauner H, Dannehl K, Gries FA. Association of elevated serum uric acid with coronary heart disease in diabetes mellitus. Diabete Metab 1993;19:159-66.

9.   Tuomilehto J, Zimmet P, Wolf E, Taylor R, Ram P, King H. Plasma uric acid level and its association with diabetes mellitus and some biologic parameters in a biracial population of Fiji. Am J Epidemiol 1988;127:321-36.

10. Bengtsson C, Tibblin E. Serum uric acid levels in women. Acta Med Scan 1974;196:93-102.

11. Okada M, Ueda K, Omae T, Takeshita M, Hirota Y. The relationship of serum uric acid to hypertension   and ischaemic heart disease in Hisayama population, Japan. J Chron Dis 1982;35:173-78.

12. Editorial.   Uric acid-a risk factor for coronary heart disease. JAMA 1993;270:378-79.

13. Goldschmitt MG, Barrett-Connor E, Edelstein SL, Wingard DL, Cohn BA, Herman WH. Dyslipidemia and ischaemic heart disease mortality among men and women with diabetes. Circulation 1994;89:991-97.

14. Walden CE, Knopp RH, Wahl PW, Beach KW, Strandness E. Sex differences in the effect of diabetes mellitus on lipoprotein triglyceride and cholesterol concentrations. N Engl J Med 1984;311:953-59.

15. DeFronzo RA, Ferranini E. Insulin resistance: a multifaceted syndrome responsible for NIDDM, obesity,   hypertension, dyslipidemia, and atherosclerosis cardiovascular disease. Diabetes Care 1991;14:173-94.

16. Modan M, Or J, Karasik A et al. Hyperinsulinemia, sex , and risk of atherosclerotic cardiovascular disease. Circulation 1991;84:1165-75.

17. Yki-Järvinen H. Sex and insulin sensitivity. Metabolism 1984;33:1011-15.
18. Krolewski AS, Warram JH. Epidemiology of diabetes mellitus. In: Marble A, Krall LP, Bradley RF, Christlieb AR, Soeldner JS, editors. Joslin's diabetes mellitus. Philadelphia: Lea & Febiger,1985:12-42.
19. Gordon T, Kannel WB, Hjortland MC, McNamara PM. Menopause and coronary heart disease: The Framingham Study. Ann Intern Med 1978;89:157-61.
20. Nabulsi AA, Folsom AR, White A, et al. Association of hormone replacement theray with various cardiovascular risk factors in postmenopausal women. N Engl J Med 1993;328:1069-75.
21. Kotake H, Sawada Y, Hoshio A, et al. Relation between serum uric acid and angiographically defined coronary artery disease in postmenopausal women. J Med 1992;23:409-15.
22. Ishihara M, Shinoda T, Aizawa T, Shirota T, Nagasawa Y, Yamada T. Hypouricemia in NIDDM patients. Diabetes Care 1988;11:796-97.
23. Herman JB, Goldbourt U. Uric acid and diabetes: Observations in a population study. Lancet 1982;2:240-43.
24. Zavaroni I, Mazza S, Fantuzzi M, et al. Changes in insulin and lipid metabolism in males with asymptomatic hyperuricaemia. J Int Med 1993;234:25-30.

CARDIOVASCULAR DISEASE PREVENTION IN THE ELDERLY

Gaetano Crepaldi and Enzo Manzato
Department of Internal Medicine
University of Padova
Via Giustiniani 2
35128 Padova
ITALY

Introduction

Epidemiologists considered contagious diseases of utmost importance during the second half of the nineteenth century and the first half of the twentieth century. Today as we approach the conclusion of the twentieth century, epidemiologists have turned their attention to chronic diseases, such as atherosclerotic cardiovascular diseases and neoplastic diseases. This change is in part due to the changing patterns in the age distribution of the populations of both developed and developing countries.

Population aging is a peculiar phenomenon characteristic not only of developed countries but also of developing nations. Italy has one of the highest percentages in the world of individuals above 70 years of age. When we compare the population composition in Italy today with that in 1951 we now have four times more individuals who are 80 or older and twice the number of persons who are 60 and older. If this trend continues we can expect to see 8 times more individuals who are 80 or older and almost 3 times more subjects 60 or older in the year 2031. The 80-year and older age group is and will have a tremendous impact on our society in terms of social, economic, and health-related expenditures [1]. The elderly presently make up the most rapidly growing segment of the population not only in Italy but also in many other countries, including both the United States and the former USSR [2].

It is generally agreed that the independent risk factors for coronary heart disease in an adult population are age, sex, family history of premature coronary heart disease, smoking, hypertension, high LDL cholesterol, low HDL cholesterol, and diabetes. When prevention of cardiovascular risk factors in the elderly is considered, first it should be determined if the risk factors for vascular disease in the elderly population are the same as those in the adult population or if other specific vascular risk factors characterize the elderly.

The mortality rate for ischemic heart disease in the Italian population as well as in other developed countries has its greatest impact on males and particularly on the older ones [3]. Therefore, age per se is responsible for a significant increase in the incidence of

A.M. Gotto et al. (eds.), Multiple Risk Factors in Cardiovascular Disease, 211-218.

cardiovascular events. Age must be considered the most important vascular risk factor, even in the elderly population. However, a distinction should be made within the elderly population between the "old adult" (between 60 and 70 years of age), the "old" (between 70 and 80 years of age), and the "very old" (above 80 years of age). In fact, different demographic, socio-economic, and psychophysical conditions characterize each of these age groups. This differentiation could also be useful in identifying different risk patterns in the different age groups within the elderly population.

Family History

It has been clearly established that a family history of vascular diseases is a significant risk factor in the adult population. Even recently, the role of family history as a vascular risk factor in older subjects has been examined.

One particular study addressed this question examining a cohort of 10,994 pairs of twins who were born between 1886 and 1925 in Sweden [4]. It was found that when one monozygotic twin died of coronary heart disease before the age of 55 in men and 65 in women, the risk of death from the same cause in the other twin was 8.1 in men and 15.0 in women higher than when a similar twin died after 55 years of age. For dizygotic twins the risk was 3.8 in men and 2.6 in women. The risk of death by coronary heart disease of one twin decreased as the age at death of the other twin increased, suggesting that the genetic susceptibility to coronary death is less important in the elderly. However, the genetic component was observed up to the age of 75 in this study. In fact, after controlling for other risk factors (such as smoking, hypertension, diabetes, body weight, etc.), a significant increase in coronary death risk was observed in one monozygotic or dizygotic twin when the other twin died before 75 years of age (in both men and women). These results seem to confirm the importance of genetic factors (as determined by family history) as vascular risk factors well into the seventh and eighth decade of life.

Apoprotein E has three common isoforms (apo E2, apo E3, apo E4) coded for by three different alleles. These isoforms have an important influence on the total and LDL cholesterol levels and may be correlated with the incidence of atherosclerotic vascular disease. Moreover, apo E4 appears to be a risk factor for Alzheimer's disease. A polymorphism of the angiotensin converting enzyme (ACE) gene is associated not only to plasma ACE concentrations but also to the risk for myocardial infarction.

It has been shown that in a population of 3,000 French centenarians the frequency of apo E4 is lower than that in a control population while the apo E2 frequency is higher [5]. The lower apo E4 frequency in centenarians might be due to an increased mortality from both heart disease and might be due to an increased mortality from both heart disease and Alzheimer's disease. It was also shown in the same group that the frequency of the ACE gene polymorphism associated with myocardial infarction is higher in centenarians. This raises the possibility that the increased frequency of this ACE gene polymorphism could be due to the potential roles of ACE outside of the cardiovascular system. Another interesting finding from this study is that the frequency of some polymorphisms of the apoprotein B gene (Xbal and ins/del polymorphism in the signal-peptide region) were similar in the centenarians to those in the controls.

Lipids

The relationship between plasma cholesterol levels and mortality (total, cardiovascular, and noncardiovascular) remains a question of debate in elderly subjects. Four prospective studies have examined the causes of death and risk factors in Italy. These are: the Brisighella Study, the Study of New Risk Factors in Rome, the Progetto Romano of the Prevention of Coronary Heart Disease, and the Italian part of the Seven Countries Study [6-9]. This last study showed that there is a direct relationship between cholesterol levels and coronary events. It was found that the longer the observation period the stronger is the relationship. Since all the subjects recruited for this study were between 40 and 59 years of age, it is evident that the cholesterol level measured at the first examination was a predictor of ischemic heart disease well into the seventh decade of life (after 25 years of follow-up).

It is well known that the association between cholesterol levels and ischemic heart disease is less evident with advancing age [10]. Based on this finding and on demographic data, which show that mortality from coronary heart disease increases considerably with age, we can safely say that the relative risk due to hypercholesterolemia is reduced in the elderly but the absolute or attributable risk is highly enhanced.

In the Framingham study in men and women with a history of myocardial infarction both before and after 65 years of age, a cholesterol level higher than 275 mg/dl was significantly associated to reinfarction [11]. This finding suggests that even in old age a high cholesterol level is a significant predictor of coronary events in those subjects already affected by coronary heart disease. A recent analysis of data obtained by the Framingham Heart Study concluded that total cholesterol levels are significantly related to coronary heart disease mortality at 40, 50, and 60 years of age [12]. There is no relationship between total cholesterol levels and coronary heart disease in subjects 70 and older. However, up until the age of 75 both LDL cholesterol (directly) and HDL cholesterol (inversely) are significantly related to coronary heart disease mortality in both men and women. There is no doubt that the relative risk for coronary heart disease due to high LDL cholesterol levels decreases with age so that by 80 it is no longer significant. It was recently demonstrated that even in very old subjects HDL cholesterol in males and LDL cholesterol in females are associated to coronary heart disease [13]. From these data we may suggest that hypolipidemic treatment should be considered a therapeutic option even in the elderly when the patient's biological age makes this intervention particularly useful.

Blood Pressure

It has been amply demonstrated that both systolic and diastolic blood pressure are associated with coronary heart diseases both in young and old subjects [14]. The results from some recent trials showed that antihypertensive treatment with β-blockers and diuretics has an important beneficial effect on cardiovascular events in the elderly [15-17]. However, the results obtained using these drugs, though impressive, may not be the final solution to the treatment of hypertension in the elderly. The purpose behind treatment of high blood pressure remains the normalization of hypertension-induced cardiovascular risk. Problems with side effects, efficacy, and compliance are also important in this type of treatment. We now have evidence suggesting that treatment of hypertension is as beneficial in the elderly as in young and middle-aged adults. The therapeutic choice in hypertensive elderly should be made on the basis of safety, efficacy, tolerability, duration of action, and the possible benefits in reducing cardiovascular morbidity and mortality.

Cigarette Smoking

The role of cigarette smoking as a vascular risk factor in the elderly has sometimes been questioned. In a five-year follow-up of more than 7,000 persons 65 years of age or older without a history of myocardial infarction, the relative risk for total mortality and cardiovascular mortality was significantly higher in both men and women who were current smokers [18]. Mortality hazards of smoking extend well into later life and suggest that cessation will continue to improve life expectancy in the elderly.

The Coronary Artery Surgery Study confirmed that in men and women who were 55 years of age and older and had angiographically documented artery disease, cessation of smoking was helpful in reducing the 6-year mortality rate, particularly in subjects in the second and third risk quartile [19]. According to this study, the benefits of smoking cessation were greatest in those subjects who were at moderate risk.

Diabetes

A low HDL cholesterol is often associated with high triglycerides, overweight, insulin resistance or type II diabetes, and hypertension. This association of vascular risk factors has been defined "syndrome X" or "plurimetabolic syndrome." It is indeed a maturity onset syndrome with important implications for cardiovascular mortality in the elderly.

Diabetes per se probably has only a small role in cardiovascular complications, that is on the risk of macroangiopathy, while the role of diabetes in the pathogenesis of microangiopathy is well established. Diabetes acts as a vascular risk factor through other associated factors such as hypercholesterolemia, small dense LDL, hypertriglyceridemia, low HDL cholesterol, microalbuminuria, and the other clinical and metabolic features mentioned in connection with the plurimetabolic syndrome [20]. In fact, in a multivariate analysis only the top quartile of the glycated hemoglobin was significantly related to cardiovascular diseases and only in women on the Framingham Study [21]. No significant relationship was found by this study between causal blood glucose and cardiovascular diseases.

In 396 men and 673 women from Kuopio (Finland) with an age range between 65 and 74, an association of several cardiovascular risk factors (high trigylcerides, low HDL, and hypertension) was noted in the subjects with hyperinsulinemia [22]. Clinical signs of coronary heart disease (angina pectoris or electrocardiographic alterations) were more frequently observed in subjects (both men and women) falling in the group with the highest insulin levels (at fasting and 2 hours after an oral glucose load). In these elderly subjects hyperinsulinemia was related to coronary heart disease and this may in part be due to the association of hyperinsulinemia with their risk factors.

An increased urinary albumin excretion rate or microalbuminuria is a strong predictor of early death (in particular due to cardiovascular disease) in both nondiabetic and diabetic patients. The association of microalbuminuria with premature death persists even when other vascular risk factors such as male sex, age, obesity, presence of coronary heart disease, hypertension, smoking, and hypercholesterolemia are taken into consideration. In a group of 216 subjects with ages between 60 and 74, it was demonstrated that the survival rate is lower in those with microalbuminuria [23]. A subsequent report by the same study group indicated that in the elderly, microalbuminuria is a short-term predictor of mortality (within 5 years) as compared to other parameters (such as HDL, hypertension, and serum creatinine) [24].

Diet

The role of diet as a vascular risk factor in the elderly certainly deserves to be mentioned. In a longitudinal study carried out in the Netherlands involving 805 men with ages ranging between 65 and 84 who were studied for five years, researchers examined the relation between baseline intake of flavonoids and subsequent coronary heart disease mortality and the incidence of myocardial infarction [25]. Flavonoids are a large group of polyphenolic antioxidants present in vegetables, fruits, and in beverages such as tea and wine. These compounds might prevent LDL oxidation. Since oxidized LDL are atherogenic and may play a role in the formation of atherosclerotic lesions, antioxidants could be considered protective factors against atherosclerosis. The Dutch study demonstrated that the dietary intake of flavonoids in elderly subjects was significantly (inversely) associated with coronary heart disease mortality.

This study further strengthened the common opinion that the dietary intake (in particular high consumption of vegetables, in this case onions, apples, and tea) may reduce the risk of coronary heart disease not only in the general population but also in elderly men.

Other Factors

Atherosclerotic vascular disease is associated with several changes in the blood-vessel wall, including abnormal vasoconstriction or vasodilation, abnormal interaction of blood cells with the vessel wall, alteration of the coagulation mechanisms, and proliferation and migration of smooth-muscle cells. The endothelium plays a crucial role in these vascular abnormalities. Endothelial cells produce nitric oxide, a potent vasodilator. Nitric oxide may also protect against thrombosis and inhibit the migration and proliferation of vascular smooth-muscle cells [26].

Several types of tests have been devised to assess the nitric oxide formation by endothelial cells. Using these tests of endothelial function it is possible to detect early vascular abnormalities in patients with cardiovascular risk factors but without clinical signs of vascular diseases. It has been demonstrated that endothelium-dependent vasodilation is impaired in patients without vascular disease but with hypercholesterolemia, hypertension, diabetes, and in smokers. It has also been demonstrated that there is an inverse relation between age and endothelium-dependent vasodilation [27-28].

Conclusions

Cardiovascular disease prevention in the elderly appears to be an important issue in the medical research area and in the clinical practice. Interesting results and new perspectives have been reported in this field during the last few years. Compressing cardiovascular morbidity and thus improving the quality of life in the elderly are today two important and achievable aims in geriatric medicine.

Acknowledgements

This work was supported in part by CNR-Italy, PF INV. 94-XXX.

References

1.   Pinella A, Golini PA, editors. Population Aging in Italy. Paris: INIA/CICRED, 1993.
2.   Kingkade WW, Torrey BB. The evolving demography of aging in the United States of America and the former USSR. Wld Hlth Statist Quart 1992;45:15-28.
3.   Maggi S, Bush TL. Fattori di rischio. Approccio epidemiologico. In: G. Crepaldi, editor. Trattato di gerontologia e geriatria. Torino:UTET, 1993:91-100.
4.   Marenberg ME, Risch N, Berkman LF, Floderus B, De Faire U. Genetic susceptibility to death from coronary heart disease in a study of twins. N Engl J Med 1994;330:1041-1046.
5.   Schachter F, Faure-Delanef F, Guénot F, et al. Genetic associations with human longevity at the APOE and ACE loci. Nature Genetics 1994;6:29-32.
6.   Descovich GC, Dormi A, Gaddi A, et al. The Brisighella Study. In: Lenzi S, Descovich GC, editors. Atherosclerosis and cardiovascular diseases. Norwell, MA: MTP Press, 1987;215-222.
7.   Spagnolo A, Menotti A, Giampaoli S, et al. High density lipoprotein cholesterol distribution and its predictive power in some Italian population studies. Eur J Epidem 1989;5:328-335.
8.   Menotti A, Farchi G, Seccareccia F, Capocaccia R, Conti S. La predizione a breve termine degli eventi coronarici nel Progetto Romano di Prevenzione della Cardiopatia Coronarica. Clin Ter Cardiov 1983;2:193-197.
9.   Italian Research Group of the Seven Countries Study. Twenty-five year incidence and prediction of coronary heart disease in two rural population samples. Acta Cardiol 1986;41:283-299.
10.   Shipley MJ, Pocock SJ, Marmot MG. Does plasma cholesterol concentration

predict mortality from coronary heart disease in elderly people? 18 year follow up in Whitehall study. BMJ 1991;303:89-92.

11. Wong ND, Wilson PWF, Kannel WB. Serum cholesterol as a prognostic factor after myocardial infarction: The Framingham Study. An Intern Med 1991;115:687-693.

12. Kronmal RA, Cain KC, Ye Z, Omenn GS. Total serum cholesterol levels and mortality risk as a function of age. Arch Intern Med 1993;153:1065-1073.

13. Zimetbaum P, Frishman WH, Lock Ooi W, et al. Plasma lipids and lipoproteins and the incidence of cardiovascular disease in the very elderly. Arteriosclerosis and Thrombosis 1992;12:416-423.

14. Castelli WP, Wilson PWF, Levy D, Anderson K. Cardiovascular risk factors in the elderly. Am J Cardiol 1989;63:12H-19H.

15. Amery A, Birkenhager W, Brixko P, et al. Mortality and morbidity results from the European Working Party on High Blood Pressure in the Elderly Trial. Lancet 1985;i:1349-1354.

16. Dahlof B, Lindhold LM, Hansson L, Schersten B, Ekborn T, Wester PO. Morbidity and mortality in the Swedish Trial in Old Patients with Hypertension (STOP-Hypertension). Lancet 1991;338:1281-1285.

17. SHEP Cooperation Research Group. Prevention of stroke by antihypertensive drug treatment in older persons with isolated systolic hypertension. Final results of the Systolic Hypertension in the Elderly Program (SHEP). JAMA 1991;265:3255-3264.

18. LaCroix AZ, Lang JM, Scherr P, et al. Smoking and mortality among older men and women in three communities. N Engl J Med 1991;324:1619-1625.

19. Hermanson B, Omenn GS, Kronmal RA, Gersh BJ. Beneficial six-year outcome of smoking cessation in older men and women with coronary artery disease. N Eng J Med 1988;319:1365-1369.

20. Crepaldi G, Manzato E, Nosadini R. Plurimetabolic syndrome or syndrome X: Is it a real syndrome? Front Diabetes 1993;12:152-164.

21. Singer DE, Nathan DM, Anderson KM, Wilson PWF, Evans JC. Association of HbA1c with prevalent cardiovascular disease in the original cohort of the Framingham Heart Study. Diabetes 1992;41:202-208.

22. Mykkanen L, Laakso M, Pyorala K. High plasma insulin level associated with coronary heart disease in the elderly. Am J Epidemiol 1993;137:1190-1202.

23. Damsgaard EM, Froland A, Jorgensen OD, Mogensen CE. Microalbuminuria as a predictor of increased mortality in elderly people. BMJ 1990;300:297-300.

24. Damsgaard EM, Froland A, Jorgensen OD, Mogensen CE. Prognostic value of urinary albumin excretion rate and other risk factors in elderly diabetic patients and non-diabetic control subjects surviving the first 5 years after assessment. Diabetologia 1993;36:1030-1036.

25. Hertog MGL, Feskens EJM, Hollman PCH, Katan MB, Kromhout D. Dietary antioxidant flavonoids and risk of coronary heart disease: The Zutphen Elderly Study. Lancet 1993;342:1007-1011.

26. Gibbons GH, Dzau V. The emerging concept of vascular remodeling. N Engl J

Med 1994;330:1431-1438.

27.   Vita JA, Treasure CB, Nabel EG, et al. Coronary vasomotor response to acetylcholine relates to risk factors for coronary artery disease. Circulation 1990;81:491-497.

28.   Zeiher AM, Drexler H, Saurbier B, Just H. Endothelium-mediated coronary blood flow modulation in humans. Effect of age, atherosclerosis, hypercholesterolemia and hypertension. J Clin Invest 1993;92:652-662.

INSULIN RESISTANCE AND CORONARY HEART DISEASE

Gerald M. Reaven
Stanford University School of Medicine
Division of Endocrinology, Gerontology, and Metabolism
and
Department of Veterans Affairs Medical Center
Palo Alto, California 94304
USA

Introduction

Insulin-mediated glucose transport varies greatly within the normal population and a substantial number of these individuals can be defined as being insulin resistant [1,2]. If they respond to this defect by secreting increased amounts of insulin, gross decompensation of glucose tolerance can be prevented. The development of impaired glucose tolerance (IGT) and/or noninsulin-dependent diabetes mellitus (NIDDM) represents the failure of the pancreas to sustain the state of compensatory hyperinsulinemia [2]. Even if the pancreas is able to maintain normal glucose tolerance in insulin-resistant individuals by sustaining the requisite degree of compensatory hyperinsulinemia, there is substantial evidence [1,2] that the combination of insulin resistance and compensatory hyperinsulinemia predisposes individuals to develop a high plasma triglyceride (TG) and low HDL-cholesterol concentration, high blood pressure, and coronary heart disease (CHD). In 1988, I suggested that this cluster of abnormalities constitutes an important clinical syndrome, designated as Syndrome X [2], and considerable evidence has been published subsequently in support of this formulation. This presentation will review the evidence that led to the initial formulation of Syndrome X, as well as summarize new information suggesting that several other abnormalities should be included under this heading.

INSULIN RESISTANCE, GLUCOSE TOLERANCE, AND COMPENSATORY HYPERINSULINEMIA

There is a more than four-fold variation in insulin-stimulated glucose uptake in individuals with normal glucose tolerance [1,2], and the defect in insulin action in many of these individuals approximates that of patients with either IGT or NIDDM. Insulin-resistant individuals with normal glucose tolerance are hyperinsulinemic when compared to an

A.M. Gotto et al. (eds.), Multiple Risk Factors in Cardiovascular Disease, 219-226.
© 1995 *Kluwer Academic Publishers and Fondazione Giovanni Lorenzini.*

insulin-sensitive control group, and it appears that it is the increase in plasma insulin concentration which permits them to overcome the defect in insulin action [1,2]. Significant fasting hyperglycemia develops when patients with NIDDM can no longer sustain a state of hyperinsulinemia [2]. Thus, resistance to insulin-mediated glucose uptake is a common phenomenon, present in the majority of individuals who are glucose intolerant, as well as a substantial proportion of an apparently healthy population [1,2]. The degree to which glucose tolerance deteriorates in insulin-resistant individuals will vary as a function of both the magnitude of the loss of *in vivo* insulin action, and the capacity of the pancreas to compensate for this defect.

INSULIN RESISTANCE, HYPERINSULINEMIA, AND DYSLIPIDEMIA

There is considerable evidence that resistance to insulin-stimulated glucose uptake leads to a compensatory increase in plasma insulin concentration, enhanced hepatic very low density (VLDL)-triglyceride (TG) secretion, and hypertriglyceridemia [2-5]. In individuals who retain insulin secretory function, there is a relatively linear relationship between measures of insulin resistance and plasma insulin concentration [1,2], i.e., the more resistant, the greater the magnitude of hyperinsulinemia. In addition, statistically significant correlations exist between resistance to insulin-stimulated glucose uptake, plasma insulin concentration, VLDL-TG secretion rate, and plasma TG concentration in both normotriglyceridemic and hypertriglyceridemic individuals [2-5]. Experimental manipulations which modify insulin action and/or plasma insulin concentration lead to predictable changes in VLDL-TG secretion rate and plasma TG concentration, i.e., weight loss is associated with a commensurate decrease in plasma insulin concentration, hepatic VLDL-TG secretion, and plasma TG concentration [6], whereas low-fat/high-carbohydrate diets lead to day-long increases in both plasma insulin and TG concentrations [7].

Once the plasma VLDL-TG pool-size increases, presumably as a result of the insulin resistance, a variety of associated abnormalities in lipoprotein metabolism develop. The association between a high plasma TG and a low high density lipoprotein (HDL)-cholesterol concentration is well-established, and there is also a relationship between hyperinsulinemia and plasma TG (direct) and HDL-cholesterol (inverse) concentrations [8]. In addition, magnitude of postprandial lipemia is accentuated in subjects with fasting hypertriglyceridemia, and higher postprandial concentrations of TG-rich lipoproteins of intestinal origin are also associated with lower HDL-cholesterol levels [9]. Finally, subjects with high TG and low HDL-cholesterol concentrations are also more likely to have smaller, denser low density lipoprotein (LDL) particles [10]. Thus, fasting hypertriglyceridemia is a marker for the concomitant existence of a low HDL-cholesterol concentration, an exaggerated degree of postprandial lipemia, and smaller, denser LDL particles.

INSULIN RESISTANCE, HYPERINSULINEMIA, AND HYPERTENSION

Patients with high blood pressure are insulin resistant, glucose intolerant, and hyperinsulinemic when compared to a matched group of normotensive individuals [2,11], and these abnormalities persist despite successful drug treatment of hypertension, and can be seen in both obese and nonobese individuals [2,11]. The fact that insulin resistance and hyperinsulinemia occur in patients with hypertension raises the possibility that these changes may play a role in regulation of blood pressure. Although the potential role of insulin resistance and hyperinsulinemia in regulation of blood pressure cannot be fully addressed in this presentation, it may be useful to summarize the main arguments, pro and con. In support of the view that changes in insulin metabolism may modulate blood pressure is the observation that as many as 50% of patients with essential hypertension appear to be insulin resistant and hyperinsulinemic [12]. Furthermore, the abnormalities of insulin metabolism can be discerned in normotensive first degree relatives of patients with high blood pressure [13], but not in patients with secondary forms of hypertension [14]. Additional support for the possibility that insulin resistance and compensatory hyperinsulinemia are involved in blood pressure regulation can be found in studies of rodent hypertension. For example, substituting fructose for the carbohydrate conventionally present in rat chow leads to insulin resistance, hyperinsulinemia, and hypertension in Sprague-Dawley rats [15]. A subsequent study showed that fructose-induced insulin resistance, hyperinsulinemia, and high blood pressure can be greatly attenuated by exercise training, an intervention well-known to enhance insulin sensitivity [16]. It has also been shown that infusing somatostatin into fructose-fed rats significantly reduced the increase in plasma insulin concentration and blood pressure associated with this dietary manipulation [17]. Hyperinsulinemia has also been demonstrated in rats with genetic hypertension, including spontaneously hypertensive, Dahl salt-sensitive, and Milano hypertensive rats [18-20]. Furthermore, resistance to insulin-stimulated glucose uptake has been demonstrated in adipocytes isolated from spontaneously hypertensive and Dahl salt-sensitive rats [18-19].

On the other hand, acute hyperinsulinemia in human beings leads to vasodilation, and blood pressure does not increase [21]. In addition, blood pressure does not change when insulin is infused into dogs for periods of up to two weeks [22]. In contrast, blood pressure does increase when rats are infused with insulin [23]. Furthermore, blood pressure has been shown to fall when insulin dose is decreased in obese, hypertensive patients with NIDDM [24], and to increase when insulin treatment is initiated in patients with NIDDM poorly controlled on oral agents [25]. It has also been argued that population studies do not always show a relationship between insulin level and blood pressure. For example, a recent report has shown that blood pressure and insulin concentration were significantly correlated in Caucasians, but in neither African-Americans nor Pima Indians [26]. On the other hand, hypertensive African-Americans are insulin resistant and hyperinsulinemic when compared to African-Americans with normal blood pressure [27,28]. This raises questions about the significance of the lack of a relationship between blood pressure and insulin levels found in African-Americans in epidemiological studies.

POSSIBLE ADDITIONS TO SYNDROME X

During the past few years evidence has appeared suggesting that other abnormalities, secondary to insulin resistance and/or compensatory hyperinsulinemia and associated with CHD, should be added to the cluster of changes initially described as comprising Syndrome X.

Hyperuricemia. Increases in serum uric acid concentration are commonly seen in patients with CHD, often present in association with glucose intolerance, dyslipidemia, and hypertension. Given the relationships described between resistance to insulin-mediated glucose uptake and the abnormalities noted to occur in association with hyperuricemia, it seemed possible that uric acid concentration might vary as a function of insulin resistance and/or hyperinsulinemia. Such a study was performed in normal volunteers [29], and demonstrated that significant correlations existed between serum uric acid concentration and both insulin resistance and the plasma insulin response to an oral glucose challenge. More recently, evidence has been published showing that healthy volunteers with asymptomatic hyperuricemia had higher plasma insulin responses to oral glucose, higher plasma TG and lower HDL-cholesterol concentrations, and higher blood pressure when compared to a well-matched group with normal serum uric acid concentrations [30].

Plasminogen Activator Inhibitor 1 (PAI-1). PAI-1 concentrations are higher in patients with CHD, and it has been suggested that this change may be a primary risk factor for myocardial reinfarction in younger males [31]. PAI-1 levels also appear to be higher in patients with NIDDM, hypertriglyceridemia, or hypertension [32]. Given the association between PAI-1 and the other features of Syndrome X, it seemed possible that PAI-I concentrations were related to insulin resistance and compensatory hyperinsulinemia. The relationship between PAI-1 and insulin resistance and hyperinsulinemia has recently been reviewed in detail. It appears that PAI-1 and plasma insulin concentration are correlated in normal subjects over a wide range of body weight, obese females, and patients with NIDDM, angina, or hypertension. Consequently, this change also seems to be highly associated with insulin resistance and/or compensatory hyperinsulinemia.

SYNDROME X: RELATIONSHIP TO OBESITY

Obesity, *per se*, can lead to a decrease in insulin-mediated glucose uptake, whereas weight loss in obese individuals is associated with enhanced *in vivo* insulin action [6]. However, level of habitual physical activity seems to be as potent as obesity in regulation of *in vivo* insulin action [33, 34]. The fact that obesity and habitual activity can modify the presentation of Syndrome X does not mean that Syndrome X is determined solely by these environmental variables. For example, in nondiabetic volunteers of European and Native American backgrounds, 50% of the total variance in insulin-stimulated glucose uptake could be attributed to the combined effects of differences in age, maximal oxygen consumption, and obesity [31]. Since all of the features of Syndrome X can develop independently of obesity, sedentary activity, etc., some descriptions of Syndrome X are misleading in that they imply that obesity is an essential attribute of the system complex being described; it simply isn't and should not be so designated.

RELATIONSHIP BETWEEN SYNDROME X AND CHD

An increase in PAI-1 also appears to be a risk factor for CHD [31, 35], presumably due to a defect in the fibrinolytic system. On the other hand, metabolic risk factors for CHD known to be associated with a increase in PAI-1, e.g., hyperinsulinemia, hypertriglyceridemia, and a low HDL-cholesterol, were not routinely measured in studies linking the fibrinolytic system to CHD, and it is possible that they also contributed to the development of ischemic heart disease.

Although emphasis is usually placed on the role played by an increase in LDL-cholesterol concentration, CHD can occur in the absence of hypercholesterolemia, and the abnormalities subsumed under the general heading of Syndrome X appear to play a major role in the etiology of CHD [35]. The importance of hypertension as a CHD risk factor is well-recognized, making somewhat confusing the evidence that little or no reduction in CHD was demonstrated when blood pressure was lowered in clinical trials [36]; possibly because no attention was directed in these trials to the abnormalities in carbohydrate and lipoprotein metabolism now known to be associated with high blood pressure and discussed earlier.

CHD is recognized as a major cause of morbidity and mortality in patients with NIDDM. However, CHD is not confined to patients with frank diabetes, and there is evidence that risk of CHD is increased among individuals with normal glucose tolerance who have the highest plasma glucose concentration post-glucose load [37,38]. Although hyperinsulinemia may maintain glucose tolerance in individuals who have a defect in insulin-stimulated glucose uptake, endogenous hyperinsulinemia has been shown to be associated with the increased risk for CHD [37].

The importance of hypertriglyceridemia as a risk factor for CHD has recently been subject to an excellent review [39], and it seems apparent that an important role for hypertriglyceridemia in the genesis of CHD cannot be easily dismissed. The combination of a high plasma TG and low HDL-cholesterol as an important risk factor for CHD has been emphasized by results from several epidemiologic studies, and there is abundant evidence implicating a low plasma HDL-cholesterol concentration as increasing risk of CHD in both nondiabetics and patients with NIDDM [40,41]. Indeed, the two lipid abnormalities most consistently associated with CHD in patients with NIDDM are a high plasma TG and a low HDL-cholesterol concentration. Finally, hypertriglyceridemic subjects tend to have smaller, denser LDL particles and an accentuation of their degree of postprandial lipemia, changes which would also increase risk of CHD.

Conclusion

Resistance to insulin-stimulated glucose uptake, and the degree to which the endocrine pancreas responds to this defect, play important roles in the development of a variety of clinical syndromes which have in common an increase in CHD. The defect in insulin action seems to be the basic abnormality in predisposing patients to develop NIDDM. Although frank diabetes can be prevented if insulin resistant individuals are able to maintain a state of chronic hyperinsulinemia, the consequences of this state of compensatory hyperinsulinemia are likely to include glucose intolerance, dyslipidemia, high blood pressure, hyperuricemia, an increase in PAI-1 activity, and CHD. Given these considerations, it seems reasonable to suggest that the various facets of Syndrome X are involved to a substantial degree in the cause and clinical course of the major diseases of civilization.

References

1.   Hollenbeck CB, Reaven GM. Variations in insulin-stimulated glucose uptake in healthy individuals with normal glucose tolerance. J Clin Endocrinol Metab 1987;64: 1169-1173.
2.   Reaven GM. Role of insulin resistance in human disease. Diabetes 1988;37:1495-1607.
3.   Reaven GM, Chen Y-DI. Role of insulin in regulation of lipoprotein metabolism in diabetes. Diabetes/Metab Rev 1988;4:639-652.
4.   Olefsky JM, Farquhar JW, Reaven GM. Reappraisal of the role of insulin in hypertriglyceridemia. Am J Med 1974;57:551-560.
5.   Tobey TA, Greenfield M, Kraemer F, Reaven GM. Relationship between insulin resistance, insulin secretion, very low density lipoprotein kinetics and plasma triglyceride levels in normotriglyceridemic man. Metabolism 1981;30:165-171.
6.   Olefsky JM, Reaven GM, Farquhar JW. Effects of weight reduction on obesity: studies of carbohydrate and lipid metabolism. J Clin Invest 1974;53:64-76.
7.   Reaven GM, Lerner RL, Stern MP, Farquhar JW. Role of insulin in endogenous hypertriglyceridemia. J Clin Invest 1967;46:1756-1767.
8.   Laws A, King AC, Haskell WL, Reaven GM. Relation of fasting plasma insulin concentration to high density lipoprotein cholesterol and triglyceride concentrations in men. Arterio Thromb 1991;11:1636-1642.
9.   Chen Y-DI, Reaven GM. Intestinally-derived lipoproteins: Metabolism and clinical significance. Diab/Metab Rev 1991;7:191-208.
10.   Krauss RM. The tangled web of coronary risk factors. Am J Med 1991;90:365-415.
11.   Reaven GM. Insulin resistance, hyperinsulinemia, hypertriglyceridemia, and hypertension: Parallels between human disease and rodent models. Diabetes Care 1991;14:195-202.
12.   Zavaroni I, Mazza S, Dall'Aglio E, Gasparini P, Passeri M, Reaven GM. Prevalence of hyperinsulinaemia in patients with high blood pressure. J Int Med 1992;231:235-240.

13. Facchini F, Chen Y-DI, Clinkingbeard C, Jeppesen J, Reaven GM. Insulin resistance, hyperinsulinemia, and dyslipidemia in nonobese individuals with a family history of hypertension. Am J Hypertens 1992;5:694-699.
14. Shamis A, Carroll J, Rosenthal T. Insulin resistance in secondary hypertension. Am J Hypertens 1992;5:26-28.
15. Hwang I-S, Ho H, Hoffman BB, Reaven GM. Fructose-induced insulin resistance and hypertension in rats. Hypertension 1987;10:512-516.
16. Reaven GM, Ho H, Hoffman BB. Attenuation of fructose-induced hypertension in rats by exercise training. Hypertension 1988;12:129-132.
17. Reaven GM, Ho H, Hoffman BB. Somatostatin inhibition of fructose-induced hypertension. Hypertension 1989;14:117-120.
18. Reaven GM, Chang H. Relationship between blood pressure, plasma insulin and triglyceride concentration, and insulin action in spontaneous hypertensive and Wistar-Kyoto rats. Am J Hypertens 1991;4:34-38.
19. Reaven GM, Twersky J, Chang H. Abnormalities of carbohydrate and lipid metabolism in Dahl rats. Hypertension 1991;18:630-635.
20. Dall'Aglio E, Tosini P, Ferrari P, Zavaroni I, Passeri M, Reaven GM. Abnormalities of insulin and lipid metabolism in Milan hypertensive rats. Am J Hypertens 1991;4: 773-775.
21. Anderson EA, Mark AL. The vasodilator action of insulin: Implications for the insulin hypothesis of hypertension. Hypertension 1993;21:136-141.
22. Hall JE, Brands MW, Kivlighn SD, Mizelle HL, Hildebrandt A, Gaillard CA. Chronic hyperinsulinemia and blood pressure. Hypertension 1990;15:519-527.
23. Brands MW, Hildebrandt DA, Mizelle HL, Hall JE. Sustained hyperinsulinemia increases arterial pressure in conscious rats. Am J Physiol 1991;260:R764-R768.
24. Tedde R, Sechi LA, Marigliano A, Palo A, Scano L. Antihypertensive effect of insulin reduction in diabetic-hypertensive patients. Am J Hypertens 1989;2:163-170.
25. Randeree HA, Omar MAK, Motala AA, Seedat MA. Effect of insulin therapy on blood pressure in NIDDM patients with secondary failure. Diabetes Care 1992;15: 1258-1263.
26. Saad M, Lillioja S, Myomba BL, et al. Racial differences in the relation between blood pressure and insulin resistance. N Engl J Med 1991;324:733-739.
27. Falkner B, Hulman S, Tennenbaum J, Kushner H. Insulin resistance and blood pressure in young black men. Hypertension 1990;16:706-711.
28. Falkner B, Hulman S, Kushner H. Insulin-stimulated glucose utilization and borderline hypertension in young adult blacks. Hypertension 1993;22:18-25.
29. Facchini F, Chen Y-DI, Hollenbeck CB, Reaven GM. Relationship between resistance to insulin-mediated glucose uptake, urinary uric acid clearance, and plasma uric acid concentration. JAMA 1991;266:3008-3011.
30. Zavaroni I, Mazza S, Fantuzzi M, et al. Changes in insulin and lipid metabolism in males with asymptomatic hyperuricaemia. J Int Med 1993;234:25-30.

31.   Hamsten A, Wiman B, Defaire U, Blomback M. Increased plasma level of a rapid inhibitor of tissue plasminogen activator in young survivors of myocardial infarction. N Engl J Med 1985;313:1557-1563.

32.   Juhan-Vague I, Alessi MC, Vague P. Increased plasma plasminogen activator inhibitor 1 levels. A possible link between insulin resistance and atherothrombosis. Diabetologia 1991;34:457-462.

33.   Rosenthal M, Haskell WL, Solomon R, Widstrom A, Reaven GM. Demonstration of a relationship between level of physical training and insulin-stimulated glucose utilization in normal humans. Diabetes 1983;32:408-411.

34.   Bogardus C, Lillioja S, Mott DM, Hollenbeck C, Reaven GM. Relationship between degree of obesity and in vivo insulin action in man. Am J Physiol 1985;248 (Endocrinol Metab 11):E286-291.

35.   Reaven GM, Laws A. Coronary heart disease in the absence of hyper-cholesterolaemia. J Int Med 1990;228:415-417.

36.   Collins R, Peto R, MacMahon S, et al. Blood pressure, stroke, and coronary heart disease. Part 2, Short-term reductions in blood pressure: Overview of randomised drug trials in their epidemiological context. Lancet 1990;335:827-838.

37.   Vaccaro O, Rivellese A, Riccardi G, et al. Impaired glucose tolerance and risk factors for atherosclerosis. Arteriosclerosis 1984;4:592-596.

38.   Pyörälä K. Relationship of glucose tolerance and plasma insulin to the incidence of coronary heart disease: Results from two populations studies in Finland. Diabetes Care 1979;2:131-141.

39.   Austin MA. Plasma triglyceride and coronary heart disease. Arterio Throm 1991;11: 2-14.

40.   Castelli WP, Doyle JT, Gordon T, et al. HDL cholesterol and other lipids in coronary heart disease. Circulation 1977;55:767-772.

41.   Laakso M, Lehto S, Penttilä I, Pyörälä K. Lipids and lipoproteins predicting coronary heart disease mortality and morbidity in patients with non-insulin-dependent diabetes. Circulation 1993;88:1421-1430, 1993.

DIABETIC DYSLIPIDEMIA: THE ASIAN PERSPECTIVE

Tong-Yuan Tai, Chih-Jen Chang, Yuan-Teh Lee
National Taiwan University Hospital
7, Chung-Shan South Road
Taipei, Taiwan 100
REPUBLIC OF CHINA

Introduction

This presentation intends to review the pattern of diabetic dyslipidemia in Taiwan as well as in other Asian countries, the differences in diabetic dyslipidemia in Caucasian and in Oriental people, and the implication of dyslipidemia to atherosclerotic diseases. The results revealed that the basic pattern of dyslipidemia was similar among various ethnic groups. The diabetic subjects showed a higher prevalence of dyslipidemia and large vessel diseases (LVD) than the nondiabetic peers.

Methods

THE CROSS-SECTIONAL STUDIES

During the epidemiological study of diabetes mellitus for those aged 40 or over conducted in 1985-6, 542 subjects with noninsulin-dependent diabetes (NIDDM) and 478 sex-matched normal subjects underwent the investigation of serum cholesterol, HDL-cholesterol (HDL-C), and the prevalence of LVD[1-6]. The ages of the two groups were 61.4 ± 9.2 and 57.4 ± 8.7, respectively ($P < 0.001$, 2-tail t-test). Among the 542 diabetics, 469 subjects took no hypolipidemic drugs, diuretics, or ß-adrenergic blocking agents. All of the 478 normal subjects did not take any of the aforementioned drugs. Another study was conducted in Chin-Shan village of Taipei prefecture in 1993. The mean values of serum lipids and the prevalence of hyperlipidemia were also present. Cholesterol, HDL-C, and triglyceride were determined with automated enzymatic methods. LDL-cholesterol was calculated by the following formula: (total cholesterol) - (HDL-C) - (VLDL-cholesterol).

THE LONGITUDINAL STUDY

A total of 479 NIDDM patients ≥ 40 years of age were recruited in July 1986 and followed

A.M. Gotto et al. (eds.), Multiple Risk Factors in Cardiovascular Disease, 227-234.
© *1995 Kluwer Academic Publishers and Fondazione Giovanni Lorenzini.*

for 4 years [6]. Blood pressure and ECG were measured, and a structured questionnaire was asked of each patient. Overnight fasting venous blood was determined for cholesterol, HDL-C, and the ratio between cholesterol and HDL-C(Chl/HDL-C) was calculated.

Statistics

Unpaired t-test was used for the comparison of lipid levels between NIDDM and normal subjects, chi-square test for the comparison of hyperlipidemic prevalence, multiple regression analysis for the association of lipid parameters to the prevalence of various LVD and Cox's proportional hazard model for the association of lipid parameters to the incidence of various LVD. Unless specified, the data were given as means and their standard deviation.

Results

Tables 1 and 2 show the prevalence of dyslipidemia of the two cross-sectional studies.

Table 1. Prevalence of dyslipidemia.

	NIDDM (N=469)		Controls (N=478)		P-value
	No.	(%)	No.	(%)	
Cholesterol ≥ 240 mg/dl	71	(15.1)	31	(6.5)	< 0.0001
HDL-Cholesterol < 35 mg/dl	120	(25.6)	76	(15.9)	< 0.0025
Chl/HDL-C ≥ 5	184	(39.2)	86	(18.0)	< 0.0001

Table 2. Prevalence of dyslipidemia*.

	Diabetic (N=308)		Nondiabetic (N=3,302)		P-value
	No.	(%)	No.	(%)	
Coronary Heart Disease	15	(4.9)	132	(4.0)	NS**
Triglyceride ≥ 250 mg/dl	79	(25.7)	215	(6.5)	< 0.0001
Cholesterol ≥ 240 mg/dl	81	(26.3)	529	(16.0)	< 0.0001
HDL-Cholesterol < 35 mg/dl	93	(30.2)	539	(16.3)	< 0.0001
LDL-Cholesterol ≥ 160 mg/dl	127	(41.2)	850	(25.7)	< 0.0001

* The survey done in Chin-Shan village of Taipei prefecture in 1993.
** NS: Not significant.

Although the prevalence of dyslipidemia among diabetics of the two studies showed a difference, diabetic patients definitely displayed higher serum triglyceride, cholesterol, and

LDL-C levels, and a lower HDL-C level (Tables 3,4). As shown in Table 5, that the diabetics had a higher cholesterol level held true for both genders. However, only female diabetics revealed a lower HDL-C level (Table 5).

Table 3. Lipid profiles of diabetic and nondiabetic subjects*.

	No. of cases	Triglyceride (mg/dl)	Cholesterol (mg/dl)	HDL-Cholesterol (mg/dl)	LDL-Cholesterol (mg/dl)
Diabetic	308	212 ± 164	212 ± 48	42 ± 12	157 ± 46
Nondiabetic	3302	118 ± 82	196 ± 45	48 ± 13	136 ± 44
P-value		< 0.0001	< 0.0001	< 0.0001	< 0.0001

* The survey done in Chin-Shan village of Taipei prefecture in 1993.

Table 4. Serum cholesterol, HDL-cholesterol, and Chl/HDL-C of NIDDM and normal subjects.

	No. of cases	Cholesterol (mg/dl)	HDL-Cholesterol (mg/dl)	Chl/HDL-C
NIDDM	469*	196 ± 44	45 ± 15	4.8 ± 1.9
Controls	478	185 ± 36	49 ± 14	4.1 ± 1.5
P-value		< 0.001	< 0.001	< 0.001

*Those who took drugs affecting lipid levels were excluded.

Table 5. Serum cholesterol, HDL-cholesterol, Chl/HDL-C of male and female NIDDM and normal subjects.

	No. of cases	Cholesterol (mg/dl)	HDL-Cholesterol (mg/dl)	Chl/HDL-C
Male				
NIDDM	219	189 ± 42	45 ± 13	4.7 ± 1.9
Controls	226	177 ± 32	46 ± 15	4.1 ± 1.4
P-value		< 0.001	NS	< 0.001
Female				
NIDDM	250	203 ± 45	46 ± 16	4.8 ± 1.8
Controls	252	193 ± 38	52 ± 15	4.0 ± 1.5
P-value		< 0.01	< 0.001	< 0.001

Urban dwellers had a higher HDL-C level than rural counterparts both in normal and diabetic subjects (Table 6).

Table 6. Serum cholesterol, HDL-cholesterol, Chl/HDL-C of normal and NIDDM subjects living in urban and rural areas.

	No. of cases	Cholesterol (mg/dl)	HDL-Cholesterol (mg/dl)	Chl/HDL-C
Normal				
Urban	206	188 ± 39	52 ± 13	3.8 ± 1.3
Rural	272	183 ± 32	47 ± 14	4.2 ± 1.5
P-value		NS	< 0.001	< 0.005
NIDDM				
Urban	260	196 ± 41	47 ± 17	4.6 ± 1.9
Rural	209	196 ± 45	42 ± 13	5.1 ± 1.8
P-value		NS	< 0.001	< 0.025

Table 7 reveals that the diabetics had a significantly higher prevalence of leg vessel disease (Leg VD) and LVD, and a borderline higher prevalence of stroke and heart vessel disease(HVD).

Table 7. Prevalence of large vessel diseases among 1,120 NIDDM and normal subjects.

	No. of cases	Stroke		HVD		Leg VD		LVD	
		No.	(%)	No.	(%)	No.	(%)	No.	(%)
NIDDM	542*	21	(3.9)	87	(16.1)	10	(1.8)	118	(21.8)
Controls	478	8	(1.7)	58	(12.2)	1	(0.2)	67	(14.0)
P-value		0.055		0.076		<0.05		<0.0025	

*Include those taking drugs influencing serum lipid levels.

Using age, gender, body mass index (BMI), mean arterial pressure, physical activity, diabetes mellitus, smoking, and living area as independent variables, multiple regression analysis of 947 diabetic and normal subjects who took no hypolipidemic drugs, diuretics, or ß - adrenergic blockers showed that females with a higher BMI and age, a lower HDL-C, and living in urban area had a higher prevalence of HVD (Table 8).

Table 8. Multiple regression analysis of HVD prevalence among 947 diabetic and normal subjects.

Variable	Comparison	ß	SE
Sex	Male vs female	0.0739	0.0235**
BMI	Every 1 kg/m^2	0.0072	0.0035*
Age	Every 1-yr increase	0.0026	0.0012*
Area	Urban vs rural	-0.0586	0.0233*
HDL-Cholesterol	1 mg/dl increase	-0.0018	0.0008*

*P < 0.05; ** P < 0.0025, based on Z test of regression coefficients.

If those who took aforementioned drugs were included for multiple regression analysis, a higher HDL-C level led to a lower prevalence of HVD and LVD(Table 9). Those with a higher cholesterol level had a lower prevalence of stroke. The victims of stroke were composed of 21 diabetics and 8 controls. In the order of serum cholesterol, HDL-C and Chl/HDL-C, the data were 192 ± 40 and 178 ± 31mg/dl (P = 0.06), 47 ± 15 and 49 ± 17 mg/dl (P = 0.521) and 4.5 ± 1.7 and 4.1 ± 1.9 (P = 0.278), respectively for stroke-free and stroke patients.

Table 9. Multiple regression analysis of vessel diseases prevalence among 1,020 diabetic and normal subjects.

Variables	Comparison	Vessel disease	ß	SE
HDL-Cholesterol	Every 1 mg/dl increase	LVD	-0.0002	0.0001*
HDL-Cholesterol	Every 1 mg/dl increase	HVD	-0.0002	0.0001*
Cholesterol	Every 1 mg/dl increase	Stroke	-0.0003	0.0001*

*P < 0.05

Univariate analysis by quartiles of lipid parameters demonstrated that only a higher mean cholesterol level was associated with a higher incidence of HVD and LVD (Table 10) [6].

Using age, sex, duration of diabetes, smoking, treatment of diabetes, hypertension, HDL-C, HbA1c, and cholesterol as independent variables, the higher mean serum cholesterol was significantly associated with a higher incidence of HVD (Table 11) and LVD(Table 12). If mean Chl/HDL-C replaced mean cholesterol and HDL-C levels, the significant association to HVD and LVD (Tables 11,12) persisted.

Table 10. Cumulative 4-year incidence rate of stroke, HVD, Leg VD, and LVD among quartiles of various lipid parameters based on Breslow's test.

Variables	Stroke	HVD	Leg VD	LVD
Mean HDL-Cholesterol (mg/dl)				
< 35	6.5 ± 2.6	25.4 ± 4.6	1.0 ± 1.0	34.7 ± 5.2
35-41	4.1 ± 1.8	24.7 ± 4.1	3.2 ± 1.6	30.4 ± 4.4
42-47	3.9 ± 1.9	18.6 ± 4.1	0.9 ± 0.9	23.8 ± 4.5
> 47	2.0 ± 1.4	25.5 ± 4.5	1.0 ± 1.0	28.4 ± 4.7
Mean Cholesterol (mg/dl)				
< 125	3.1 ± 1.8	17.0 ± 3.9*	1.0 ± 1.0	22.1 ± 4.4*
125-135	3.5 ± 1.7	19.0 ± 3.8	0.9 ± 1.0	24.3 ± 4.3
136-145	6.4 ± 2.5	24.7 ± 4.5	1.0 ± 1.0	30.4 ± 4.9
> 145	3.5 ± 1.7	33.8 ± 4.8	3.4 ± 1.7	39.8 ± 5.0
Mean Chl/HDL				
< 2.837	1.8 ± 1.3	16.5 ± 3.6	1.9 ± 0.9	18.4 ± 3.7
2.837-3.308	1.8 ± 1.3	14.6 ± 3.4	0	16.4 ± 3.5
3.309-3.873	5.5 ± 2.0	18.4 ± 3.3	2.8 ± 1.3	22.9 ± 4.0
> 3.873	6.4 ± 2.0	20.9 ± 3.9	2.7 ± 1.6	25.4 ± 4.2

Table 11. Lipid parameters associated with HVD based on Cox's proportional hazard model.

Variables	Comparison	Regression Coefficient	SE	Relative Risk	P-value
HDL-Cholesterol	Every 1-mg/dl increment	-0.01	0.01	0.996	0.53
Cholesterol	Every 1-mg/dl increment	0.01	0.01	1.016	0.04*
Chl/HDL-C*	Every 1 increment in ratio	0.25	0.12	1.279	0.04*

*P < 0.05; ** If Chl/HDL-C replaced cholesterol and HDL-cholesterol.

Discussion

Basically, the pattern of diabetic dyslipidemia is similar between Caucasians and oriental people, and is characterized by higher serum triglyceride, cholesterol, and LDL-C levels, and a lower HDL-C level [7]. Among Asian countries, there is much diversity in the levels of economic development as well as nutritional status, thus leading to differences in the

Table 12. Lipid parameters associated with LVD based on Cox's proportional hazard model.

Variables	Comparison	Regression Coefficient	SE	Relative Risk	P-value
HDL-Cholesterol	Every 1-mg/dl increment	-0.02	0.01	0.958	0.13
Cholesterol	Every 1-mg/dl increment	0.01	0.01	0.013	0.01*
Chl/HDL-C**	Every 1 increment in ratio	0.27	0.11	1.306	0.02*

* P <0.05; ** If Chl/HDL-C replaced cholesterol and HDL-cholesterol.

absolute value and prevalence of dyslipidemia. Nevertheless, the prevalence and extent of dyslipidemia both in normal and NIDDM subjects in Taiwan were similar to those reported from Thailand, Korea, and Japan [8-11]. The values of cholesterol [11] and the prevalence of hypercholesterolemia seemed lower among Asians as compared with Caucasians [12]. However, the prevalence of high LDL cholesterol levels ($\geq$ 160mg/dl) among NIDDM patients was very similar between Taiwanese and American inhabitants [13]. The prevalence of high cholesterol and LDL-C levels among NIDDM individuals greatly outnumbered those of the normal subjects [13].

The phenomenon of higher HDL-C levels among normal females disappeared in female NIDDM patients; however, in the latter the high cholesterol characteristic of the female gender persisted (Table 5). This might account for the fact that female patients with NIDDM are at the same risk as their male counterparts to atherosclerotic diseases [14-16].

Despite heavier body build and less daily exercise of urban dwellers [2], they had higher HDL-C levels than rural controls both for normal and NIDDM subjects. Other factors such as diet, smoking, drugs etc. will be explored.

Although the results of the cross-sectional study do not identify the causal relationship, the fact that those with higher HDL-C levels had fewer cases with HVD or LVD was worth noting (Tables 8,9). However, in the longitudinal study, cholesterol levels and Chl/HDL-C played a more important role than HDL-C in the development of LVD. (Tables 11,12)

The fact that those with high cholesterol levels had a lower prevalence of stroke was hard to explain. An effort to define the nature of stroke and the follow up study with more patients might clarify this issue.

Acknowledgements

This study was supported by grants DOH75-0299-25, DOH 76-22, DOH 77-25, DOH 78-11 and DOH 79-19 from the Department of Health, Executive Yuan, Taiwan, Republic of China.

Reference

1.   Tai TY, Yang CL, Chang CJ, et al. Epidemiology of diabetes mellitus among adults in Taiwan, R.O.C. J Med Assoc Thai, 1987;70 (Suppl.2):42-8.

2.   Tai TY, Yang CL, Chang CJ, et al. Epidemiology of diabetes mellitus in Taiwan, R.O.C. - Comparison between urban and rural areas. J Med Assoc Thai 1987;70 (Suppl.2):49-53.

3.   Jarrett RJ, Keen H, Grabauskas V. The WHO multinational study of vascular disease in diabetes 1. General description. Diabetes Care 1979;2:175-186.

4.   Diabetes Drafting Group. Prevalence of small vessel and large vessel disease in diabetic patients from 14 centers: the World Health Organization Multinational Study of Vascular Disease in Diabetics. Diabetologia 1985;28(Suppl.):615-640.

5.   Tai TY, Chuang LM, Chen CJ, Lin BJ. Link between hypertension and diabetes mellitus - Epidemiological study of Chinese adults in Taiwan. Diabetes Care 1991;14:1013-1020.

6.   Fu CC, Chang CJ, Tseng CH, et al. Development of macrovascular diseases in NIDDM patients in northern Taiwan. Diabetes Care 1993;16:137-143.

7.   Stern MP, Mitchell BD, Haffner SM, Hazada HP. Does glycemic control of Type 2 diabetes suffice to control diabetic dyslipidemia. Diabetes Care 1992;15:638-644.

8.   Serirat S, Santhornthepvarakuel T, Makaxasara C, Deerochanawong C, Phongviratchai S. Lipid disorder in Thai diabetic patients at Rajavithi Hospital. J Med Assoc Thai 1992;75:215-216.

9.   Chang MY. Cardiovascular diseases in diabetes mellitus. In: Goto Y, Lee TH, Kaneko T, Shigeta Y, editors. Prevention and treatment of NIDDM. Sendai, Japan: Smith-Gordon and Nishimura 1992:231-238.

10. Kim BI, Lee HY, Jeon WK, Lee MH, Lee SJ. In Goto Y, Lee TH, Kaneko T, Shigeta Y, editors. Prevention and treatment of NIDDM. Sendai, Japan: Smith-Gordon and Nishimura 1992:239-244.

11. Mimura G, Nakamasu J, Irie M. Incidence of hyperlipidemia in diabetics in Okinawa and its relation to ischemic heart disease. Tohoku J Exp Med 1983;141(Suppl.):611-617.

12. Pacy PJ, Dodson PM, Kubicki DA, Fletcher RF. Differences in lipid and lipoprotein levels in white, black and Asian non-insulin dependent (Type 2) diabetics with hypertension. Diabetes Research 1987;4:187-193.

13. Harris MI. Hypercholesterolemia in individuals with diabetes and glucose intolerance in the U.S. population. Diabetes Care 1991;14:366-374.

14. Janka HU. Five year incidece of major macrovascular complications in diabetes mellitus. Horm Metab Res 1985;15(Suppl.):15-19.

15. Kannel EB, McGee DL. Diabetes and glucose tolerance as risk factors for cardiovascular disease: The Framingham study. Diabetes Care 1979;2:120-126.

16. Standl E. Die Angiopathien des Typ II-Diabetes. Verh Dtsch Ges Inn Med 1986;92:579-586.

THERAPEUTIC INTERVENTION IN DIABETIC DYSLIPIDEMIA

Antonio M. Gotto, Jr.
Department of Medicine
Baylor College of Medicine
The Methodist Hospital
6550 Fannin, M.S. SM-1423
Houston, Texas 77030
USA

Introduction

Both insulin-dependent diabetes mellitus (IDDM) and noninsulin dependent diabetes mellitus (NIDDM) are associated with a several-fold increase in risk for coronary heart disease (CHD). This increased risk is somewhat greater in women than in men, effectively negating the 6–10 year delay in CHD onset in women compared with men. Furthermore, NIDDM and poorly controlled IDDM are frequently associated with the presence of other CHD risk factors, such as elevated triglyceride, low high-density lipoprotein (HDL) cholesterol, hypertension, and obesity. Because of this frequent clustering of CHD risk factors in diabetes, and because 75–80% of all deaths in diabetics are due to CHD, cerebrovascular disease, or peripheral vascular disease, it is essential that diabetic dyslipidemia be identified and managed aggressively.

Management

The epidemiology and metabolic basis of insulin resistance and diabetic dyslipidemia have already been discussed in detail. Diabetic dyslipidemia may reflect a number of abnormalities of lipoprotein metabolism: overproduction or decreased clearance of very-low-density lipoprotein (VLDL), overproduction or decreased clearance of low-density lipoprotein (LDL), or decreased clearance of chylomicrons. Low HDL is usually associated with increased clearance of this lipoprotein. Other lipid abnormalities reported in diabetes include elevated apolipoprotein B levels, a predominance of small, dense LDL believed more atherogenic than normal LDL, and an increased susceptibility of LDL to oxidation.

Although treatment guidelines for dyslipidemia emphasize the significance of diabetes as a risk factor, there is no clear consensus regarding cutpoints for initiating therapy. This is in part due to the paucity of clinical trail data in diabetics. Because

A.M. Gotto et al. (eds.), Multiple Risk Factors in Cardiovascular Disease, 235-238.

dyslipidemia may greatly improve with aggressive treatment of hyperglycemia, particularly in IDDM, the first approach of therapy should be optimization of diabetes control with diet, exercise, and where indicated, antihyperglycemic agents or insulin therapy. Antilipidemic drug therapy should be reserved for those who remain at high total risk.

The Adult Treatment Panel II [1] (ATP II) of the U.S. National Cholesterol Education Program (NCEP) does not give separate serum lipid cutpoints for patients with diabetes, although the panel acknowledges that more aggressive therapy may be justified in diabetics and that clinical judgment should be used. The ATP emphasizes LDL cholesterol as the primary target of therapy, although triglyceride and HDL cholesterol influence the choice of therapy. Diabetes is counted as a risk factor when determining follow-up according to the ATP II algorithm.

In primary prevention, the ATP II recommends that dietary therapy be initiated if LDL cholesterol is ≥ 160 mg/dL (4.1 mmol/L), or ≥ 130 mg/dL (3.4 mmol/L) if two or more other risk factors are present. Drug therapy should be considered if LDL cholesterol remains ≥ 190 mg/dL (4.9 mmol/L), or ≥ 160 mg/dL (4.1 mmol/L) if two or more other risk factors are present, after an adequate trial of intensive dietary therapy. Clinical judgment must be used to determine whether drug therapy would be sufficiently beneficial if LDL cholesterol remains between the initiation levels for dietary and drug therapy.

In secondary prevention, LDL cholesterol ≤ 100 mg/dL (2.6 mmol/L) is considered optimal, although individualized hygienic measures should be instituted in all patients with CHD, regardless of serum lipid levels. Drug therapy should be considered if LDL cholesterol remains ≥ 130 mg/dL, or, if the clinician deems that sufficient benefit would be obtained, if LDL cholesterol remains between 100–130 mg/dL (2.6–3.4 mmol/L).

The European Atherosclerosis Society (EAS) guidelines [2] also state that therapy for dyslipidemia is not in principle different for diabetics, but add that treatment should be vigorous because of the high global risk. Because the EAS places equal emphasis on triglyceride and LDL cholesterol, its recommendations are somewhat different from the ATP II. The EAS considers triglyceride > 2.3 mmol/L (200 mg/dL), LDL cholesterol > 3.5 mmol/L (135 mg/dL), and HDL cholesterol < 0.9 mmol/L (35 mg/dL) matters of concern in diabetes.

In 1993, the American Diabetes Association (ADA) convened a consensus development conference to review the management of dyslipidemia in individuals with diabetes mellitus [3]. The panel concluded that the low HDL cholesterol and elevated serum triglyceride common in diabetics are intrinsically related to the abnormal physiology of the disease. Consequently, the panel recommended that a fasting lipoprotein analysis be obtained annually if diabetes is present, and that treatment of diabetic dyslipidemia focus on HDL cholesterol and triglyceride as well as LDL cholesterol. In primary prevention, ADA treatment goals are 130 mg/dl (3.4 mmol/L) for LDL cholesterol and 200 mg/dl (2.3 mmol/L) for triglyceride; corresponding goals in secondary prevention are 100 mg/dl (2.6 mmol/L) and 150 mg/dl (1.7 mmol/L), respectively. In agreement with the ATP II and the EAS guidelines, the ADA defines low HDL cholesterol to be < 35 mg/dL (0.9 mmol/L).

Dietary therapy entails the restriction of total fat, saturated fat, and cholesterol in the diet, as well as increased physical activity and weight reduction if necessary. The initial level of dietary therapy recommended by the NCEP is the STEP I Diet, which limits total fat to ≤ 30% of calories, saturated fat to 8–10% of calories, and cholesterol to < 300 mg/d. Carbohydrate and protein should constitute 55% and 15% of calories, respectively. If response is inadequate, the more intensive Step II Diet should be instituted. The Step II Diet lowers the portion of calories derived from saturated fat to < 7%, and further restricts cholesterol to < 200 mg/d. In general, these goals should be achieved by substituting complex carbohydrate for fat and by avoiding cholesterol-rich foods. The ratio of monounsaturated fat to saturated fat in the diet should also be increased.

The assistance of a registered dietician is often of great value in tailoring a dietary regimen that maximizes adherence and ensures proper nutrition. The latter is of particular concern if the patient is elderly or if the Step II Diet is prescribed. A dietician can help individualize food choices according to patient preference and identify less obvious sources of fat and cholesterol in the diet.

Weight reduction is an important goal in all obese diabetics, and the physician should emphasize the importance of increased exercise and an appropriate caloric intake in maintaining a height-proportionate body weight. Additionally, these measures often effectively lower serum triglyceride and raise HDL cholesterol, and have other cardioprotective benefits such as lowered blood pressure. There is evidence that abdominal obesity is more closely associated with increased CHD risk than gluteofemoral obesity [4]; distribution of body fat should therefore be considered when defining goals of therapy. If significant weight loss is expected, sufficient time should be allowed for changes in serum lipid levels to become apparent before changes in therapy are made. Rapid weight loss should be discouraged.

Restriction of alcohol intake should be considered if triglyceride is elevated. The physician should also be aware that certain antihypertensive drugs and other medications worsen glucose tolerance or serum lipid levels, which may necessitate changes in dose or selection of alternative agents.

If response to diet, exercise, and glucose control is inadequate after a sufficient trial, pharmacologic therapy may be initiated to supplement, but not replace, dietary therapy. The fibric-acid derivatives (bezafibrate, ciprofibrate, clofibrate, fenofibrate, and gemfibrozil) are first-line pharmacotherapy in diabetes because of their efficacy in lowering triglyceride and raising HDL cholesterol. Triglyceride is lowered 40–60% depending on initial levels, and HDL cholesterol is raised 10–25%. If initially elevated, LDL cholesterol is lowered approximately 10% by the drugs. However, LDL cholesterol may be raised significantly if initially at normal levels. Additionally, bezafibrate [5], ciprofibrate [6], fenofibrate [7], and gemfibrozil [8] have been shown to alter the composition of LDL, producing less dense and presumably less atherogenic particles.

An HMG-CoA reductase inhibitor (fluvastatin, lovastatin, pravastatin, or simvastatin) is preferred if LDL cholesterol is the predominant lipid elevated; in addition to lowering LDL cholesterol 20-40%, this class of drugs lowers triglyceride moderately and mildly increases HDL cholesterol. Although bile-acid resins are also effective in lowering LDL cholesterol, they often raise triglyceride. If both LDL and triglyceride are elevated, the combination of a fibric-acid derivative and a bile-acid resin may be considered. Nicotinic acid is not recommended as first-line drug therapy in diabetes because it frequently worsens glucose intolerance.

The metabolic abnormalities of diabetes are complex and patients receiving pharmacologic therapy should be monitored closely. Adherence to hygienic measures should continue to be assessed and encouraged.

Summary

Although there is consensus that diabetes mellitus increases risk for CHD and that aggressive therapy for diabetic dyslipidemia is justified, guidelines differ somewhat on type and intensity of therapy. Glucose control and hygienic measures remain first-line therapy. Antilipidemic drugs should be considered if the patient remains at high risk; the fibric-acid derivatives or the HMG-CoA reductase inhibitors are preferred, depending on phenotype. More clinical trial data are needed to clarify the benefit of antilipidemic interventions in this population.

References

1.   National Cholesterol Education Program. Second report of the Expert Panel on Detection, Evaluation, and Treatment of High Blood Cholesterol in Adults (Adult Treatment Panel II). Circulation 1994;89:1329–1445.

2.   International Task Force for the Prevention of Coronary Heart Disease. Prevention of coronary heart disease. Scientific background and new clinical guidelines. Nutr Metab Cardiovasc Dis 1992;2:113–156.

3.   Detection and management of lipid disorders in diabetes. Consensus statement. Diabetes Care 1993;16:106–112.

4.   Bjorntorp P. Metabolic implications of body fat distribution. Diabetes Care 1993;14:1132–1143.

5.   Homma Y, Ozawa H, Kobayashi T, et al. Effects of bezafibrate therapy on subfractions of plasma low-density lipoprotein and high-density lipoprotein, and on activities of lecithin:cholesterol acyltransgerase and cholesteryl ester transfer protein in patients with hyperlipoproteinemia. Atherosclerosis 1994;106:191–201.

6.   Bruckert E, Dejager S, Chapman MJ. Ciprofibrate therapy normalises the atherogenic low-density lipoprotein subspecies profile in combined hyperlipidemia. Atherosclerosis 1993;100:91–102.

7.   Caslake MJ, Packard CJ, Gaw A, et al. Fenofibrate and LDL metabolic heterogeneity in hypercholesterolemia. Arterioscler Thromb 1993;13:702–711.

8.   Mantarri M, Koskinen P, Manninen V, Huttunen JK, Frick MH, Nikkila EA. The effect of gemfibrozil on the concentration and composition of serum lipoproteins. A controlled study with special reference to initial triglyceride levels. Atherosclerosis 1990;81:11–17.

RED BLOOD CELL CATION HETEROEXCHANGE AND CARDIO-VASCULAR RISK

Andrea Semplicini, Giulio Ceolotto, Marcella Felice, Annalisa Gebbin,
Alessandra Fontebasso, Roberto Valle, Luca Serena, Cesare Dal Palù
Clinica Medica I
University of Padua
ITALY

Introduction

An abnormal cell cation homeostasis could contribute to the development of hypertension and of its cardiovascular complications. In this field, the cation transporter that has received the greatest attention is the Na^+/H^+ exchanger (NHE), a transmembrane protein which exchanges intracellular H^+ with extracellular Na^+. The aim of the present report is to summarize the kinetic abnormalities of NHE associated with hypertension, to provide possible explanations for them, and to show how they could contribute to the development of hypertension and of its cardiovascular complications. We propose that the activity of NHE can be regarded as an indicator of cardiovascular risk.

Kinetic Properties of Na^+/H^+ Exchange

It has been established that there are different isoforms of NHE [1]. NHE-1 is a housekeeping protein, involved in the control of cell pH and cell volume. Moreover, it has a permissive role in the cell response to hormones, growth factors, and mitogens. It is amiloride sensitive and it is present in all the eukariotic cells. Other isoforms (NHE-2 to NHE-4) are present in polarized epithelia, are involved in Na^+ transport, and are insensitive to or only partially inhibited by amiloride and its derivatives.

NHE-1 is present also in human red cells [2], where it exchanges Na^+ for H^+, Na^+ for Li^+, Li^+ for H^+, and even Na^+ for Na^+ [3]. The transporter has a specific affinity for each cation, which is translocated with a different velocity. Therefore, it is wrong to identify one transport mode with the others.

The most widely investigated transport modes are Na^+/H^+ exchange and Na^+/Li^+ exchange or countertransport. For each transport mode the kinetic properties should be fully characterized to avoid discrepancies in results and thus confusion.

Na^+/H^+ exchange can be measured as the H^+ driven Na^+ influx. Therefore

239

A.M. Gotto et al. (eds.), Multiple Risk Factors in Cardiovascular Disease, 239-244.
© 1995 *Kluwer Academic Publishers and Fondazione Giovanni Lorenzini.*

maximal velocity of translocation, K_m for internal protons, and number of Hill (n_{app}) should be assessed because of the existence of a proton regulatory site and of a positive cooperation between the transport units. Na^+/Li^+ exchange is most commonly assessed as the Na^+ stimulated Li^+ efflux from Li^+ loaded cells: maximal velocity and affinity for external Na^+ should be defined.

In our laboratory we have assessed the kinetic properties of Na^+/H^+ and Na^+/Li^+ exchange in hypertensive subjects. The results, summarized in Table 1, show that both transport modes display abnormal kinetic properties in essential hypertensives in comparison with normotensive controls.

Table 1. Kinetic properties of Na^+/H^+ and Na^+/Li^+ exchange according to blood pressure status.

	Normotensives	Hypertensives	P
Na^+/H^+ exchange			
V_{max}	44 ± 27 (57)	60 ± 34 (86)	0.003
$K_m H_i$	0.38 ± 0.34 (36)	0.46 ± 0.36 (49)	n.s.
n_{aap}	2.2 ± 1.0 (36)	1.7 ± 0.5 (49)	0.005
Na^+/Li^+ exchange			
V_{max}	0.30 ± 0.12 (19)	0.42 ± 0.16 (27)	0.008
$K_m Na_o$	34 ± 23 (19)	53 ± 31 (27)	0.029

Note: mean ± SD (n), V_{max}: maximal transport rate (mMol/L cell x h), K_m: concentration for half-maximal activation (H_i, internal H^+, µMol/L, Na_o, external Na^+, mMol/L), n.s.: not significant.

Na^+/Li^+ exchange is weakly but significantly correlated to Na^+/H^+ exchange (r=0.22, n=143, P=0.005). We did not investigate the K_m for external Na^+ of Na^+/H^+ exchange and the K_m for internal Li^+ of Na^+/Li^+ exchange.

Posttranslational Effects of Protein Kinase C, Insulin, and Lipids on Red Cell Cation Heteroexchange

Mutations of the gene encoding for NHE or expression of different isoforms of NHE could account for kinetic abnormalities of red cell cation heteroexchange in hypertensives. However, Lifton has excluded mutations [4] and isoform heterogeneity has not yet been reported. Other possibilities are: posttranslational effects of intracellular calcium [5]; phosphorylation of the transport protein; insulin; different lipid composition and fluidity of the cell membrane, which can affect cation transport.

According to our recent experiments in red cells, protein kinase C activation with phorbol esters decreases the K_m for protons (from 0.42 ± 0.05 µmol/L to 0.23 ± 0.04, P < 0.02). V_{max} and n_{app} are not affected. However, in immortalized lymphoblasts incubation of the cells with phorbol ester significantly reduces the sigmoidicity of the activation curve of the Na^+/H^+ exchange and n_{app} [6], an abnormality similar to the one that can be observed in hypertensives.

Insulin can account for some kinetic abnormalities of the countertransport, since it has profound effects on cation transport [7] and insulin sensitivity is negatively correlated to countertransport [8]. Chronic insulin administration to insulin-dependent diabetics increases countertransport in comparison with nondiabetic controls and nondiabetic hypertensives [9]. The effect is similar in normotensive and hypertensive diabetics, suggesting that insulin can only amplify the countertransport abnormality associated to hypertension.

Insulin affects also the affinity for external Na. Acute insulin exposure, *in vitro* [10] and *in vivo* after feeding [11], doubles the K_m for external Na^+ of countertransport in comparison with fasting conditions. Similarly, long-term exposure to insulin reduces the affinity for Na^+ of the external site. As already mentioned, K_m for sodium and V_{max} of countertransport are higher in hypertensives than in normotensives. In collaboration with Dr. Canessa in Boston, we have shown that the difference of V_{max} and K_m is greater in hyperinsulinemic hypertensives than in normoinsulinemic ones (Table 2).

Table 2. Kinetic properties of red cell Na^+/Li^+ exchange according to blood pressure and fasting insulin.

	Normotensives		Hypertensives	
	insulin (µU/mL)		insulin (µU/mL)	
	< 10	> 10	< 10	> 10
n	22	6	13	12
V_{max}	0.31 ± 0.07	0.32 ± 0.03	0.41 ± 0.05	$0.57 \pm 0.05^*$
$K_m Na_o$	28 ± 3	36 ± 5	$46 \pm 4^{**}$	$73 \pm 9^{***}$

Note: Abbreviations as in Table 1; *p < 0.05 versus both groups of normotensives; **p < 0.05 versus normoinsulinemic hypertensives; ***p < 0.05 versus both groups of normotensives and normoinsulinenic hypertensives.

Finally, correction of insulin sensitivity in insulin-resistant hypertensives with short-term metformin administration, reduces fasting insulin and increases K_m for H_i of Na^+/H^+ exchange even if it does not reduce blood pressure [12].

The whole of these data underlines the wide range of kinetic effects of insulin on NHE. It reduces the affinity on the sodium site and increases that on the internal proton site, which is necessary for an efficient cation translocation, while increasing the V_{max}.

Plasma lipids are also correlated with countertransport in many studies [9]. Na^+/Li^+ exchange is positively correlated to triglycerides and negatively correlated to HDL cholesterol. Since blood lipids are in equilibrium with membrane lipids, this correlation could be due either to a direct effect of membrane lipids on cation transport or to increased membrane fluidity. Alternatively, it could be created by the correlation of insulin with blood lipids, on one hand, and with the kinetic properties of the antiporter, on the other. The reverse could also be true. In fact a reduction of polyunsaturated fatty acids in the red cell membrane, if associated to defective delta 5-desaturase, decreases the arachidonic acid content of the cell membrane and this hampers insulin sensitivity [13]. The ensuing hyperinsulinemia and hyperlipidemia may affect the kinetic properties of cell membrane cation heteroexchange.

Red Cell Cation Heteroexchange and Cardiovascular Risk

Whichever their cause, abnormal kinetic properties of NHE may favor the development of hypertension and its cardiovascular complications. They may in fact increase stimulus-response coupling, vascular smooth muscle cell resting tone, and total peripheral resistances. Moreover, they may favor cell proliferation and growth, thereby contributing to the cardiovascular remodelling of the hypertensive patient [14]. Evidence has been gathered that they may also favor reperfusion arrhythmias [15], postischemic contractile dysfuntion [16] and sodium retention [17].

As for the pathogenesis of hypertension, two large genetic studies [18,19] have shown that a biometrically inferred single gene with a large effect on countertransport is able to predict the future development of hypertension. The genotype associated with high countertransport predicts the development of high blood pressure at a young age. On the other hand, the increase in pressure makes a later appearance with alternate genotypes and phenotypes. However, high countertransport is associated with a greater prevalence of severe hypertension and drug-resistant hypertension.

High countertransport is also associated with cardiac and vascular hypertrophy. In hypertensives with high countertransport, left ventricular mass and relative wall thickness are greater than in normotensive controls and in hypertensives with low countertransport, despite similar demographic characteristics [20]. The same is true also for insulin-dependent diabetics: high countertransport even in normotensive diabetics is associated to an early development of cardiac hypertrophy [21]. This suggests that countertransport can be used to pick up the subjects at risk of developing the cardiac complications of hypertension and diabetes.

In hypertensives with increased countertransport, kidney volume, glomerular filtration, and proximal sodium reabsorption are increased in comparison to normotensive controls and hypertensives with normal countertransport [20]. The increase of kidney volume is favored by the activation of NHE, while glomerular hyperfiltration is probably due to intrarenal activation of the renin - angiotensin system [22].

Activation of NHE may favor cell sodium and calcium accumulation during ischemia and reperfusion and it may delay restoration of cardiac contractility, which can be prevented by pretreatment with amiloride analogs [16].

Finally, among the members of a large family affected by familial hypertrophic cardiomyopathy, abnormal red cell cation heteroexchange was correlated to a more severe septal hypertrophy and to significant left ventricular diastolic dysfunction, as assessed by transmitral flow velocity [23].

In conclusion, experimental evidence from various laboratories suggests that the abnormal kinetic properties of red cell cation heteroexchange may reflect both the phenotypic expression of a major gene encoding for high countertransport, and posttranslational effects of insulin, lipids, and agonists acting through protein kinase C. The abnormal kinetic properties of cell cation heteroexchange may amplify the effects of other cardiovascular risk factors, epistatically. High countertransport should therefore be regarded as a marker of increased cardiovascular risk because it is associated to high blood pressure, reduced insulin sensitivity, glomerular hyperfiltration, remodelling of the cardiovascular system, and increased risk of developing diabetic and hypertensive nephropathy.

References

1. Wakabayashi S, Sardet C, Fafournoux P, et al. Structure function of the growth factor-activatable Na+/H+ exchanger (NHE1). Rev Physiol Biochem Pharmacol 1992;119:157-186.

2. Corry DB, Tuck ML, Nicholas S, Weinman EJ. Increased Na/H antiport activity and abundance in uremic red blood cell. Kidney Int 1993;44:574-578.

3. Canessa M, Morgan K, Semplicini A. Genetic differences in lithium-sodium exchange and regulation of the sodium-hydrogen exchanger in essential hypertension. J Cardiovasc Pharmacol 1988;12(Suppl.3):S92-S98.

4. Lifton RP, Hunt SC, Williams RR, Pouyssegur J, Lalouel JM. Exclusion of the Na-H antiporter as a candidate gene in human essential hypertension. Hypertension 1991;17:8-14.

5. Escobales N, Canessa M. Ca2+-activated Na+ fluxes in human red cells: amiloride sensitivity. J Biol Chem 1985;260:11914-11923.

6. Rosskopf D, Fromter E, Siffert W. Hypertensive sodium-proton exchanger phenotype persists in immortalized lymphoblasts from essential hypertensive patients. A cell culture model for human hypertension. J Clin Invest 1993;92:2553-2559.

7. Moore RD. Stimulation of Na/H exchange by insulin. Biophys J 1981;33:203-210.

8. Doria A, Fioretto P, Avogaro A, et al. Insulin resistance is associated with high sodium-lithium countertransport in essential hypertension. Am J Physiol 1991;261:E684-E691.

9. Semplicini A. The Li+/Na+ countertransport in hypertension. In: Coca A, Garay

RP, editors. Ionic transport in hypertension. Boca Raton: CRC Press, 1994:89-117.

10. Canessa M, Zerbini G. Insulin modulation of Na+/Li+ countertransport: impact on hypertension and diabetes. Acta Diabetol 1992;29:186-190.

11. Pontremoli R, Zerbini G, Rivera A, Canessa M. Insulin activation of red blood cell Na+/H+ exchange decreases the affinity of sodium sites. Kidney Int 1994;46; 365-375.

12. Semplicini A, Del Prato S, Giusto M, et al. Short term effects of metformin on insulin sensitivity and sodium homeostasis in essential hypertensives. J Hypertension 1993;11(Suppl.5):S276-S277.

13. Borkman M, Storlien LH, Pan DA, Jenkins AB, Chisholm DJ, Campbell LV. The relation between insulin sensitivity and the fatty-acid composition of skeletal-muscle phospholipids. N Engl J Med 1993;328:238-244.

14. Rosskopf D, Dusing R, Siffert W. Membrane sodium-proton exchange and primary hypertension. Hypertension 1993;21:607-617.

15. Gambassi G. Stimolazione dei recettori α1-adrenergici durante riperfusione simulata dopo acidosi miocardica. Evidenza di un ruolo dello scambiatore Na/H. Cardiologia 1993;38:25-36.

16. Moffat MP, Karmazyn M. Protective effect of the potent Na/H exchange inhibitor methylisobutyl amiloride against post-ischemic contractile dysfunction in rat and guinea pig hearts. J Mol Cell Cardiol 1993;25:959-971.

17. Semplicini A, Ceolotto G, Massimino M, et al. Interactions between insulin and sodium homeostasis in essential hypertension. Am J Med Sci 1994;307(Suppl. 1):S43-S46.

18. Hunt SC, Stephenson SH, Hopkins PN, Hasstedt SJ, Williams RR. A prospective study of sodium-lithium countertransport and hypertension in Utah. Hypertension 1991;17:1-7.

19. Rebbeck TR, Turner ST, Sing CF. Sodium-lithium countertransport genotype and the probability of hypertension in adults. Hypertension 1993;22:560-568.

20. Nosadini R, Semplicini A, Fioretto P, et al. Sodium-lithium countertransport and cardio-renal abnormalities in essential hypertension. Hypertension 1991;18:191-198.

21. Semplicini A, Lusiani L, Marzola M, et al. Erythrocyte Li+/Na+ and Na+/H+ exchange, cardiac anatomy and function in insulin dependent diabetes. Eur J Clin Invest 1992;22:254-259.

22. Semplicini A, Serena L, Valle R, et al. Red blood cell Li+/Na+ countertransport (CT) and hypotensive and renal response to ACE inhibitors (ACEI) in essential hypertensives (HT). J Hypertension 1994;12(Suppl.3):S47.

23. Semplicini A, Mozzato MG, Bongiovì S, et al. Red blood cell sodium heteroexchange in familial primary hypertrophic cardiomyopathy. Eur. Heart J. 1994;15:328-334.

HYPERTENSION IN THE ELDERLY: WITH SPECIAL FOCUS ON SIDE EFFECTS

L.H. Lindholm
Health Sciences Centre
Lund University
S-240 10 Dalby
SWEDEN

It is generally accepted that high blood pressure is a major risk factor for cardiovascular morbidity and mortality in middle-aged subjects [1]. Does this also hold true for the elderly? In some studies the answer to this question is yes [1-3], but in some other studies there is an inverse relation [4,5], and in others there is no relation between blood pressure and risk [6]. Furthermore, in some studies the systolic blood pressure (SBP) is a better predictor than diastolic blood pressure (DBP) [1,3], while in some others the reverse has been found [7]. To further complicate the situation, several workers have demonstrated U- or J-shaped relations between blood pressure and risk [8,9]. The relation between blood pressure and cardiovascular risk seems to be more complex in the elderly and could at least in part be due to selection mechanisms during earlier years.

In summary, several studies of high quality have demonstrated an increased risk of cardiovascular disease (CVD) in relation to high blood pressure in the younger elderly, whereas the risk seems to decline with age in the older elderly.

Efficacy of Treatment in the Elderly on Mortality and Morbidity

One of the first studies was the Veterans Administrations Cooperative Study Group on Antihypertensive Agents initiated in 1963. In an analysis of subgroups [10] it was shown that the patients aged 60 and above (20%) benefited from treatment in a similar way to the younger ones (approximately 50% reduction of morbid events). Those 20% over 60 accounted for half of the morbid events in the whole group.

In the Hypertension Detection and Follow-up Program (HDFP) 10,940 persons with high blood pressure were either randomized to a special systematic antihypertensive treatment program (Stepped Care; SC) or referred to a usual community medical therapy (Referred Care; RC) [11]. In those aged 60-69 the reduction in mortality was 16% in the SC group. In this age group the reduction in stroke was 45% lower in the SC group.

A.M. Gotto et al. (eds.), Multiple Risk Factors in Cardiovascular Disease, 245-250.
© *1995 Kluwer Academic Publishers and Fondazione Giovanni Lorenzini.*

In the Australian National Blood Pressure Study an on-treatment analysis of those over 60 years at entry showed a reduction of 39% of trial end-points (p<0.025) (27 active versus 42 placebo) [12].

In the European Working Party of Hypertension in the Elderly (EWPHE), 840 patients over the age of 60 (mean age 72) with a DBP of 90-119 mmHg and a SBP of 160-239 mmHg were randomly allocated to active treatment (hydrochlorothiazide [HCTZ] + triamterene and if necessary, methyldopa) [13]. Over the study period more than 15% of the patients were lost to follow-up. The overall analysis, on the intention-to-treat principal, revealed a significant reduction in cardiovascular mortality of 27% (p=0.037), which was mainly due to a reduction in cardiac mortality (38%, p=0.036). There was also a nonsignificant reduction in cerebrovascular mortality (32%, p=0.16). Practically no benefit from treatment could be demonstrated with intention-to-treat analysis in patients over the age of 74 years (n = 294) of whom a great majority were women.

The Randomised Trial of the Treatment of Hypertension in Elderly Patients in Primary Care (HEP study) [14] showed a significant reduction of fatal stroke by 30%, and all stroke by 58% compared to the untreated group. The incidence of myocardial infarction and total mortality was unaffected by treatment. The 884 patients aged 60-79 (mean age 69) were recruited from 13 general practitioners in England and Wales, and randomized to either atenolol or no treatment. An analysis of a subset of patients aged 70-79 years showed a similar reduction in total stroke, but the study was not large enough in this age-group to give a significant result.

The Systolic Hypertension in the Elderly Program (SHEP) was set up to test the efficacy of antihypertensive treatment on patients with isolated systolic hypertension [15]. The main objective of the study was to assess the ability of antihypertensive drug treatment to reduce the risk of nonfatal and fatal stroke in isolated systolic hypertension, defined as SBP 160-219 mmHg and DBP < 90 mmHg. In this multicenter study, almost half a million people aged over 60 were screened and finally 4,736 (1.06%) were randomized to either placebo or active therapy, basically chlortalidone. If the blood pressure goal was not reached, medication was increased in steps from 12.5 mg chlorthalidone o.d. (30%), to 25 mg o.d. (16%), with a further addition of 25 mg o.d. atenolol (11%), to 50 mg atenolol o.d. (12%). Active treatment resulted in significant reductions of 5-year incidence of total stroke by 36% (p=0.0003), nonfatal myocardial infarction plus coronary death by 27%, and major cardiovascular events by 37%. The 5-year cumulative stroke rates in the active group were 5.2 per 100 participants and 8.2 in the placebo group.

In the Swedish Trial in Old Patients with Hypertension (STOP-Hypertension), 1627 patients (mean age 76; mean blood pressure 195/102 mmHg) from 116 Swedish health centers were randomized double-blindly to placebo or active treatment (ß-blockers or diuretic). At the end of the study the average blood pressure reduction was 20/8 mmHg in the actively treated group compared to placebo. The mean follow-up was 2.1 years. No patient was lost to follow-up [10]. Compared with placebo, active treatment significantly reduced the number of primary endpoints (55.5 versus 33.5 per 1000 person-years; p=0.0031), the stroke morbidity and mortality (31.3 versus 16.8; p=0.0081), and the total mortality (35.4 versus 20.2; p=0.0079). There was a clear effect of active treatment on the incidence of stroke in women (31.1 versus 11.7); in men, this effect was less impressive (31.6 versus 25.8). The effect also seemed to diminish with age and was nonexistent after 84.

Thus, both the EWPHE trial [13]and the HEP study [14] in the 1980s provided evidence of benefit in treating high blood pressure in the elderly at least up to the age of 70-74. These results have been confirmed recently [15,16], also including older patients (STOP) [16] and isolated systolic hypertension (SHEP) [15]. Therefore, drug treatment with ß-blockers and diuretics should be considered in hypertensive men and women aged 70 and above. It should also be remembered that elderly hypertensives often have other diseases as well and that the drug treatment should be adjusted accordingly.

Adverse Effects of Blood Pressure Lowering Drugs

The frequency and type of side effects reported in different studies depend greatly on the drugs used, and on the method of collecting this information. The results should be given as net effects with the placebo effects deducted. Adverse effects or side effects could in principle be of two kinds. Firstly, they could be symptoms or signs reported by the patient or discovered by the doctor, or secondly changes in the metabolism revealed as changes in different laboratory variables.

In the EWPHE study [13] a HCTZ plus triamterene combination was the basic drug. One third received additional methyldopa. Symptoms of dry mouth, nasal stuffiness, and diarrhea were reported significantly more often by the actively treated patients. There was also a rise in the serum creatinine level and a decrease in serum potassium, and more reports of gout and diabetes in the actively treated ones [17].

In the HEP study [14] the principal antihypertensive agents were atenolol with supplementation of bendrofluazide in 75% of the actively treated patients. There were no significant difference between the groups in reporting symptoms by self-administered questionnaires. About a quarter of the patients discontinued treatment due to side effects, mainly general fatigue, muscular weakness, and breathlessness when exercising.

The drugs used in SHEP [15] was chlorthalidone, a diuretic without potassium-sparing properties, and if needed additional atenolol was given. In the actively treated group there were more reports of chest pain, cold or numb hands, ankle swelling, trouble with memory/concentration, and change of bowel habits. Serum potassium, uric acid, glucose, and cholesterol levels out of specified ranges were reported more frequently in the actively treated group.

In STOP-Hypertension, no unexpected, serious, or previously unknown side effects were evident during the study. Fifty-eight patients on active treatment and 47 on placebo discontinued randomized treatment because of subjective side effects not classified as any specific clinical event (difference not significant). Congestive heart failure was less common in the actively treated group than in the placebo group, 19 versus 39 cases [16]. The only significant differences found in the prevalence of symptoms at the two-month visit (active treatment compared with placebo in mono-therapy) were more dryness in the mouth (atenolol), less swollen ankles (metoprolol CR, HCTZ + Amiloride), more muscle discomfort/cramp (pindolol), more reduced heart rate (atenolol), and less irregular heart beat (HCTZ + Amiloride). At the twelve-month visit (65% with supplementary treatment), the findings were similar with a few exceptions [18].

Active Antihypertensive Treatment and Laboratory Variables

The changes in laboratory values over time were limited in all studies using a ß-blocker together with a low-dose diuretic with a potassium-sparing component [18]. At the twelve-month visit in STOP, however, both serum creatinine and serum urate were increased, regardless of treatment group.

In conclusion, drug treatment with ß-blockers and diuretics in hypertensive men and women aged 70 and above confers highly significant and clinically relevant reductions in cardiovascular (especially stroke) morbidity and mortality. This satisfactory effect is not impaired by a low tolerability of the drugs used. The clinical implication of this is that blood pressure lowering therapy should be considered in elderly hypertensives, at least up until they are 80 years old.

References

1.   Kannel WB. Prevalence, incidence and hazards of hypertension in the elderly. Ger Cardiovasc Med 1988;1:5-10.
2.   Holme I, Waaler HT. Five-year mortality in the city of Bergen, Norway, according to age, sex and blood pressure. Acta Med Scand 1976;200:229-39.
3.   Agner E. Predictive value of arterial blood pressures in old age. A ten-year prospective study of men and women born in 1897 and examined at the age of 70 and 80 years. Acta Med Scand 1983;214:285-94.
4.   Fry J. Natural history of hypertension. A case for selective non-treatment. Lancet 1974;ii:431-3.
5.   Mattila K, Haavisto M, Rajala S, Heikinheimo R. Blood pressure and five year survival in the very old. Br Med J 1988;296:887-9.
6.   Anderson F, Cowan NR. Survival of healthy older people. Brit J Prev Soc Med 1976;30:231-2.
7.   Landahl S, Lernfelt B, Sundh V. Blood pressure and mortality in old age. Eleven years' follow-up of a 70-year-old population. J Hypertension 1987;5:745-8.
8.   Staessen J, Bulpitt C, Clement D, et al. Relation between mortality and treated blood pressure in elderly patient with hypertension: report of the European Working Party on High Blood Pressure in the Elderly. BMJ 1989;298:1552-6.
9.   Coope J, Warrender TS, McPherson K. The prognostic significance of blood pressure in the elderly. J Human Hypertension 1988;2:79-88.
10.   Veterans Administration Cooperative Study Group on Anti-Hypertensive Agents. Effects of treatment on morbidity in hypertension. III. Influence of age, diastolic blood pressure, and prior cardiovascular disease. Further analysis of side effects. Circulation 1972;45:991-1004.

11. Hypertension and Detection and Follow-up Program Cooperative Group. Five-year findings of the Hypertension Detection and Follow-up Program. I. Reduction in mortality of persons with high blood pressure, including mild hypertension. JAMA 1979;242:2562-71.

12. Management Committee. Treatment of mild hypertension in the elderly. The National Heart Foundation of Australia. Med J Aust 1981;2:398-402.

13. Amery A, Birkenhäger W, Brixko P, et al. Efficacy of antihypertensive drug treatment according to age, sex, blood pressure, and previous cardiovascular disease in patients over the age of 60. Lancet 1986;ii:589-92.

14. Coope J, Warrender TS. Randomised trial of teatment of hypertension in elderly patients in primary care. BMJ 1986;293:1145-51.

15. SHEP Cooperative Research Group. Prevention of stroke by antihypertensive drug treatment in older persons with isolated systolic hypertension. Final results of the Systolic Hypertension in the Elderly Program (SHEP). JAMA 1991;265:3255-64.

16. Dahlöf B, Lindholm LH, Hansson L, Scherstén B, Ekbom T, Wester PO. Morbidity and mortality in the Swedish Trial in Old Patients with Hypertension (STOP-Hypertension). Lancet 1991;338:1281-5.

17. Fletcher AE. Adverse treatment effects in the trial of the European Working Party on High Blood Pressure in the Elderly. Am J Med 1991;90(Suppl. 3A):S42-S44).

18. Ekbom T, Dahlöf B, Hansson L, Lindholm LH, Scherstén B, Wester PO. Antihypertensive efficacy and side effects of three beta-blockers and a diuretic in elderly hypertensives - a report from the STOP-Hypertension Study. J Hypertens 1992;10:1525-30.

DRUGS DIRECTLY AFFECTING THE ARTERIAL WALL

Rodolfo Paoletti and Maurizio R. Soma
Institute of Pharmacological Sciences
University of Milan
Via Balzaretti 9
20133 Milan
ITALY

Great progress has been made over the last 3 decades in identifying the most important risk factors for cardiovascular disease (CVD), and we have learned to apply measures that successfully lower the incidence of this disease. The interest focused on smoking in the late 1960s and on hypertension in the 1970s while the 1980s saw increasing attention paid to the diagnosis and management of hypercholesterolemia. The declining rates of CVD mortality and morbidity throughout the industrialized world during the same period clearly reflect the identification and proper management of these three major risk factors [1]. The recent advances in epidemiological, clinical, and basic research on primary and secondary dyslipidemias have allowed both investigators and physicians to gain new insights into the pathogenesis and clinical management of CVD [2]. Atherosclerosis can be viewed as the result of a multiplicity of complex interactions that involve repeated injury with healing or restorative responses. Atherosclerosis plays a crucial role in many cardiovascular diseases, including myocardial infarction and cerebrovascular insufficiency [3], and has been involved, together with other mechanisms, in restenosis after successful coronary angioplasty [4]. This latter emerges as a critical clinical problem for the future, in view of the explosive growth of coronary angioplasty [5], the continuing high rate of restenosis, and the poor efficacy of current treatments [6].

Therapeutic strategies for the prevention of "spontaneous" or induced atherosclerosis in man are essentially based on the correction of major risk factors, either elevated plasma lipids or arterial blood pressure. Such interventions have been successful in reducing cardiovascular risk following long-term treatment and can induce a regression of existing lesions. However, it appears that the prevention of cardiovascular disease in the future will also involve the direct pharmacological control of the processes occurring in the arterial wall [7]. For these reason, more attention must be paid to the development and clinical use of drugs acting directly on the arterial walls. Calcium antagonists and HMG-CoA reductase inhibitors (statins) will be discussed in this chapter.

A.M. Gotto et al. (eds.), Multiple Risk Factors in Cardiovascular Disease, 251-258.
© *1995 Kluwer Academic Publishers and Fondazione Giovanni Lorenzini.*

Calcium Antagonists

The calcium antagonists show several important antiatherosclerotic activities *in vitro* and *in vivo*. In cultured cells these drugs protect arterial smooth muscle cells (SMC) against cholesterol deposition and control cellular proliferation. In addition the matrix synthesis by SMC is reduced. In *in vivo* models calcium antagonists protect against lesions induced by cholesterol feeding, endothelial injury, and experimental calcinosis [8].

The antiatherosclerotic effect of calcium antagonists does not involve a reduction of plasma cholesterol or blood pressure thus indicating a direct effect on the arterial wall [8]. In a series of animal experiments the influence of calcium antagonists on calcium deposition within the vessel wall and on the development of artificially induced atherosclerosis proved to be favorable [9-11]. Two randomized, placebo-controlled studies [12,13] have reported on the effects of calcium antagonists on atheroma in the coronary arteries. The first study is the International Nifedipine Trial on Antiatherosclerotic Therapy (INTACT). Four hundred twenty-five patients were controlled and randomized to treatment with nifedipine. The study lasted for three years. No regression, or at least lack of progression, was reported, but a 28% reduction in the number of new lesions could be recorded. In the second study, by Waters et al. [13] 383 patients were randomized to treatment with nicardipine. The study lasted for two years and the findings were essentially the same of those reported in the INTACT study: no effect on the regression or progression of established coronary lesions, but a reduction in the progression of small or new lesions. In both studies the inhibitory effect on progression of new lesions was accomplished without a correlated effect on blood lipid levels. The results of these studies indicate that some as yet unidentified biological processes in the early development of atheromatous lesions are sensitive to calcium antagonists. While the efficacy of calcium antagonists as coronary and peripheral vascular dilators can be accounted for in terms of their inhibitory effects on calcium influx throughout the voltage-sensitive calcium channels, their ability to act as antiatherosclerotic agents is less well understood. Several calcium-dependent processes contribute to the atherogenesis, including lipid infiltration and oxidation, endothelial injury, action of chemotactic and growth factors, and smooth muscle cell migration and proliferation.

Proliferation of vascular smooth muscle cells is an early and key event in the formation of an atherosclerotic lesion. Smooth muscle cells accumulate in the intima in atherogenic conditions. In response to experimental arterial injury, SMC migrate from the media into the intima, where they proliferate and secrete large amounts of extracellular matrix. This reaction results in rapid neointimal hyperplasia, a convenient means for studying proliferative atherosclerotic lesions and stenotic processes frequently observed in patients undergoing percutaneous transluminal coronary angioplasty (PTCA) [14].

An *in vivo* model for the study of SMC in the carotid walls of rabbits has been used in our laboratory [4]. To characterize the antiatherogenic activity of the new calcium antagonist lacidipine, we studied the effect of this drug on the atherosclerotic response of the hypercholesterolemic rabbit carotid artery 14 days after perivascular manipulation of the vessel. This model, described by Booth et al. [15], allows the direct following, *in vivo* and independently of other factors, of the effect of a drug on arterial myocyte proliferation in normotensive hypercholesterolemic rabbits.

The use of lacidipine, a lipophylic dihydropyridine, clearly indicates that it and similar calcium antagonists may be used as protective agents against lesions to the arterial walls (Table 1).

Table 1. Effect of lacidipine (3 mg/kg/day) on proliferative lesions induced by perivascular manipulation of hypercholesterolemic normotensive rabbit carotid arteries.

Treatment	I:M	SD	% of control	p value
Control	0.56	0.11	-	-
Sham	0.03	0.02	5	-
Lacidipine	0.32	0.10	57	0.01

Ten rabbits each in the control and lacidipine treatment groups; 20 rabbits in the sham group.
I:M, intimal:medial tissues ratio (mean ± SD); SD, standard deviation; p value, lacidipine versus control treatment.

The availability of quantitative procedures to assess in man the thickening of the carotid arterial walls in pathological condition, also opens the way for clinical studies leading to the protection of the carotid artery in presence of one or more major risk factors and not only in hypertensive patients.

HMG-CoA Reductase Inhibitors (Statins)

In recent years the development of drugs that inhibit cholesterol synthesis, thus lowering plasma cholesterol levels, has to a large degree centered on controlling the HMG-CoA reductase activity. However, since mevalonic acid, the product of the enzyme reaction, is the precursor of numerous metabolites, inhibition of HMG-CoA reductase has the potential of resulting in pleiotropic effects. These possibilities are supported by several *in vivo* and *in vitro* observations which have shown how some HMG-CoA reductase inhibitors can in fact inhibit cellular proliferation and modulate changes in the cell cycle and cell morphology [4,16-18]. Based on these findings this class of drugs has received increasing attention as a pharmacological tool for controlling abnormal pathological cell growth, such as in tumors and in proliferative processes contributing to atherosclerosis.

Pharmacological approaches using vastatins to inhibit smooth muscle cell proliferation, an early event in atherogenesis, have already been tried. Simvastatin inhibits smooth muscle cell growth *in vitro* [19]. Aggressive lipid-lowering treatment with lovastatin prevented restenosis after balloon angioplasty in hypercholesterolemic rabbits [20] and humans [21]. However, no correlation between serum cholesterol and restenosis was found in percutaneous transluminal coronary angioplasty patients.

Several vastatins have been tested in our laboratory in order to establish if they directly affect neointimal formation in the carotid arteries of normocholesterolemic rabbits independent of the lowering of plasma cholesterol concentration. For this purpose, we have used a scheme for the drug-treatment regimen that did not modify the plasma cholesterol level in normolipidemic rabbits. Intimal thickening was induced by inserting a flexible extra-arterial collar around the common carotid artery, as previously described.

The effect of vastatins was evaluated 14 days after collar insertion. The sham-operated contralateral arteries showed no thickening of the intima either in positive control or drug-treated rabbits (Table 2). A marked increase in intimal thickness (mostly cellular) was evident in the carotid arteries with the collar of untreated animals (positive control group). The mean value of intimal carotid thickening in the positive control group, expressed as the I/M ratio, was 12 times greater than that observed in the contralateral sham-operated carotid artery (Table 2).

Table 2. Effect of different vastatins on intimal thickening induced by perivascular manipulation of rabbit carotid arteries after 2 weeks.

Treatment	I/M (mean)	± SD	% of control	p value
Positive control	0.36	0.04	-	-
Sham	0.03	0.02	3	-
Pravastatin	0.32	0.03	89	NS
Lovastatin	0.24	0.03	67	0.001
Simvastatin	0.20	0.03	56	0.001
Fluvastatin	0.17	0.03	47	0.001

I/M, intimal/medial layer ratio; SD, standard deviation; NS, not significant; n=12. The sham value is the mean ± SD of all 60 rabbits.

The levels of total plasma cholesterol measured before surgery and at the time the animals were killed (14 days later) did not change, and the values were comparable in positive control and vastatin-treated animals throughout the study (Table 3).

Figure 1 reports the effect of the different vastatins on thickening induced in the carotid intimas of rabbits: all drugs at the dose of 20 mg/kg body wt per day limited the increase of the I/M ratio (when compared with the positive-control-group mean value). Fluvastatin was the most effective drug in this regard, followed by simvastatin, lovastatin, and pravastatin in decreasing order. Differences versus positive controls were statistically highly significant for all drugs with the exception of pravastatin (Table 2). In all rabbits treated with vastatins, the inhibition of hyperplasia consisted of fewer layers of intimal cells.

Table 3. Total plasma cholesterol levels through the study in control and vastatin-treated groups.

Treatment	Total cholesterol before surgery	Total cholesterol at sacrifice
Positive control	28.4 ± 3.6	31.5 ± 4.2
Pravastatin	26.5 ± 4.8	24.6 ± 6.3
Lovastatin	29.6 ± 5.2	27.8 ± 6.4
Simvastatin	29.7 ± 12.5	31.1 ± 7.8
Fluvastatin	32.6 ± 7.7	28.9 ± 5.5

Values are in milligrams per decilitre and are mean ± SD.

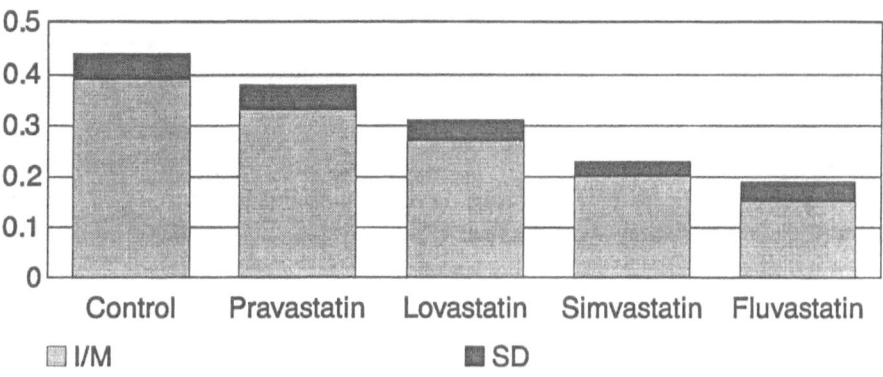

Statins effect on neointimal formation

normocholesterolemic rabbits

Figure 1. Bar graph of vastatins' effect on neointimal formation induced by perivascular manipulation of normocholesterolemic rabbit carotid arteries. Vastatins were administered for 3 weeks mixed with food at a daily dose of 20 mg/kg body weight starting on the day of collar placement.

The inhibition of SMC proliferation induced by statins is totally abolished by local infusion of mevalonate (Table 4).

Table 4. Effect of mevalonate on arterial SMC proliferation inhibited by fluvastatin.

	Control	Fluva	Fluva + MVA
I/M	0.22	0.12	0.20
LI	3.6	1.6	3.1

Fluva = Fluvastatin 5 mg/kg/day IP/or 5 days.
MVA = Sodium mevalonate 8 mg/kg/day (local delivery) for 5 days.
I/M = Intimal/medial tissue (ratio).
LI = Labelling index (INTIMA * MEDIA)

These *in vivo* data are more in accordance with an antiproliferative action of statins than a cholesterol lowering effect.

Conclusions

The examples of two classes of drugs which protect arterial walls even in presence of risk factors or after endothelial and SMC damage show new ways to prevent atherosclerosis and its cardiovascular consequences.

New clinical approaches using quantitative and repeated observations of the arterial wall thickness and the progression and regression of plaques in man are needed to study those and newly developed drugs at the clinical level.

Combinations of two drugs (such as a calcium antagonist and a statin) may be tested in human subjects with a variety of risk factors (hypertension, dyslipoproteinemias and diabetes). This new approach is needed to avoid multiplication of drugs which affect individually each risk factor without a well-demonstrated global impact on the atherosclerotic disease.

References

1. Paoletti R, Soma MR. Pharmacological approach of individual and combined risk factors. In: Van Zwieten PA, Mancia G, Brodde OE, editors. Hypertension, atherosclerosis, and lipids. London: Royal Soc Med Serv, 1992;27-34.
2. Ross R. The pathogenesis of atherosclerosis: A perspective for the 1990s. Nature 1993;362:801-809.
3. Corsini A, Mazzotti M, Raiteri M, et al. Relationship between mevalonate pathway and arterial myocyte proliferation: In vitro studies with inhibitors of HMG-CoA reductase. Atherosclerosis 1993;101:117-125.
4. Soma MR, Donetti E, Parolini C, et al. HMG-CoA reductase inhibitors: In vivo

effects on carotid intimal thickening in normocholesterolemic rabbits. Arterioscl Thromb 1993;13:571-578.

5.   Goldstein JL, Brown MS. Regulation of the mevalonate pathway. Nature 1990;343:425-430.

6.   Maltese WA, Sheridan KM. Isoprenoid synthesis during the cell cycle. J Biol Chem 1988;263:10104-10110.

7   Faust JR, Goldstein JL, Brown MS. Synthesis of ubiquinone and cholesterol in human fibroblast: Regulation of branched pathway. Arch Biochem Biophys 1979;192:86-99.

8.   Soma MR, Donetti E, Parolini C, et al. Effect of lacidipine on the carotid intimal thickening induced by cuff injury. J Cardiovasc Pharmacol 1994;23(Suppl.5):S71-S74.

9.   Schmitz G, Hankovitz J, Kovacs EM. Cellular processes in atherogenesis: Potential targets of calcium channel blockers. Atherosclerosis 1991;88:109-132.

10.   Fronek K. Calcium antagonists and experimental atherosclerosis. Cardiovasc Drug Rev 1990;8:229-237.

11.   Scheneider W, Kober G, Roebruck P, et al. Retardation of development and progression of coronary atherosclerosis: A new indication for calcium antagonists? Eur J Clin Pharmacol 1990;39:S17-S23.

12.   Lichtlen PR, Hugenholtz PG, Hecker H, Jost S, Deckers JW. Retardation of angiographic progression of coronary artery disease by nifedipine. Results of international nifedipine trial on atherosclerotic therapy (INTACT). Lancet 1990;335:1109-1113.

13.   Waters D, Lespérance J, Francetich M, et al. A controlled clinical trial to assess the effect of calcium channel blocker on the progression of coronary atherosclerosis. Circulation 1990;82:1940-1953.

14.   Popma JJ, Califf RM, Topol EJ. Clinical trials of restenosis after coronary angioplasty. Circulation 1991;84:1426-1436.

15.   Booth RGF, Martin JF, Honey AC, Hassall DG, Beesley JE, Moncada S. Rapid development of atherosclerotic lesions in the rabbit carotid artery induced by perivascular manipulation. Atherosclerosis 1989;76:257-268.

16.   Soma MR, Baetta R, De Renzis R, Mazzini G, Davegna C, Magrassi L, Butti G, Pezzotta S, Paoletti R, Fumagalli R. In vitro and in vivo enhanced anti-tumor activity of carmustine (BCNU) by simvastatin, a hypocholesterolemic drug. Cancer Research 1995, in press.

17.   Soma MR, Baetta R, Paoletti R, et al. Effect on cell cycle of hypocholesterolemic drugs. Eur J Histochem 1993;37(Suppl.):88, Abstract.

18.   Soma MR, Pagliarini P, Butti G, Paoletti R, Paoletti P, Fumagalli R. Simvastatin, an inhibitor of cholesterol biosynthesis, shows synergistic effect with N,N'-Bis(2-chloroethyl)-N-nitrosourea and beta interferon on human glioma cells. Cancer Res 1992;52:1-9.

19.   Corsini A, Raiteri M, Soma MR, Fumagalli R, Paoletti R. Simvastatin but not pravastatin inhibits the proliferation of rat aorta myocytes. Pharm Res 1991;23:173-

180.

20. Gellman J, Ezekowitz MD, Sarembock IJ, et al. Effect of lovastatin on intimal hyperplasia after balloon angioplasty. A study in an atherosclerotic hypercholesterolemic rabbit. J Am Coll Cardiol 1991;17:251-259.

21. Sahni R, Maniet AR, Voci G, Banka VS. Prevention of restenosis by lovastatin after successful coronary angioplasty. Am Heart J 1991;121:1600-1608.

THE POSCH TRIAL: IMPORTANCE OF CHOLESTEROL LOWERING IN REDUCING CORONARY HEART DISEASE PROGRESSION

Christian T. Campos, Henry Buchwald, and the POSCH Group
Division of Cardiothoracic Surgery
New England Deaconess Hospital
Harvard Medical School
Boston, Massachusetts
and
Department of Surgery
University of Minnesota
Minneapolis, Minnesota
USA

The Program on the Surgical Control of the Hyperlipidemias (POSCH) examined the effects of intensive cholesterol lowering by partial ileal bypass (PIB) on overall mortality and other cardiovascular endpoints, including subsequent need for percutaneous transluminal coronary angioplasty (PTCA) or coronary artery bypass surgery (CABG) in hypercholesterolemic survivors of a single myocardial infarction (MI). During POSCH (1975-1990), the PIB-treated group (n=421) total plasma cholesterol was 23.3% lower, the LDL cholesterol was 37.7% lower, and the HDL cholesterol was 4.3% higher versus the diet-treated control group (n=417). There were 62 control-group deaths and 49 PIB-group deaths (21.7% risk reduction, p=0.164). The combined endpoint of coronary heart disease (CHD) death or definite nonfatal MI occurred in 125 control-group patients and in 82 PIB-group patients (35.0% risk reduction, p < 0.001). Post-trial follow-up until September 30, 1992 (mean follow-up = 11.8 years) revealed a 52% decrease in the performance of PTCA and a 60% decrease in the performance of CABG in PIB-treated patients. The decision to perform PTCA or CABG was made by referring physicians according to standard clinical criteria acting independently of POSCH. Arteriographic progression of CHD occurred more frequently in the control group; whereas, arteriographic stabilization or regression of CHD was observed more frequently in the PIB group. The results of the POSCH trial provide the most compelling evidence todate supporting the beneficial effects of intensive cholesterol lowering therapy for the secondary prevention of CHD.

A.M. Gotto et al. (eds.), Multiple Risk Factors in Cardiovascular Disease, 259-266.
© *1995 Kluwer Academic Publishers and Fondazione Giovanni Lorenzini.*

The Program on the Surgical Control of the Hyperlipidemias (POSCH)

The Program on the Surgical Control of the Hyperlipidemias (POSCH) was a multi-centered, prospective, randomized, controlled, clinical trial designed to ascertain whether reductions in total plasma cholesterol and LDL cholesterol induced by the PIB operation would reduce overall mortality and the mortality and morbidity due to coronary heart disease in survivors of a single myocardial infarction. Detailed descriptions of the design and methodology of POSCH [1], of the enrollment experience [2], and of the baseline patient characteristics [3] have been published.

Between 1975 and 1983, 838 survivors of a single enzyme- and electro-cardiographically-documented myocardial infarction were entered into POSCH: 417 were randomly assigned to treatment with American Heart Association (AHA) Phase II diet instruction only (control group) and 421 were randomly assigned to treatment with identical dietary instruction plus a partial ileal bypass (surgery group). Patients were males or females between 30 and 64 years of age. After at least six weeks on the AHA Phase II diet, they were required to have a total plasma cholesterol level of at least 220 mg/dl (5.7 mmol/L) or a LDL cholesterol level of at least 140 mg/dl (3.6 mmol/L) if their total plasma cholesterol level was between 200 and 219 mg/dl (5.17-5.66 mmol/L). Potentially confounding major atherosclerosis risk factors such as hypertension (systolic blood pressure $\geq$ 180 mm Hg or diastolic blood pressure $\geq$ 105 mm Hg), obesity, or diabetes were causes for exclusion. Other exclusion criteria included: greater than 75% stenosis of the left main coronary artery, no measurable coronary artery stenosis on the prerandomization arteriogram, and previous CABG or PTCA. Cigarette smokers were eligible and were distributed by the randomization process.

Partial ileal bypass was performed as previously reported [4-6]. Briefly, under general anesthesia, the small bowel length is measured along the mesenteric border, allowing 25 cm for the duodenal length. The small intestine is divided 200 cm proximal to the ileocecal valve or at a distance one-third of the total small bowel length from the ileocecal valve if the total length is greater than 600 cm. The distal end of the divided ileum is closed, and the proximal end is anastomosed, in end-to-side fashion, into the anterior taenia of the cecum. The appendix is removed routinely. The closed end of the bypassed ileum is sutured to the anterior taenia of the cecum, between the anastomosis and the appendiceal stump, to prevent intussusception of this segment, and the mesenteric defects are closed to prevent internal herniation. The PIB procedure is illustrated in Figure 1.

All patients were followed by means of clinic visits and telephone contacts according to a uniform protocol. Serial lipid analyses were performed at the POSCH Central Lipid Laboratory at baseline, three months after randomization, and at every clinic visit (annual visits during the first five years and one visit at either seven or ten years). Coronary arteriograms were obtained at baseline, three years, five years, and at either seven years (for patients enrolled on or after June 1, 1980) or ten years (for patients enrolled before June 1, 1980). The formal POSCH trial ended, with the vital status of all 838 patients known, in July of 1990 with an average follow-up of 9.7 years (range: 7-14.8 years). Since the conclusion of the formal POSCH trial in July of 1990, all surviving patients have been followed by annual detailed telephone interviews (the POSCH Long-Term Follow-Up Study).

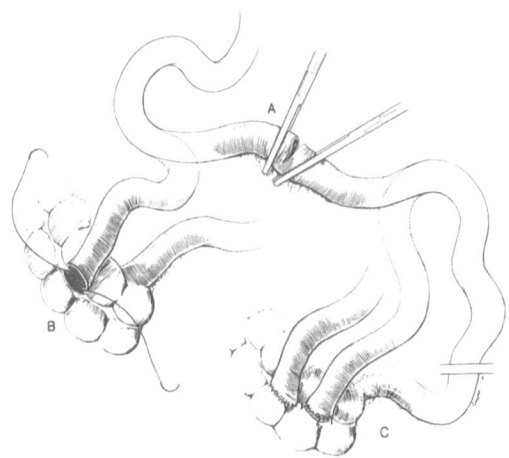

Figure 1. Partial Ileal Bypass.
A. Division of the ileum 200 cm proximal to the ileocecal valve or one-third of the total small bowel length proximal to the ileocecal valve if the total small intestinal length is greater than 600 cm.
B. End-to-side anastomosis of the proximal segment into the anterior taenia of the cecum, 6 cm distal to the appendiceal stump.
C. Tacking of the closed distal segment to the anterior taenia of the cecum midway between the anastomosis and the appendiceal stump.

Determination of the specific cause of death was based upon a blinded review of all available records by the POSCH Mortality Review Committee. The diagnosis of MI during the trial was made following a blinded review of all available records by a POSCH cardiologist. The sequential coronary arteriography assessments were performed by two-member teams from the POSCH Arteriography Review Panel. No team member was from the clinic from which the arteriograms originated. The films were interpreted in pairs, with the reviewers blinded to the patient's treatment assignment and to the temporal sequence of the films. With use of an evaluation protocol virtually identical to that employed by the Cholesterol Lowering Atherosclerosis Study (CLAS), a global evaluation of the severity of the coronary artery disease was derived by consensus. An eight-point scale was used to grade the change between two sets of films (-3, -2, -1, -0, +0, +1, +2, and +3; -3 = much worse and +3 = much better).

POSCH LIPID AND LIPOPROTEIN RESULTS

Five years after randomization [7], the surgery group, as compared with the control group, had a 23.3 ± 1.0 (mean ± S.E.)% lower total plasma cholesterol level (p < 0.0001), a 37.7 ± 1.2% lower LDL cholesterol level (p < 0.0001), a 4.3 ± 1.8% higher HDL cholesterol level (p=0.02), an 18.3 ± 7.5% higher very low density lipoprotein (VLDL) cholesterol level (p=0.02), and a 19.8 ± 6.5% higher triglyceride level (p=0.003). The five-year total plasma cholesterol and LDL cholesterol results are presented in Figures 2 and 3.

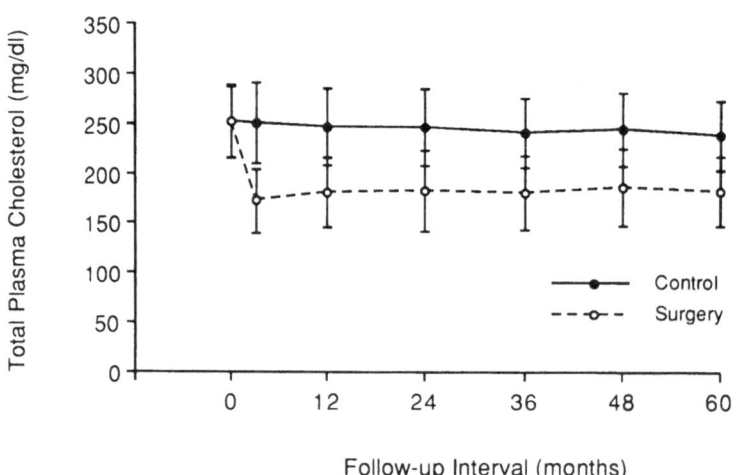

Follow-up Interval (months)

Figure 2. Five-year total plasma cholesterol results presented as mean ± S.D. The differences between groups were statistically significant (p < 0.0001) at each follow-up interval.

The ratio of HDL cholesterol to total plasma cholesterol was 37.8 ± 2.8% higher, and the ratio of HDL cholesterol to LDL cholesterol was 71.8 ± 4.3% higher in the surgery group. Determinations of apolipoprotein and HDL subfraction levels were added to the POSCH protocol in June of 1985. In the subset of patients with five-year apolipoprotein and HDL subfraction determinations, a significantly higher HDL subfraction 2 level (10.4 ± 6.6 mg/dl [0.27 ± 0.17 mmol/L] versus 8.1 ± 5.8 mg/dl [0.21 ± 0.15 mmol/L]; p < 0.0001), a significantly higher apolipoprotein A-I level (118.7 ± 22.4 mg/dl [3.07 ± 0.58 mmol/L] versus 106.0 ± 20.5 mg/dl [2.74 ± 0.53 mmol/L]; p < 0.0001), and a significantly lower apolipoprotein B-100 level (92.8 ± 20.5 mg/dl [2.40 ± 0.53 mmol/L] versus 123.4 ± 21.7 mg/dl [3.19 ± 0.56 mmol/L]; p < 0.0001) were observed in the surgery group.

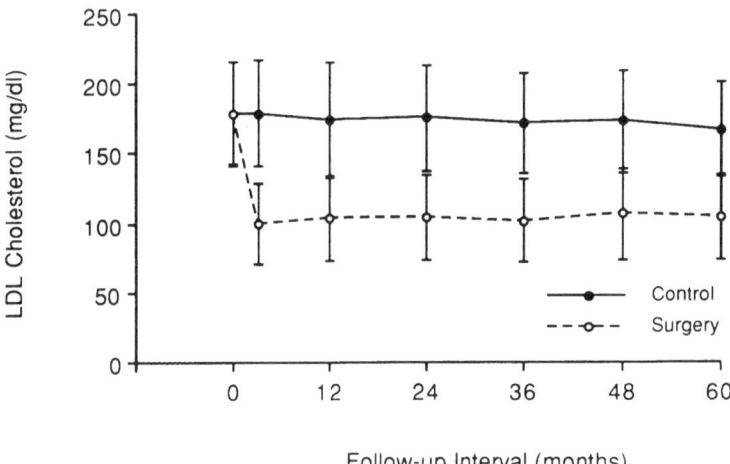

Figure 3. Five-year LDL cholesterol results presented as mean ± S.D. The differences between groups were statistically significant (p < 0.0001) at each follow-up interval.

POSCH OVERALL AND CAUSE-SPECIFIC MORTALITY

During the mean 9.7-year follow-up period of the formal POSCH trial, there were 62 deaths in the diet-treated control group and 49 deaths in the PIB-treated intervention group [7]. This 21.7% reduction in overall mortality in the surgery group did not, however, achieve statistical significance (two-sided p = 0.164). The mortality due to atherosclerotic coronary heart disease was reduced by 28% (p = 0.113), with 44 atherosclerotic coronary heart disease deaths among controls and 32 similar deaths in the surgery group patients.

In a subgroup analysis dividing the POSCH population into two groups: patients with a left ventricular ejection fraction ≥ 50% and patients with a left ventricular ejection fraction < 50%, no significant difference in overall mortality between the control and surgery group patients with a depressed resting left ventricular ejection fraction (< 50%) was observed. However, in the patients with a normal left ventricular ejection fraction following a myocardial infarction (≥ 50%), there were 39 deaths in the control group and only 24 deaths in the PIB group, a reduction of 36% (p = 0.052 by Mantel-Haenszel test, and p = 0.021 by Gehan test). This result suggests that aggressive lipid modification may be of benefit in increasing survival in hypercholesterolemic survivors of a myocardial infarction with preserved resting left ventricular function. This was the first demonstration of a significant overall mortality effect from lipid intervention observed during a clinical trial of the lipid-atherosclerosis theory.

Since the conclusion of the formal POSCH trial in July of 1990, all surviving patients have been followed by means of annual, detailed telephone interviews (the POSCH Long-Term Follow-Up Study). Event documentation, myocardial infarction analysis, and cause of death determinations are performed according to procedures identical to those employed during the formal POSCH trial. With post-trial follow-up extended until September 30,

1992 (mean follow-up = 11.8 ± 2.0 years), there have been 76 deaths in the control group and 56 deaths in the intervention group (p = 0.052). This overall mortality difference approaches statistical significance. In the subgroup of patients with a left ventricular ejection fraction ≥ 50%, there have been 49 control group deaths and 27 intervention group deaths (p = 0.011), an overall mortality difference that is statistically significant.

ATHEROSCLEROSIS ENDPOINTS COMBINED WITH OVERALL MORTALITY

Analysis of the combined endpoint of death due to coronary heart disease or definite nonfatal myocardial infarction [7] disclosed 125 such events in the control group and 82 occurrences in the surgery group, a 35 percent risk reduction (p < 0.001). This is the endpoint employed by the Lipid Research Clinics Coronary Primary Prevention Trial (LRC-CPPT) and several other trials of the lipid-atherosclerosis theory. Rather than relying on a one-sided test of significance to demonstrate a statistically significant result as in the LRC-CPPT, the POSCH results were statistically significant at the p < 0.001 level using a more rigorous two-sided test of statistical significance. All combinations of overall mortality with other clinical atherosclerosis events (definite nonfatal myocardial infarction, suspected nonfatal myocardial infarction, or the occurrence of unstable angina) demonstrated highly significant reductions (p < 0.001) in the group undergoing partial ileal bypass compared with the group receiving dietary therapy alone as treatment for hypercholesterolemia.

POSCH SEQUENTIAL CORONARY AND PERIPHERAL ARTERIOGRAPHY

In POSCH, the percentage of patients with angiographic progression of coronary artery disease increased in both groups as follow-up continued [7]. However, the percentage of patients with progression (global change score = -3, -2, or -1) was consistently greater in the diet-treated control group compared with the PIB-treated intervention group: 41% versus 28% at three years, 65% versus 38% at five years, 77% versus 48% at seven years, and 85% versus 55% at ten years (p < 0.001 for all comparisons). These decreases in the rate of angiographic coronary artery disease progression were associated with a marked decline in the occurrence of clinical atherosclerotic coronary artery disease events. This is the first such demonstration by a lipid-atherosclerosis intervention trial. Furthermore, statistically significant evidence (p < 0.01) for angiographic coronary artery disease regression was observed at five- and seven-year follow-up. The proportion of POSCH patients free of peripheral vascular disease assessed angiographically was consistently higher in the surgery group compared with the control group, a difference that approached statistical significance after 10 years of follow-up (p = 0.09).

CORONARY ARTERY BYPASS SURGERY, PERCUTANEOUS TRANSLUMINAL CORONARY ANGIOPLASTY, AND HEART TRANSPLANTATION

One of the important observations in the POSCH trial was the demonstration that aggressive lipid modification can limit the clinical progression of coronary atherosclerosis to the point requiring interventional therapy [7,8]. In POSCH, the decision to perform coronary artery bypass surgery (CABG), percutaneous transluminal coronary angioplasty (PTCA), or heart transplantation was made by each patient's personal physician acting independently of the POSCH trial and without prior discussion with the POSCH investigators or clinic personnel. Copies of the reports of coronary arteriograms performed according to POSCH protocol, without any clinical recommendations by the angiographer or by the POSCH clinic physicians or personnel, were forwarded to the patients' personal physicians as a courtesy. Aside from these routine arteriographic summaries, no contact was made with POSCH patients' personal physicians during the formal POSCH trial or during the POSCH Long-Term Follow-Up Study, except in the context of event documentation interviews conducted by the clinic personnel.

With post-trial follow-up extended until September 30, 1992 (mean follow-up = 11.8 ± 2.0 years), 42 control group patients and 23 intervention group patients had undergone a first PTCA (p = 0.01). Eleven control group patients and 4 intervention group patients had undergone a second PTCA (p = 0.07), and two control group patients had undergone a third PTCA (p = 0.2). There was, therefore, a 52% reduction in PTCA performance in the POSCH intervention group.

During the mean 11.8 ± 2.0 year follow-up period, 149 control group patients and 62 intervention group patients underwent a first CABG (p < 0.001). Twelve control group patients and two intervention group patients underwent a second CABG during the follow-up period (p = 0.007). There was, therefore, a 60% decrease in CABG performance in the POSCH intervention group.

Four control group patients and three intervention group patients underwent heart transplantation for end-stage ischemic cardiomyopathy during the follow-up period (p = 0.7). The total number of interventional cardiac procedures (PTCA, CABG, or heart transplantation) was 58% lower (94 versus 221) in the PIB-treated intervention group in POSCH.

Summary and Conclusions

The clinical and arteriographic results of the Program on the Surgical Control of the Hyperlipidemias (POSCH) have provided clear and convincing evidence supporting the beneficial effects of cholesterol lowering in hypercholesterolemic survivors of a myocardial infarction [7]. Even though overall mortality as a single endpoint was not significantly reduced, a favorable trend toward improved overall survival in patients undergoing aggressive lipid modification was observed, and in the *post hoc* subgroup of patients with preserved left ventricular ejection fractions (≥ 50%) following a myocardial infarction, a statistically significant improvement in overall survival was noted. With extended post-trial follow-up until September 30, 1992, the reduction in overall mortality in the PIB-treated intervention group approaches statistical significance. For the combined endpoint of atherosclerotic coronary heart disease mortality and subsequent confirmed nonfatal MI, the POSCH results clearly demonstrate a significant reduction in the intervention group. In POSCH, the 35% reduction in atherosclerotic coronary heart disease mortality or definite nonfatal myocardial infarction was significant at the $p < 0.001$ level using a two-sided test of significance. The POSCH arteriographic results demonstrate decreased arteriographic coronary artery disease progression, and increased arteriographic stabilization and even regression of coronary artery disease, in the intervention group undergoing effective cholesterol reduction. These arteriographic results are correlated with decreased coronary heart disease event rates in the intervention group [9]. Dramatic reductions in subsequent need for percutaneous transluminal coronary angioplasty (PTCA) and coronary artery bypass surgery (CABG) have been observed in the PIB-treated intervention group [8]. Thus, the POSCH clinical and arteriographic results provide the strongest evidence todate supporting the beneficial effects of effective cholesterol lowering in hypercholesterolemic patients with clinically evident coronary heart disease.

References

1.   Buchwald H, Matts JP, Fitch LL, et al. Program on the Surgical Control of the Hyperlipidemias (POSCH): Design and methodology. J Clin Epidemiol 1989; 42:1111-1127.
2.   Buchwald H, Matts JP, Hansen BJ, Long JM, Fitch LL, and the POSCH Group. Program on the Surgical Control of the Hyperlipidemias (POSCH): Recruitment experience. Controlled Clin Trials 1987; 8:(Suppl.4):94S-104S.
3.   Matts JP, Buchwald H, Fitch LL, et al. Program on the Surgical Control of the Hyperlipidemias (POSCH): Patient entry characteristics. Controlled Clin Trials 1991; 12:314-339.
4.   Buchwald H. Intestinal bypass for hypercholesterolemia. In: Nyhus LM, Baker RJ, editors. Mastery of surgery. Boston: Little, Brown and Co., 1984:901-907.
5.   Buchwald H, Campos CT. Partial ileal bypass for control of hyperlipidemia and atherosclerosis. In: Sabiston DC Jr, Spencer FC, editors. Surgery of the chest. 5th edition. Philadelphia: W.B. Saunders, Co., 1990:1799-1820.
6.   Buchwald H, Campos CT, Fitch LL. Partial ileal bypass for hypercholesterolemia. In: Scott HW Jr, Sawyers JL, editors. Surgery of the stomach, duodenum, and small intestine. Boston: Blackwell Scientific Publications, Inc., 1992:903-924.
7.   Buchwald H, Varco RL, Matts JP, et al. Effect of partial ileal bypass surgery on mortality and morbidity from coronary heart disease in patients with hyper-cholesterolemia. Report of the Program on the Surgical Control of the Hyperlipidemias (POSCH). N Engl J Med 1990; 323:946-955.
8.   Campos CT, Nguyen P, Buchwald H, and the POSCH Group. Effect of cholesterol lowering on PTCA, CABG, and heart transplantation rates: POSCH Long-Term Follow-Up Study (abstr). Circulation 1993; 88 (Suppl.I):I-386.
9.   Buchwald H, Matts JP, Fitch LL, et al. Changes in sequential coronary arteriograms and subsequent clinical events. JAMA 1992; 268:1429-1433.

THREE-DIMENSIONAL RECONSTRUCTION OF INTRACORONARY ULTRASOUND IMAGES: TECHNICAL APPROACHES, CLINICAL APPLICATIONS, AND CURRENT LIMITATIONS IN THE ASSESSMENT OF VESSEL DIMENSIONS

Clemens von Birgelen, Carlo Di Mario, Wenguang Li, Francesco Prati, Nicolaas Bom, Jos R.T.C. Roelandt, and Patrick W. Serruys
Thoraxcenter
Division Cardiology
University Hospital Rotterdam-Dijkzigt and Erasmus University
Rotterdam
THE NETHERLANDS

Summary

Three-dimensional (3-D) reconstruction of intracoronary ultrasound (ICUS) images is a technique, which provides directly spatial information on the longitudinal architecture and pathology of coronary arteries. The technical method requires sequential procedural steps, including image acquisition and segmentation, which are most crucial concerning the final quality of the 3-D reconstruction.

After optimization of the image quality, the basic images are acquired by a slow and uniform speed pull-back. Use of ECG-gating during continuous or step-wise withdrawal of the imaging catheter is now available. A new device, which senses the insertion depth of ICUS catheters, permits reliable measurements even during manual withdrawal of the imaging catheter. During the segmentation step, discrimination between the blood-pool inside the lumen and structures of vessel wall has to be performed in the digitized images. This can be achieved by two principal approaches.

A blood-speckle identification method detects the blood-pool by statistical pattern recognition, but no quantitative information on the plaque dimensions are provided. The system can be used on-line even in very irregular lumen shapes without user interaction; however, image quality may limit the feasibility of this technique. In contrast to this approach, a contour detection method performs the segmentation by the application of a contour detection algorithm, permitting measurement of coronary lumen and plaque. Particularly in very irregular lumen shapes some user interaction is required. Therefore on-line use of this technique could not yet be achieved.

Both complementary methods of segmentation provide specific advantages and

A.M. Gotto et al. (eds.), Multiple Risk Factors in Cardiovascular Disease, 267-287.

limitations, defining their application in the clinical arena. During and after intracoronary interventions, on-line 3-D ICUS can be very helpful in displaying the characteristics of coronary plaques and in guiding interventions. Since off-line 3-D reconstruction of the basic ICUS images provides accurate and reproducible area and volume measurements of coronary lumen and plaque, the method permits the quantification of volumetric changes in coronary plaque during progression-regression studies of atherosclerosis or studies of interventional techniques.

Three-dimensional ICUS has the capability to address several questions which are of fundamental interest. Current clinical experience suggests despite some remaining limitations that the application of 3-D ICUS techniques is practical and scientifically rewarding.

Introduction

Introduction of two-dimensional conventional intracoronary ultrasound (ICUS) in the clinical arena has been a milestone in the assessment of extent, distribution, and treatment of coronary atherosclerosis. Information on the spatial relationship of vessel wall structures, however, could only be obtained by simultaneous fluoroscopy, providing information on the position of the ICUS catheter tip. Intracoronary ultrasound provides an unrivaled tomographic visualization of coronary lumen and wall and their structural [1] or functional pathology [2]. Great effort has currently been invested in new technical developments, providing an improved 3-D reconstruction of ICUS [3-6]. 3-D reconstruction systems provide several new display modalities and suggest a variety of clinical applications, which the pioneers of this technique recently began to explore. Specimens of coronary and peripheral arteries were successfully reconstructed and quantitatively assessed, showing good correlation with histology and biplane quantitative angiography [7,8]. *In vivo* acquired images of coronary and peripheral arteries showed reliable reconstruction results with remarkable image quality and value in clinical use [9,10].

Three-dimensional reconstruction of ICUS has the capability to address several questions of fundamental interest, but some technical limitations still remain [11]. The technical method of 3-D reconstruction requires sequent procedural steps. The correct acquisition of the basic images, and even more particularly the segmentation, are the most crucial steps in the process of 3-D reconstruction of ICUS.

Image Acquisition

Before the basic images are acquired, zoom and gain settings have to be optimized. The gain settings are crucial since most of the 3-D reconstruction programs allow display of full gray scale information (volume rendered display). The ICUS catheter is withdrawn from distal to proximal through the coronary segment, which is supposed to be reconstructed. To acquire the basic tomographic images, several pull-back methods are available, which operate either at a uniform speed using a continuous motorized pull-back or on withdrawal by an ECG-gated step-motor [12]. Alternatively the linear motion of the ICUS catheter can be monitored by a catheter sensing device which allows either a manual or a motorized pull-back of the ICUS catheter [13].

UNIFORM SPEED PULL-BACK

The uniform pull-back speed results in an equidistant spacing of adjacent images. Side-branches or spots of calcium are used as topographic landmarks, allowing an accurate matching of serial studies of the same coronary segment. During withdrawal in tortuous arteries the speed of the catheter tip can be checked by fluoroscopy.

A recently introduced imaging system is equipped with a transparent distal sleeve, in which several pull-backs can be performed without any direct contact of imaging core and vessel wall. This design reduces the risk of a nonuniform pull-back speed of the imaging catheter. At the start of a pull-back with uniform speed the first 5-10 seconds are usually required to straighten the imaging core. After this short period of time the pull-back reaches a constant speed of withdrawal.

ECG-GATED VIDEO LABELING AND WITHDRAWAL

An ECG-triggered video label can be added to the video image before it is recorded on the video tape. Images can be labeled at the time of the R-wave and defined images can thus be used for the three-dimensional reconstruction. The vessel dimensions can be displayed and measured for instance at end-diastole or end-systole. Since the technique of ECG-labeling permits a selection of images for reconstruction, which were acquired with a defined and constant timing, cyclic artifacts can be minimized.

Alternatively a step-motor, which is gated by an ECG-signal, is used for a non-uniform step-withdrawal. The resolution of the final reconstruction depends on the size of steps. The ECG-gated pull-back of the ICUS catheter is another way to overcome the problem of cyclic movement artifacts.

CATHETER DISPLACEMENT SENSING DEVICE

A catheter displacement sensing device has recently been validated in femoral arteries [13]. The method is based upon a continuous measurement of the insertion depth of ICUS catheters. Thus, images can be matched with their real location in a reconstructed vessel segment by using the data, which are provided by the catheter displacement sensing device. This technique can be applied to a multitude of different types of ICUS catheters. A motorized pull-back devices can be used or the withdrawal can be performed manually.

Image Segmentation Methods

The subsequent step in the 3-D reconstruction process is the segmentation of the digitized images, which discriminates between the blood-pool inside the lumen and structures of the vessel wall. Segmentation influences directly the quality of reconstruction and the accuracy of quantitative analyses. This can be achieved by application of either a speckle identification algorithm [3] or a contour detection algorithm [14,15]. These 3-D reconstruction systems are at present frequently used in our Intracoronary Imaging Laboratory or Heart Catheterization Laboratory. The speckle identification provides distinction between blood pool and vessel wall by a statistical pattern recognition algorithm (EchoQuant ™, CVIS, Sunnyvale, CA, USA). The second method has been developed at the Thoraxcenter, Erasmus University, Rotterdam. It is based on a minimum cost algorithm for contour detection, which permits identification of both lumen-intima and media-adventitia boundaries.

BLOOD SPECKLE IDENTIFICATION METHOD

This statistical pattern recognition system has recently been validated in normal rabbit aortas [3]. It requires an Intel 80486 50 Hz or a Pentium personal computer and the OS/2 operating system and can be used either on-line or off-line. The ICUS images are digitized with a rate of 8.5 images/s.

The data of the images are then transferred into the computer memory. In the current version of the system a maximum capacity of 255 basic ICUS images can be stored. Since the image acquisition rate is fixed, the length of the reconstructed coronary segment will be determined by the pull-back speed. If a pull-back speed of 1 mm per second is used, a segment of 30 mm of length can be reconstructed.

The backscatter pattern of flowing blood cells shows more variation in time than the pattern of the vessel wall [16]. The speckle identification algorithm is able to distinguish between these two patterns (Figure 1) and detects as a result the interface between blood and intima. Segmentation is performed by removing the blood pool, which is identified in all the ICUS images. The quality of segmentation can be visually checked by displaying the pixels identified as part of the blood pool in red. The settings of several parameters which determine the speckle identification process can be modified by the user. This option is particularly valuable in ICUS images of limited quality. The system furthermore offers options which help to remove catheter artifacts and allow manual correction of the computer defined blood-intima boundary.

In order to obtain a three-dimensional model, volumetric units are used (voxel modeling method). A selected transverse image, a longitudinal reconstructed image, and a 3-D view of the coronary segment are displayed on the output screen. In the 3-D view the coronary segment is presented in a cylindrical format, which is opened longitudinally with both halves tilted back. This "clam-shell" view of the reconstructed coronary segment can be rotated perpendicular to the longitudinal axis of the vessel in order to provide insight from different angles. The cross-sectional luminal area in each transverse image is measured and the results are displayed in a diagram. Scrolling along the reconstructed coronary segment, the measurements can be checked in the individual transverse images (Figure 2).

The current version of the program provides an option, which allows one to draw manually the external elastic membrane in transverse images and thus to measure the plaque area in a particular image of interest, as, for example, in the image of the minimal luminal cross-sectional area or the reference.

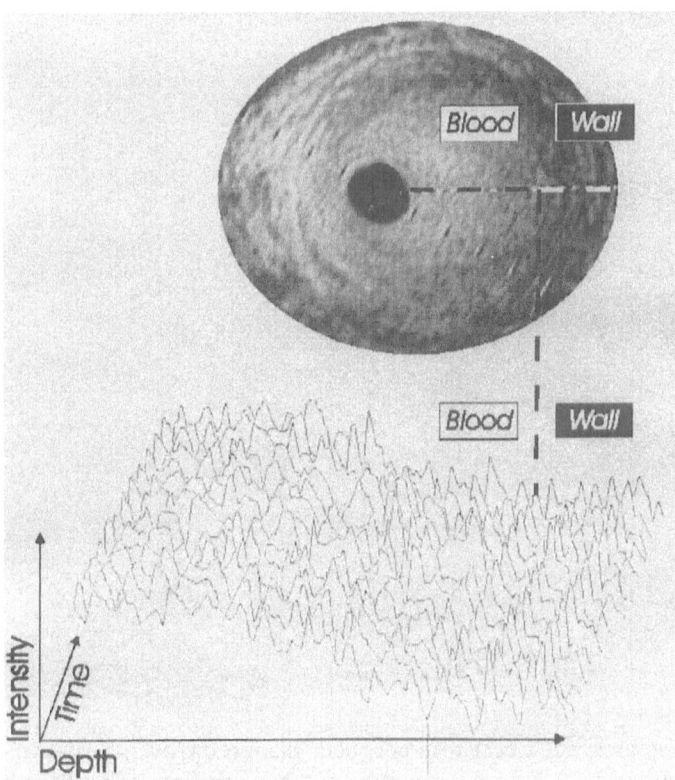

Figure 1. Backscatter pattern of flowing blood (BLOOD) shows more variation in time (z-axis) than the vessel wall (WALL), which has a much more stable pattern. This difference permits discrimination between blood pool and vessel wall by application of a speckle identification algorithm.

Relative Advantages And Limitations Of This Method. The method allows distinction between vessel lumen and wall. No geometric assumption on the lumen shape is required and the program may therefore provide accurate segmentation in irregular shapes of the lumen as well (Table 1). Application of the algorithm, however, may be hampered by the quality of the ICUS images. The blood-speckle algorithm is not able to detect the external boundary of the plaque and is thus not capable of providing quantitative information on the coronary plaque (Table 2). The reconstruction of the blood speckle identification system is performed within 2 minutes and so on-line use is feasible. The option to rotate the 3-D image offers a good insight into spatial proportions of vessel wall structures.

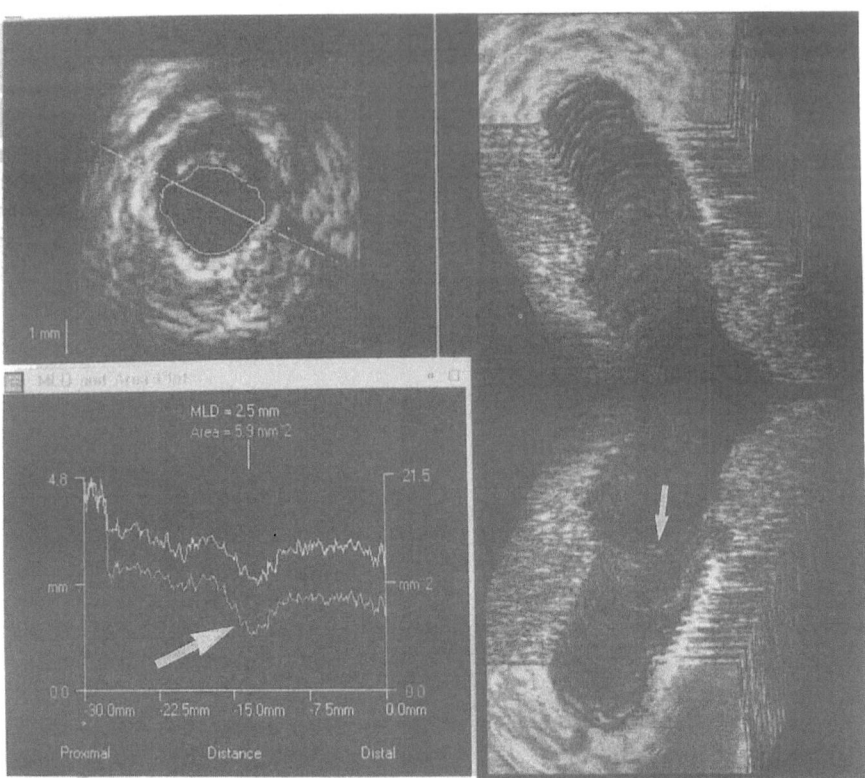

Figure 2. A circumscribed eccentric coronary plaque (arrows) is shown in a selected transverse image and a 3-D view, reconstructed by the application of the blood speckle identification algorithm. Luminal cross-sectional area and minimal luminal diameter of each transverse image are measured and the results are displayed (left lower panel). The measurements can be checked in the individual transverse images by scrolling a cursor along the reconstructed coronary segment.

CONTOUR DETECTION METHOD

Application of this method requires a Pentium personal computer (60 MHz) with 16 Mbytes of internal RAM and a frame-grabber, which digitizes a user-defined region of interest of a maximum of 200 tomographic images at a resolution of 800 x 600 x 8 Bits. The images can be processed either on-line or off-line from a video tape.

The length of the reconstructed coronary segment is defined by the pull-back speed and the acquisition rate, which can be determined by the user (maximum of 25 images/s). A pull-back speed of 1 mm per second and processing of 5 images per second (= 0.2

mm/image) results for instance in a reconstructed segment length of 4 cm. The program allows removal of the catheter artifacts and thus improves the image quality.

The semiautomatic contour detection procedure consists of three steps (Figure 3). First, the sequence of the ICUS images is modeled in a voxel space [17] and two perpendicular cut planes which are parallel to the longitudinal axis of the vessel are interactively selected. Data located at the interception of these cut planes and the voxel volume are derived to reconstruct two longitudinal images of the vessel segment. Angle and location of the cut planes can be changed interactively by the user in order to optimize the image quality of the longitudinal images.

Secondly, the contours of the lumen and plaque are semiautomatically defined, based on the application of a minimum cost algorithm. This algorithm has previously been validated [18-21]. During the interactive contour detection process the user is allowed to add points to the initial contours, which are detected automatically. These points enforce upon the contours to pass through the defined spots. During this user interaction process the optimal path of the contours is updated serially, using dynamic programming techniques.

The computer-screen of the program displays three windows. In two of them the two reconstructed longitudinal views are shown, which may be zoomed to full-screen size. In the third window the transverse images are presented, through which the user may scroll. The xy-coordinates of the contours are displayed on each transverse image, permitting inspection of the contour detection in both the longitudinal and the transverse images. Thus, two contours of the lumen-intima and the media-adventitia boundaries are interactively detected for each longitudinal image.

Finally, a contour detection is performed in all of the transverse images, employing information derived from the longitudinal contours. The contours of the longitudinal images are transformed into four defined edge points for each of both contours in each individual transverse image. These points serve as landmarks and guide the path of the contours, detected by the application of a minimum cost algorithm. The accuracy of the final contour detection can be visually checked in all the longitudinal and transverse images and, if necessary, manual correction of the transverse contours can be performed (Figure 4).

Then, quantitative analysis of lumen and plaque is performed. Each transverse image represents a thin slice of the coronary segment and thus volumetric measurements can be obtained by multiplication of the cross-sectional areas with the thickness of the total number of slices. The transverse image, corresponding to the minimal luminal cross-sectional area, is given automatically. For the whole series of transverse images areas and mean diameters of the total vessel, determined by the external elastic membrane, the lumen and the plaque are measured. The results are displayed in two diagrams, presenting also a diameter and an area-stenosis function. Preliminary results of a validation study *in vitro* and *in vivo* suggest that the contour detection method yields accurate and reproducible results [14,15].

Relative Advantages And Limitations Of This Method. The contour detection program provides quantitative information on both coronary lumen and plaque (Table 2). The method depends less on the image quality since it operates interactively. Reliable

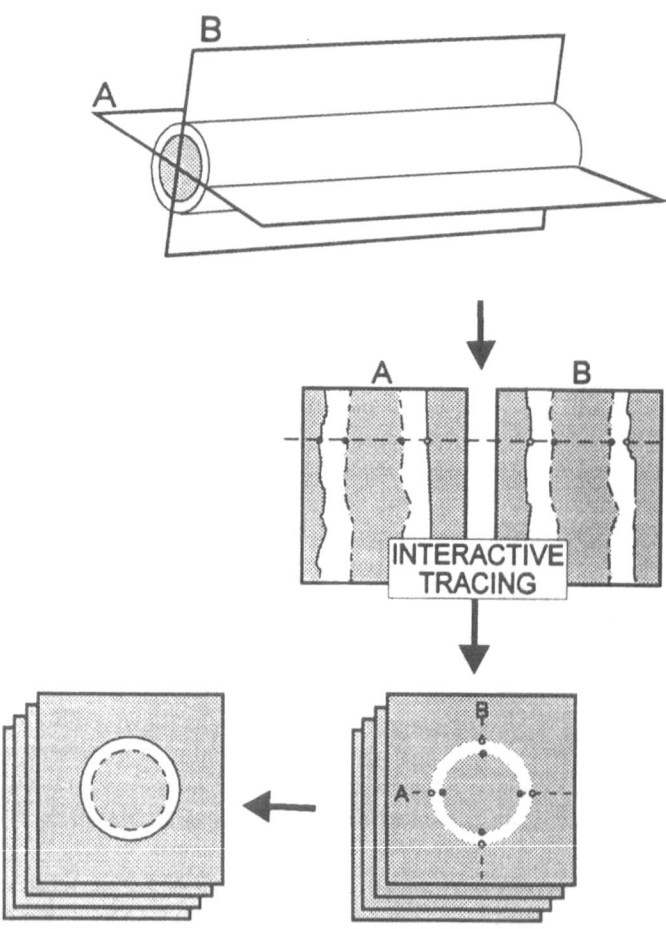

Figure 3. *Contour Detection Method:* The basic images are modeled in a voxel space and two perpendicular cut planes are selected, which are parallel to the longitudinal axis of the reconstructed coronary segment. In the two derived longitudinal views contours of lumen and plaque are semiautomatically traced (interactive tracing) by the application of a minimum cost algorithm and use of dynamic programming techniques. Four edge points are derived from the longitudinal contours for each contour and each individual transverse image. These points serve as landmarks and guide the path of the contours, detected by the application of a minimum cost algorithm. The transverse contours can be checked in each individual transverse image and manual correction is possible. Finally, the measures are displayed.

segmentation and 3-D reconstruction remains possible even when the image quality is not optimal. However, more user interaction is required in the presence of very irregular lumen shapes. As a result of the user interaction, the contour detection system requires more time and an on-line use is to date not yet practicable (Table 1). Since the program allows removal of artifacts it is able to improve the off-line contour detection. Thus, the edited images can then be used for 3-D reconstruction by application of the contour detection method or the blood speckle identification algorithm.

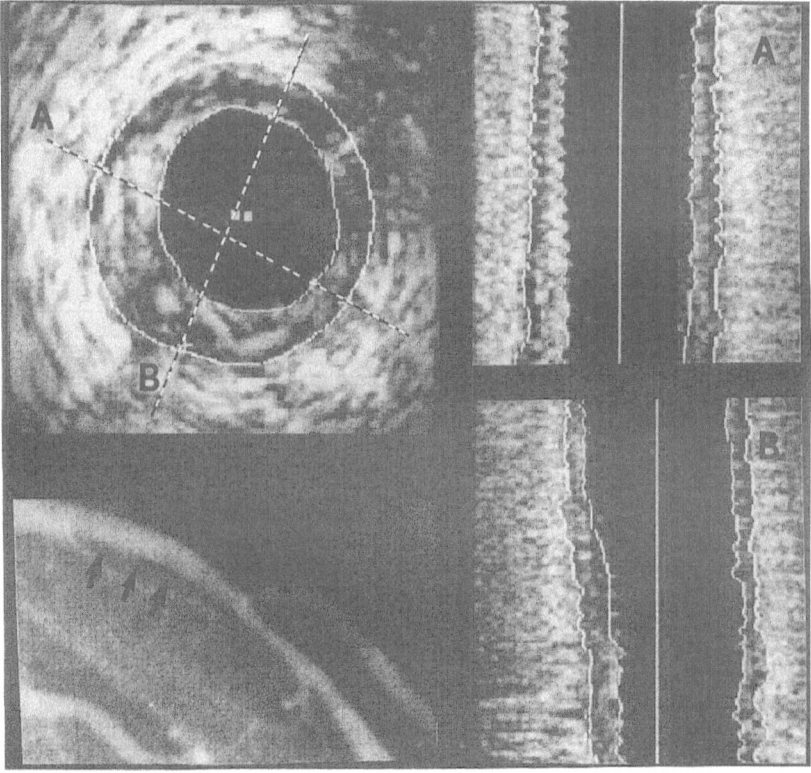

Figure 4. After reconstruction by the contour detection method, a nonsignificant intimal atherosclerosis was found in this angiographically normal segment (see arrows) of a left anterior descending coronary artery. The contours of the lumen-intima and media-adventitia boundaries are displayed in the two longitudinal views (right upper and lower panels), derived from two perpendicular longitudinal cut planes (A and B, left upper panel), and all the transverse images.

Table 1. Relative Advantages and Limitations of the 2 Principal Methods of 3-D ICUS: Applicability and On-line Use.

	Speckle Identification	Contour Detection
Applicability	• No geometric assumption on the lumen shape • May provide accurate segmentation even in irregular lumen shape • Applicability depends clearly on the image quality	• Assuming a fairly elliptic lumen shape • More user interaction is required in very irregular lumen shapes • Applicability depends less on the image quality
On-Line Use	• On-line use is feasible	• The time, required for user interaction, prevents on-line use

Table 2. Relative Advantages and Limitations of the 2 Principal Methods of 3-D ICUS: Visualization and Quantification.

	Speckle Identification	Contour Detection
Visualization	• Transverse and longitudinal image and a 3-D view • Limited capability to compensate artifacts	• Transverse and two longitudinal images • Artifacts can be removed to obtain a better visualization and quantification
Quantification	• Detects the lumen-plaque boundary; therefore quantitative information on the lumen, but not on the plaque, are provided	• Detects the contours of the lumen-plaque and plaque-adventitia boundaries; thus measurements of both lumen and plaque are provided

Examples of Clinical Applications

ASSESSMENT OF VESSEL DIMENSIONS DURING INTERVENTIONS

Use of ICUS before and after balloon dilatation is a remarkable help in analyzing the operative mechanism of this interventional technique. Wall stretching and wall dissection were reported as the main operative mechanism of balloon angioplasty in both coronary and peripheral arteries [22,23]. However, recently a significant plaque compression with reduction of plaque area was detected by ICUS [24]. An important problem and limitation of these serial pre/post studies is the fact that the two sites, where measurements are performed, do not match well. This can be explained by the lack of the third dimension in two-dimensional ICUS images. 3-D reconstruction of ICUS images permits serial assessment of cross-sectional areas at the same site of the coronary artery and measurement of plaque volume along the entire segment of angioplasty can provide more reliable studies of plaque geometry. During on-line studies by 3-D ICUS, measurements of the target lesion and the reference segment can immediately be obtained by simply moving a cursor along the longitudinal axis of the reconstructed longitudinal view. Thus, from the on-line use of

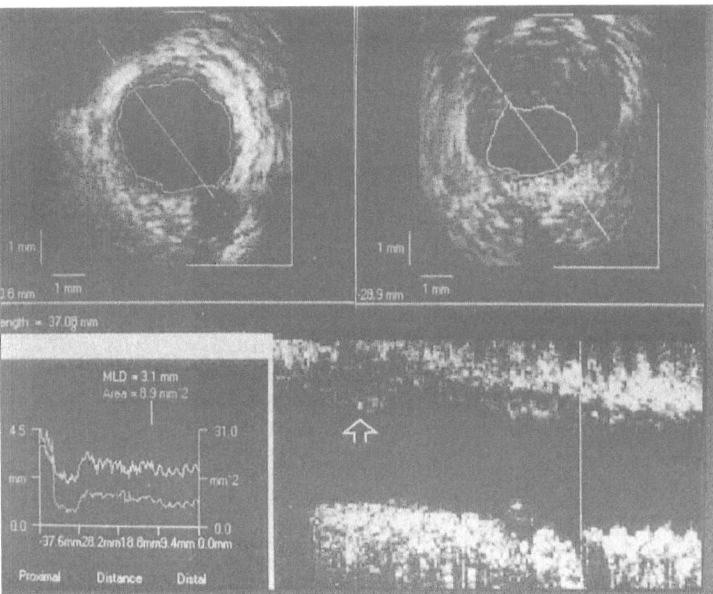

Figure 5. Three-dimensional reconstruction of a soft eccentric plaque prior to directional atherectomy. The plaque which is visible in the left region of the longitudinal image (arrow) causes narrowing of the proximal left anterior descending coronary artery. The measurements of cross-sectional luminal area and minimal luminal diameter (MLD) are presented in the left lower panel. They indicate clearly this circumscribed stenosis. In two transverse images cross-sections of the normal and the stenotic segment (left and right upper panel) are displayed. A contour indicates the lumen-intima boundary, automatically detected by application of the blood speckle identification algorithm. Note the side-branch (left upper and right lower panels), which is helpful in comparison of serial ICUS studies of the same coronary artery segment.

3-D ICUS, essential information on the ideal type and size of balloon or interventional device can be derived (Figure 5).

ANALYSIS OF PLAQUE COMPOSITION

ICUS has the unique potential to provide information on plaque composition. It detects calcification of the target lesion in 80% of the patients undergoing coronary angioplasty [25,26]. Information on calcification of the target stenosis is significant, as increased incidence, depth and circumferential extension of dissection after balloon dilatation has been reported in calcification of plaques [26-28].

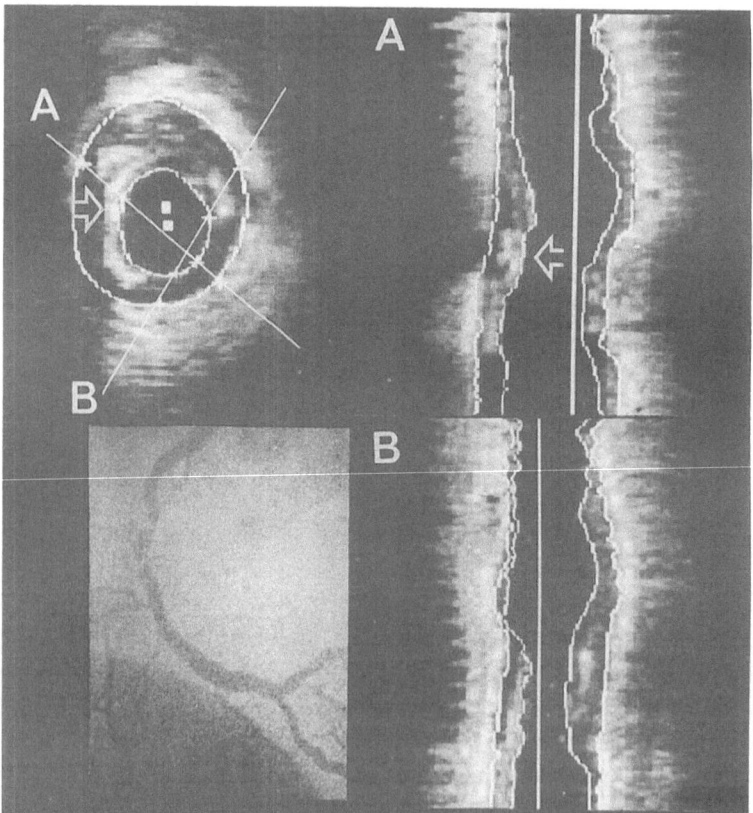

Figure 6. This stenotic segment of a right coronary artery shows target-lesion calcium (arrows). In the selected transverse image (left upper panel) the arc of calcium (approximately 120°) is displayed, shadowing the vessel wall. Information on the longitudinal distribution of the calcium can be obtained from the midpart of the longitudinal image A (right upper panel), reconstructed by use of the contour detection method.

After directional coronary atherectomy, a higher incidence of complications and a smaller amount of retrievable material can be observed in the presence of diffuse subendothelial calcification [29]. Three-dimensional ICUS allows visualization and quantification of the length of calcification in an entire coronary segment (Figure 6). It is superior to coronary angiography in detecting calcium and better than two-dimensional ICUS in showing the real extent of calcification in coronary plaques.

EVALUATION OF DISSECTIONS AFTER INTERVENTIONS

Diffuse disruption of the atherosclerotic plaque is one of the predominant mechanisms of lumen enlargement after balloon dilatation [30], but even in the presence of complex intraluminal flaps, angiographic filling defects are reported only in a minority of cases. Intravascular ultrasound is more sensitive in the detection of dissections after interventions [1,31-33]; however, the longitudinal extent of complex flaps cannot be displayed by conventional ICUS. As dissection plays has an important prognostic value in predicting immediate outcome and restenosis [34], studies of vessel trauma are of great clinical interest. From studies in peripheral and coronary arteries, it is known that the reconstruction of a longitudinal image facilitates the analysis of dissections [8,9]. Excellent agreement has been described between 3-D reconstruction of ICUS images and pathologic findings in the evaluation of length and depth of dissections after balloon angioplasty in arteries without diffuse intimal calcification [35]. On-line 3-D reconstruction of ICUS allows immediate assessment of the vessel wall changes such as dissection and plaque rupture induced by the operative mechanism of intracoronary interventions. Thus, 3-D ICUS can prove the need for adjunctive therapy as coronary stenting in extensive coronary dissection.

ASSESSMENT OF STENTING AND DIRECTIONAL ATHERECTOMY

Recent reports [36,37] have emphasized the usefulness of intravascular ultrasound in identifying true lumen and dissection length before stenting. Three-dimensional reconstruction of ICUS after stenting allows analysis of the dimensions of stents after implantation [38]. Detection of a moderate residual stenosis inside the stented coronary segment is difficult by angiography, but it carries potentially a higher risk of turbulence inside the stent, leading to thrombosis and long-term restenosis. The optimization of stent deployment by use of ICUS, however, practically eliminates the risk of acute or subacute stent thrombosis [39]. Detection of an incomplete stent deployment is facilitated by use of 3-D ICUS (Figure 7). Thus, segments of incomplete stent deployment with an increased risk of thrombosis can be much more easily identified.

Intravascular ultrasound is a clinically useful device in guidance of directional atherectomy or laser interventions [29,40,41]. 3-D reconstruction of ICUS facilitates the orientation of the cutter in relation to side-branches and the detection of deep or spiral cuts [42]. The clinical value of intravascular ultrasound in planning and guiding several trans-catheter techniques and the specific usefulness of on-line 3-D reconstruction has recently been reported [43].

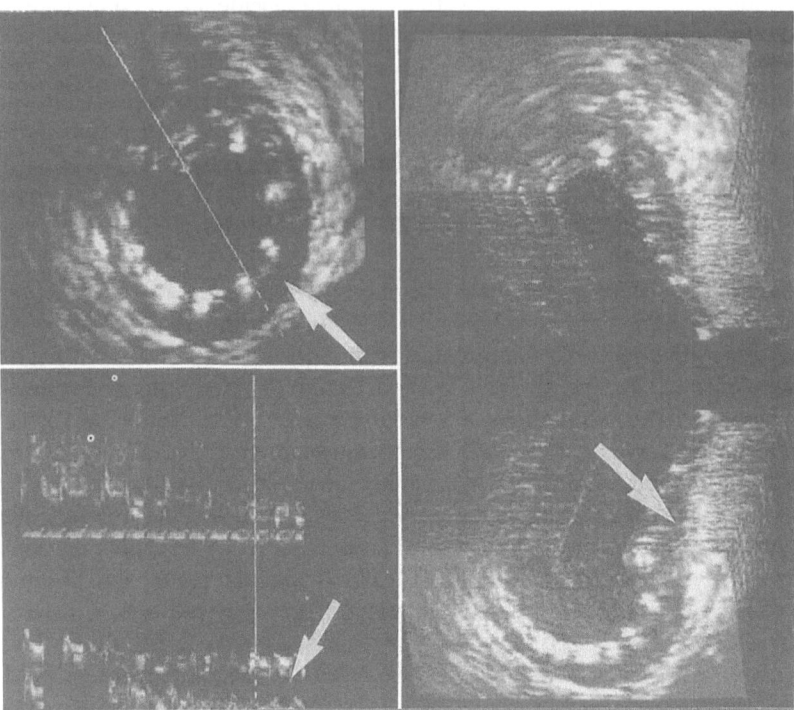

Figure 7. Three-dimensional reconstruction of intravascular ultrasound images can be used to visualize incomplete stent deployment, as shown in this example of a Wallstent in a left anterior descending coronary artery. The space between the struts of the stent and the vessel wall (arrows) has low echogenicy and is visible in the transverse image (left upper panel), the longitudinal image (left lower panel) and the 3-D view (right panel). Only the longitudinal image and the 3-D view show clearly that the incomplete stent deployment is limited to a part of the reconstructed vessel segment. A good result was achieved after balloon inflation at this site. Note the longitudinal strut artifact inside the lumen in the reconstructed longitudinal image (left lower panel, top) and the 3-D view (right panel, left side), which can now be avoided by use of a new 2.9 F ICUS catheter which is operating by use of a flexible rotating imaging cable.

PLAQUE ANALYSIS IN PROGRESSION / REGRESSION STUDIES

Volumetric ICUS measurement of lumen [7,14,15] and plaque [14,15,44] can be used for studies of changes in atherosclerotic plaques during progression/regression studies [45,46]. Using two-dimensional ICUS images, reliable evaluation of progression or regression depends critically on the correct matching of the sequentially acquired images. Application of 3-D reconstruction techniques, however, facilitates the analysis and promises to improve significantly the precision of serial measurements.

Limitations

The quality of three-dimensional reconstruction of ICUS images may be hampered by several circumstances, which are listed in Table 3. General limitations of ICUS as well as specific problems of 3-D reconstruction may render 3-D reconstruction difficult.

Table 3. Limitations of Three-Dimensional Reconstruction.

General Limitiations of Intracoronary Ultrasound

- Incomplete or poor definition of the lumen-plaque or plaque-adventitia boundaries is caused by high blood echogenicy or absence of a hypoechoic media
- Shadowing by calcium hides a part of the vessel wall
- Resolution properties of the current transducers are still limited
- Nonuniform rotation of the transducer may cause inaccuracies
- Noncoaxial position of the cathereter may cause elliptical image distortion
- Eccentric position of the transducer may distort the shape of the vessel lumen
- Plaques may be compressed by catheters, especially at vessel curvatures

---

Specific Limitations of 3-D Reconstruction

- Catheter bends affect precision of pull-back, causing discrepancies between the pull-back speed of the proximal part of the catheter and the transducer tip
- Cyclic (saw-fish) movement artifacts hamper the longitudinal contour detection
- Prolonged acquisition time is required in ECG-gated image acquisition
- Vessel curvatures create artificial curvatures in the longitudinal reconstruction
- An artificially straightened disiplay of the 3-D view is provided by some 3-D programs
- Rotation of the cathether during pull-back creates mismatch between structures, visible in adjacent intracoronary ultrasound images

---

QUALITY OF THE BASIC IMAGES AND THE IMAGE ACQUISITION

The quality of the basic two-dimensional ICUS images is (as mentioned above) crucial. An insufficient or incomplete circumferential representation of the lumen-plaque boundary or the plaque-adventitia interface hampers volumetric measurements of lumen and plaque. Calcium may conceal a part of the vessel wall [47]. Current ultrasound probes show a good lateral resolution in the near field, but it deteriorates rapidly in the far field. The lateral and out-of-plane resolution is furthermore limited by the dimensions of the piezoelectric crystal [48]. The use of a limited number of cross-sections for reconstruction of a longitudinal plane further reduces the accuracy of the 3-D reconstruction. Image distortions by nonuniform rotation of the ICUS transducer or by a noncoaxial position of the catheter inside the coronary artery are able to create complex artifacts in the 3-D ICUS images [11].

        During acquisition of the basic conventional ICUS images, another inaccuracy can be caused by the motorized pull-back. Motorized pull-back devices or sensors, which measure the catheter displacement, are used in order to yield an equal space between adjacent two-dimensional ICUS images. However, this cannot perfectly be achieved, since the presence of bends of the ultrasound catheter may induce differences between the movement of the distal transducer and the proximal end of the ICUS catheter.

PLAQUE COMPRESSION AND CYCLIC MOVEMENT ARTIFACTS

Compression of plaques by the ICUS catheter at a vessel curvature may result in an underestimation of the measurements from the 3-D reconstructed image. Use of a new forward locking transducer could help to overcome this limitation [6], but application of these device is still limited by low resolution and large dimensions of the transducer.

        The movement of the ICUS catheter during the cardiac cycle and systolic-diastolic changes in vessel dimensions create a typical saw-fish aspect of the vessel wall, which is more evident in arteries with large mobility such as mid-right coronary artery and bypass grafts. However, the extent of these artifacts differs from one patient to the other. Since the movement of a coronary artery is usually more intense in a certain plane, differences in the amplitude of the movement artifact can be found even in the reconstructed longitudinal 3-D view of the same coronary artery, which depend indeed on the selected orientation of the longitudinal cut-plane. Thus, rotation of the longitudinal cut-plane may sometimes improve the quality of the displayed longitudinal 3-D image.

ECG-GATED METHODS

ECG-gated pull-back devices and ECG-gated off-line image acquisition from a continuously recorded video tape provide the potential to minimize these artifacts [11]. In order to avoid a reduction of resolution, it will presumably be required to reduce the speed of the pull-back Resulting prolongation of image acquisition and subsequent myocardial ischemia may not be tolerated before intervention in some critically symptomatic patients with very severely obstructed coronary arteries.

SPATIAL ORIENTATION AND ROTATION OF THE ICUS CATHETER

The vessel curvatures cause a distortion of the 3-D image which is reconstructed along a straight line, passing through the individual center of the lumen in the cross-sectional images. Thus, certain over- or underestimation of plaque regions may be caused by catheter bending. Other 3-D reconstruction systems display the coronary segment in an artificially straightened way. Combined use of simultaneously performed biplane angiography and ICUS may help to improve the control of the spatial orientation of the catheter tip and to overcome these problem in the future.

Rotation of the ICUS catheter during pull-back can also cause a mismatch between the orientation of sequential images. As a potential method for the assessment of the catheter orientation, a miniaturized receiving antenna, fixed at the distal tip of the ICUS catheter, and an external electromagnetic transmit antenna, which should be in a plane perpendicular to the ICUS catheter axis, have been suggested [41].

Conclusions

Three-dimensional reconstruction of ICUS images requires a sequence of procedural steps, including image acquisition and segmentation, which are the most crucial steps concerning the quality of the final reconstruction. Image acquisition and quality can be improved by ECG-gating. During the segmentation step, discrimination between the blood-pool inside the lumen and structures of the vessel wall is performed in the digitized images. This can be achieved by two principal approaches. A blood-speckle identification method detects the blood-pool by statistical pattern recognition, but no quantitative information on the plaque dimensions are provided. The system can be used on-line even in very irregular lumen shapes without user interaction; however, image quality may limit the feasibility of this technique. In contrast to this approach, a contour detection method performs the segmentation by the application of a minimum-cost algorithm, permitting measurement of coronary lumen and plaque. Particularly in very irregular lumen shapes some user interaction is required. Therefore on-line use of this technique could not yet be achieved. Both complementary methods of segmentation provide specific advantages and limitations, defining their favored application in clinical practice. During and after intracoronary interventions on-line 3-D ICUS can be very helpful in displaying the characteristics of coronary plaques and guiding interventions. Since off-line 3-D reconstruction of the basic ICUS images provides accurate and reproducible area and volume measurements of coronary lumen and plaque, the method permits quantification of volumetric changes in coronary plaque during progression-regression studies of atherosclerosis or scientific studies on intracoronary interventions. Development of ICUS imaging systems with higher resolution and less artifacts is an important challenge for the future, since it will facilitate the application of segmentation algorithms for blood subtraction and detection of coronary lumen and plaque but also increase the accuracy of ICUS assessment. Although several limitations of ICUS and the 3-D reconstruction remain to be solved in the coming years, 3-D ICUS has the capability of addressing several questions of fundamental interest. Clinical experience indicates even now a great potential and usefulness, as 3-D ICUS provides both unique visualization and measurement of coronary plaque and/or lumen.

References

1.   Nissen SE, Gurley JC, Grines CL, et al. Intravascular ultrasound assessment of lumen size and wall morphology in normal subjects and patients with coronary artery disease. Circulation 1991;84:1087-99.

2.   Ge J, Erbel R, Rupprecht H-J, et al. Comparison of intravascular ultrasound and angiography in the assessment of myocardial bridging. Circulation 1994;89:1725-32.

3.   Hausmann D, Friedrich G, Sudhir K, et al. 3D intravascular ultrasound imaging with automated border detection using 2.9 F catheters. J Am Coll Cardiol 1994;23:174A.

4.   Koch L, Kearney P, Erbel R, et al. Three-dimensional reconstruction of intracoronary ultrasound images: Roadmapping with simultaneously digitised coronary angiograms. IEEE Proc Comp Cardiol 1993;89-91.

5.   Li W, Bosch JG, Zhong Y, et al. Image segmentation and 3D reconstruction of intravascular ultrasound images. Acoustic Imaging 1993;20:489-96.

6.   Ng K-H, Evans JL, Vonesh MJ, et al. Arterial imaging with a new forward-viewing intravascular ultrasound catheter, II. Three-dimensional reconstruction and display of data. Circulation 1994;89:718-23.

7.   Matar FA, Mintz GS, Douek PC, Leon MB, Popma JJ. Three-dimensional intravascular ultrasound: A new standard for vessel lumen volume measurements? J Am Coll Cardiol 1992;19:382A.

8.   Rosenfield K, Kaufman J, Losordo DW, Isner JM. Lumen cast analysis: a quantitative format to expedite on-line analysis of 3D-intravascular ultrasound images. J Am Coll Cardiol 1992;19:115A.

9.   Rosenfield K, Kaufman J, Pieczek A, Langevin RE, Razvi S, Ilsner JM. Real-time three-dimensional reconstruction of intravascular ultrasound images of iliac arteries. Am J Cardiol 1992;70:412-15.

10. Rosenfield K, Losordo DW, Ramaswamy K, Isner JM. Three-dimensional reconstruction of human coronary and peripheral arteries from images recorded during two-dimensional intravascular ultrasound examination. Circulation 1991;84:1938-56.

11. Roelandt JRTC, Di Mario C, Pandian NG,et al. Three-dimensional reconstruction of intracoronary ultrasound images: Rationale, approaches, problems and directions. Circulation 1994;90:1044-55.

12. Mintz GS, Keller MB, Fay FG: Motorized IVUS transducer pull-back permits accurate quantitative axial measurements. Circulation 1992;86:I-323.

13. Gussenhoven EJ, van der Lugt A, van Strijen M, et al. Displacement sensing device enabling accurate documentation of catheter tip position. In: Roelandt JRTC, Gussenhoven EJ, Bom N, editors. Intravascular Ultrasound. Dordrecht: Kluwer Academic Publishers, 1993:157-66.

14. von Birgelen C, Di Mario C, Li W, et al. Volumetric quantification in intracoronary ultrasound: validation of a new automatic contour detection method with integrated

user interaction. Circulation 1994;90:I-550.

15. Li W, von Birgelen C, Di Mario C, et al. Semi-automatic contour detection for volumetric quantification of intracoronary ultrasound. In: Computers in Cardiology 1994. Los Alamitos: IEEE Computer Society Press, 1994; in press.

16. Li W, Gussenhoven EJ, Zhong Y, et al. Temporal averaging for quantification of lumen dimensions in intravascular ultrasound images. Ultrasound in Med & Biol 1994;20:117-22.

17. Kitney R, Moura L, Straughan K. 3-D visualization of arterial structures using ultrasound and voxel modelling. Int J Cardiac Imag 1989;4:135-43.

18. Di Mario C, The SHK, Madretsma S, et al. Detection and characterization of vascular lesions by intravascular ultrasound: An in-vitro correlative study with histology. J Am Soc Echocardiogr 1992;19:135-46.

19. Di Mario C, Wilson R, Gussenhoven EJ, Serruys PW, Verdouw PD, Roelandt JRTC. Norepinephrine-induced decrease in large artery compliance. Eur Heart J 1992;13:394.

20. Li W, Bosch JG, Zhong Y, et al. Image segmentation and 3D reconstruction of intravascular ultrasound images. Acoustic Imaging 1993;20:489-96.

21. Li W, Gussenhoven EJ, Zhong Y, et al. Validation of quantitative analysis of intravascular ultrasound images. Int J Cardiac Imag 1991;6:247-54.

22. The SHK, Gussenhoven EJ, Zhong Y, et al. Effect of balloon angioplasty on femoral artery evaluated with intravascular ultrasound imaging. Circulation 1992; 86:483-93.

23. Tenaglia AN, Buller CE, Kisslo KB, Stack RS, Davidson CJ. Mechanisms of balloon angioplasty and directional coronary atherectomy as assessed by intracoronary ultrasound. J Am Coll Cardiol 1992;20:685-91.

24. Losordo DW, Rosenfield K, Pieczek A, Baker K, Harding M, Isner JM. How does angioplasty work? Serial analysis of human iliac arteries using intravascular ultrasound. Circulation 1992; 86:1845-58.

25. Mintz GS, Douek P, Pichard AD, et al. Target lesion calcification in coronary artery disease. J Am Coll Cardiol 1992;20:1149-55.

26. Honye J, Mahon DJ, White CJ, et al. Morphological effects of coronary balloon angioplasty in vivo assessed by intravascular ultrasound imaging. Circulation 1992; 85:1012-25.

27. Fitzgerald PJ, Ports TA, Yock PG. Contribution of localized calcium deposits to dissection after angioplasty. An observational study using intravascular ultrasound. Circulation 1992;86:64-70.

28. Potkin BN, Keren G, Mintz GS, et al. Arterial response to balloon coronary angioplasty: An intravascular ultrasound study. J Am Coll Cardiol 1992;20:942-51.

29. Kimura BJ, Fitzgerald PJ, Sudhir K, Amidon TM, Strunk BL, Yock PG. Guidance of directional coronary atherectomy by intracoronary ultrasound imaging. Am Heart J 1992;124:1365-1369.

30. Waller BF. Coronary balloon artery dissections: "The good, the bad and the ugly." J Am Coll Cardiol 1992;20:701-06.

31. Tobis JM, Mallery JA, Mahon D, et al. Intravascular ultrasound imaging of human arteries in vivo. Circulation 1991;83:913-26.

32. Werner GS, Sold G, Buchwald A, Wiegand V. Intravascular ultrasound imaging of human coronary arteries after percutaneous transluminal angioplasty: Morphologic and quantitative assessment. Am Heart J 1991;122:212-20.

33. Gussenhoven WJ, Frietman P, The SHK, et al. Assessment of medial thinning in atherosclerosis with intravascular ultrasound. Am J Cardiol 1991;68:625-32.

34. Tenaglia AN, Buller CE, Kisslo KB, Phillips HR, Stack RS. Intracoronary ultrasound predictors of adverse outcomes after coronary artery interventions. J Am Coll Cardiol 1992;20:1385-90.

35. Coy KM, Park JC, Fishbein MC, et al. In vitro validation of three-dimensional intravascular ultrasound for the evaluation of arterial injury after balloon angioplasty. J Am Coll Cardiol 1992;20:692-700.

36. Cavaye DM, White RA, Lerman RD, et al. Usefulness of intravascular ultrasound imaging for detecting experimentally induced aortic dissection in dogs and for determining the effectiveness of endoluminal stenting. Am J Cardiol 1992;69:705-7.

37. Schryver TE, Popma JJ, Kent KM, Leon MB, Mintz GS. Use of intracoronary ultrasound to identify the true coronary lumen in chronic coronary dissection treated with intracoronary stenting. Am J Cardiol 1992;69:107-8.

38. Mintz GS, Leon MB, Popma JJ, Kent KM. Three-dimensional reconstruction of endovascular stents. J Am Coll Cardiol 1992;19:224A.

39. Colombo A, Hall P, Almagor Y, et al. Results of intravascular ultrasound guided coronary stenting without subsequent anticoagulation. J Am Col Cardiol 1994:335A.

40. Yock PG, Fitzgerald PJ, Linker DT, Angelsen BAJ. Intravascular ultrasound guidance for catheter-based coronary interventions. J Am Coll Cardiol 1991;17:39B-45B.

41. Aretz HT, Gregory KW, Martinelli MA, Gregg RE, Ledet EG, Haase WC. Ultrasound guidance of laser atherectomy. Int J Cardiac Imag 1991;6:231-37.

42. Smucker ML, Kil D, Sarnat WS, Howard PF. Is three-dimensional reconstruction a gimmick or a useful clinical tool? Experience in coronary atherectomy. J Am Coll Cardiol 1992;19:115A.

43. Mintz GS, Leon MB, Satler LF, Kent KM, Pichard AD. Pre-intervention ultrasound imaging influences transcatheter coronary treatment strategies. Circulation 1992;86:I-323.

44. Galli FC, Sudhir K, Kao AK, Fitgerald PJ, Yock PG. Direct measurement of plaque volume by three-dimensional ultrasound: potential and pitfalls. J Am Coll Cardiol 1992;19:115A.

45. Gupta M, Connolly AJ, Zhu BQ, et al. Quantitative analysis of progression and regression of atherosclerosis by intravascular ultrasound: Validation in a rabbit model. Circulation 1992;86:I-518.

46. Lassetter JE, Krall RC, Moddrelle DS, Jenkins RD. Morphologic changes of the arterial wall during regression of experimental atherosclerosis. Circulation

1992;86:I-518.

47.   Di Mario C, Madrestma S, Linker D, et al. The angle of incidence of the ultrasonic beam: A critical factor for the image quality in intravascular ultrasound. Am Heart J 1993;125:442-48.

48.   Benkeser PJ, Churchwell AL, Lee C, Abouelnasr DM. Resolution limitations in intravascular ultrasound imaging. J Am Soc Echocardiogr 1993;6:158-65.

METABOLIC BASIS OF THE ATHEROGENIC LIPOPROTEIN PHENOTYPE

C.J. Packard and J. Shepherd
Institute of Biochemistry
Glasgow Royal Infirmary
Glasgow, GF OSF
UNITED KINGDOM

Introduction

Plasma triglyceride exhibits a strong positive association over the normal range with low density lipoprotein (LDL) cholesterol and an equally strong negative association with high density lipoproteins (HDL). These relationships, the result of metabolic links that exist between all lipoproteins in the circulation, confound classical statistical analyses and in her elegant study Austin [1] explains how the statistical approach used in multivariate regression cannot distinguish the relative importance of closely related variables, especially when one--plasma triglyceride--is measured with much less precision than the other--HDL. More recent epidemiological surveys [2] find that plasma triglyceride persists as a risk marker even when confounding factors are taken into account and the emerging consensus view which has been incorporated into new guidelines from the European Atherosclerosis Society (EAS) for the prevention of coronary disease [3] is that moderately elevated triglycerides associated with a low HDL cholesterol level predispose to increased risk of coronary disease. Furthermore the Helsinki Heart Study demonstrated that the lowering of triglyceride levels with an attendant rise in HDL cholesterol results in clinical benefit [4]. Plasma triglyceride is thought to increase CHD risk through both direct and indirect mechanisms. Examples of the former are the observations that chylomicrons and VLDL promote thrombosis and when incubated with endothelial cells *in vitro* cause dysfunction and toxicity. The discussion which follows explores the metabolic links between triglyceride-rich lipoproteins, LDL, and HDL and seeks to explain how even a moderate plasma triglyceride elevation can lead indirectly to enhanced atherogenesis.

Impact of Raised Plasma Triglyceride Levels on High Density Lipoprotein Metabolism

A considerable body of evidence indicates that low plasma levels of HDL cholesterol are associated with increased risk of atherosclerosis. However, the metabolic processes that

A.M. Gotto et al. (eds.), Multiple Risk Factors in Cardiovascular Disease, 289-294.

result in a low HDL level are unclear. As noted above, the concentration of the lipoprotein is inversely correlated with plasma triglyceride and explanations of this relationship have been sought for a number of years. HDL is partly derived from the metabolism of chylomicrons and VLDL and it has been postulated that in hypertriglyceridemic individuals failure of lipolysis leads to decreased synthesis of HDL particles. However, there is little evidence to support this hypothesis. HDL apoprotein A production is normal in people with raised triglyceride levels [5,6] and it is the enhanced fractional catabolic rate (FCR) of apoAI and apoAII that causes a reduction in the HDL concentration. The recent, elegant work by Brinton et al. [6] confirmed in our own studies [7] of normal and diabetic men demonstrated that a number of plasma-lipid parameters were related to the FCR of apoA1, in particular the HDL cholesterol:total apoA ratio. This is an index of HDL particle size and is related to the HDL subfraction distribution, a higher HDL cholesterol:apoA ratio being a reflection of higher HDL_2 levels. A scheme showing current concepts of the relationship between plasma triglyceride and HDL metabolism is given in Figure 1.

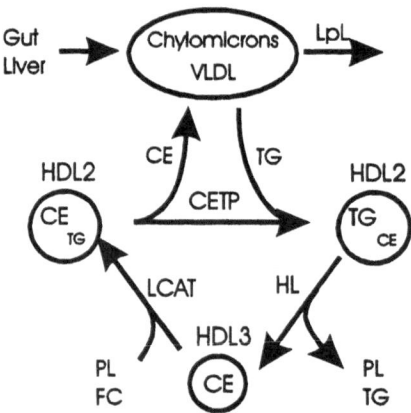

Figure 1. Triglyceride-rich lipoproteins, lipases, and HDL metabolism.

LpL is the key enzyme regulating the hydrolysis of triglyceride in chylomicrons and VLDL. In people with high LpL activity the plasma levels of triglyceride-rich lipoproteins are low and this limits the extent of neutral-lipid exchange occurring in the circulation. Thus HDL remains large (i.e. increased HDL_2 levels), relatively cholesterol-rich, and has (for as yet unknown reasons) a reduced catabolic rate. When LpL activity is low or the synthesis of large triglyceride-rich VLDL particles is stimulated, increased CETP-mediated exchange generates triglyceride-enriched HDL which are a better substrate for hepatic lipase (HL). The action of this enzyme removes lipid from the core of HDL reducing its size and results in the conversion of HDL_2 to HDL_3 [8]. Smaller HDL are catabolized more rapidly than their larger counterparts and plasma concentration falls. Lecithin:cholesterol acyl transferase (LCAT) acts in the opposite direction. When lipolysis is active, for example, in a person with high LpL, redundant surface components, phospholipid and unesterified cholesterol are shed by triglyceride-rich lipoproteins into the HDL density range. LCAT generates cholesteryl esters from these components, expands the core of HDL, and favors the formation of HDL_2 from HDL_3. Thus the triglyceride synthesis rate and the activities of LpL, HL, and LCAT control HDL size, the HDL_2:HDL_3 ratio, HDL apoprotein plasma-clearance rates, and hence the amount of this lipoprotein present in the bloodstream to mediate the process of reverse cholesterol transport.

Impact of Raised Plasma Triglyceride Levels on Low Density Lipoprotein Metabolism

VLDL is the metabolic precursor to LDL. Through a series of delipidation steps the former loses its triglyceride core and most of its surface phospholipid and apolipoproteins (apoC and apoE but not apoB which remains with the lipoprotein). Concomitantly, the particle gains cholesteryl ester via a process of neutral lipid exchange so that the end-product is a complex of solubilized cholesterol and apolipoprotein B. Not surprisingly the metabolism of LDL is closely linked to that of VLDL; however, the relationship is not that of a simple precursor and product. Both species are heterogeneous and different forms of VLDL give rise to varying LDL products which appear to have distinct structural and metabolic properties.

In a recent study [9] we examined the metabolic basis of the 50% rise in LDL cholesterol as plasma triglyceride levels increase from the bottom (0.5 mmol/l) to the top (2.3 mmol/l) of the normal range. When the results of LDL turnovers were derived by standard methods it appeared that as plasma triglyceride levels rose, the catabolic rate of the lipoprotein (i.e. the fractional catabolic rate or FCR in pools per day) fell. However, a more detailed analysis using multicompartmental modelling of both the plasma and the urine data revealed a different, more complex picture. It was found that LDL exhibited metabolic heterogeneity that could be explained by the presence in plasma of two pools of independent behavior. Pool A was cleared rapidly, probably by the specific cell membrane LDL receptor, whereas pool B LDL was removed relatively slowly. As plasma triglyceride rose, the proportion of pool B LDL increased in the circulation and thus the overall fractional catabolic rate (i.e. of A + B) fell. This rise in pool B LDL was due to an increase in its production. In separate experiments [10] investigating the VLDL to LDL conversion we noted that LDL derived from large, triglyceride-rich VLDL exhibited a slow FCR while that produced from the delipidation of small VLDL had a rapid clearance rate. Combining this finding with the earlier observations we hypothesized that in normal subjects when hepatic triglyceride synthesis is enhanced, an increased amount of large triglyceride-rich VLDL is produced and plasma triglyceride levels rise. As this VLDL is converted to an LDL which is inefficiently removed, LDL cholesterol levels rise also.

The impact of triglyceride lowering on LDL metabolic heterogeneity has also been investigated recently in our laboratory [11]. Turnovers were performed on subjects with moderately elevated plasma cholesterol and triglyceride levels in the untreated state and then after eight weeks of fibrate (fenofibrate) therapy. The drug reduced plasma triglyceride by 35% and decreased the proportion of pool B LDL from 63% to 51% of the total by inhibiting its synthesis. This action of fibrates was postulated to arise from their ability to inhibit the production of large triglyceride-rich VLDL.

It is likely that the metabolic heterogeneity observed in these studies is caused by an underlying structural heterogeneity. Krauss [12] has shown that LDL can be separated by size into three or four species. In some individuals large LDL predominates (Pattern A) whereas in others smaller particles are most abundant (Pattern B). The latter profile has been shown [13] to be associated with moderately elevated plasma triglycerides and a low HDL cholesterol in a dyslipidemic syndrome, termed the atherogenic lipoprotein phenotype (ALP). Case-control studies indicated that the presence of Pattern B profile for LDL was associated with an increased risk of myocardial infarction regardless of the plasma cholesterol level [13].

Indeed an ALP was one of the commonest lipid abnormalities seen in patients with angiographically proven CHD. Recent investigations [12,14,15] have begun to uncover the factors that predispose to the generation of small, dense LDL in the circulation. Plasma triglyceride is the major controlling factor and when this reaches a level in excess of 1.5 mmol/l, pattern B becomes the rule rather than the exception. The activities of lipoprotein lipase and hepatic lipase are also important (Figure 2).

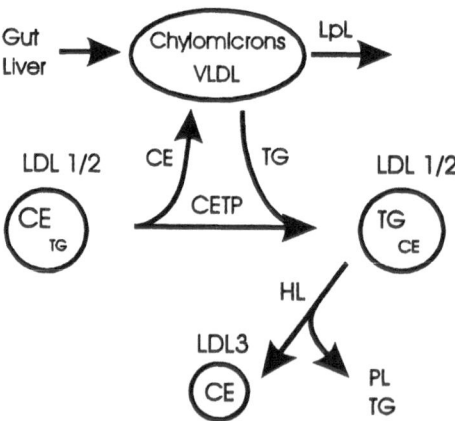

Figure 2. Triglyceride-rich lipoproteins and LDL remodelling. As plasma triglyceride levels rise, transfer via CETP to larger, cholesteryl-ester-rich LDL results in the latter becoming a better substrate for hepatic lipase. Action of the enzyme causes loss of core lipid and shrinkage of the LDL to a small, dense species.

When the latter is high there is increased concentration of small, dense LDL even at lower plasma triglyceride concentrations. Thus the metabolic basis of an ALP is increased $VLDL_1$ synthesis and/or increased HL activity leading to the generation of small, dense LDL with a slow clearance rate and small, dense HDL with a rapid clearance rate.

The LDL subfraction profile is perturbed by lipid-lowering and other drugs in a predictable manner depending on their actions on lipoprotein and hepatic lipase, plasma triglyceride levels and LDL receptors (Figure 2). Drugs that lower plasma triglyceride levels, e.g. nicotinic acid [6] and fibrates (e.g. fenofibrate [11]), shift the spectrum towards less dense particles. In contrast, activation of LDL receptors by statins or bile acid sequestrant resins tends to reduce LDL-I and LDL-II specifically due to increased receptor-mediated clearance of these subfractions [17].

Clinical Importance of an ALP

In the moderate hypercholesterolemia range (cholesterol 6.5-8.0 mmol/l) plasma and LDL cholesterol are not particularly good predictors of CHD. Measurement of plasma triglyceride and HDL levels and, when possible, the LDL subfraction profile can greatly improve the identification of subjects at risk. Austin et al. [13] found that the existence of Pattern B LDL profile was associated with a three-fold risk of an MI and in our own study [18], an LDL-III concentration in excess of 100 mg/dl was associated with a seven-fold increase in risk even at plasma cholesterol levels of 6.0 mmol/l, which would otherwise be unremarkable. Current arguments about the benefits and potential risks of treating relatively modest elevations in plasma and LDL cholesterol center around the fact that these parameters are poor predictors. Better discrimination of those at-risk enables a more rational approach to primary and secondary prevention of CHD.

Acknowledgements

We acknowledge the excellent secretarial assistance of Mrs. Nancy Thomson in the preparation of this manuscript. The authors' cited research was supported by a grant from the British Heart Foundation (190/1242).

References

1. Austin MA. Plasma triglyceride and coronary heart disease. Arterioscler Thomb 1991;11:2-14.
2. Bainton D, Miller NE, Bolton CH, et al. Plasma triglyceride and high-density-lipoprotein cholesterol as predictors of ischaemic heart disease in British men. Br Heart J 1992;68:60-66.
3. European Atherosclerosis Society: Prevention of coronary heart disease. Scientific background and new clinical guidelines. Nutr Metab Cardio Dis 1992;2:113-156.
4. Manninen V, Elo O, Frick H, et al. Lipid alterations and decline in the incidence of coronary heart disease in the Helsinki Heart Study. JAMA 1988;260:641-651.
5. Shepherd J, Packard CJ. High-density lipoprotein apolipoprotein metabolism. In: Miller NE, Miller GJ, editors. Clinical and metabolic aspects of high density lipoproteins. Amsterdam: Elsevier Publishers, 1984:247-274.
6. Brinton EA, Eisenberg S, Breslow JL. Increased apo AI and AII fractional catabolic rate in patients with low high-density lipoprotein cholesterol with or without hypertriglyceridaemia. J Clin Invest 1991;87:536-544.

7.   Taskinen M-R, Kahri J, Koivisto V, et al. Metabolism of HDL apolipoprotein A-I
        and A-II in type 1 (insulin dependent) diabetes mellitus. Diabetologia 992;35:347-
        356.
8.   Shepherd J, Packard CJ. Effects of diet and drugs on high-density lipoprotein
        metabolism. Atherosclerosis Rev 1987;16:181-206.
9.   Caslake MJ, Packard CJ, Series JJ, et al. Plasma triglyceride and low-density
        lipoprotein metabolism. Europ J Clin Invest 1992;22:96-104.
10.   Demant T, Bedford D, Packard CJ, et al. Influence of apolipoprotein E
        polymorphism on apolipoprotein B100 metabolism in normolipaemic subjects. J
        Clin Invest 1991;88:1490-1501.
11.   Caslake MJ, Packard CJ, Gaw A, et al. Fenofibrate and LDL metabolic
        heterogeneity in hypercholesterolaemia. Arterioscler Thromb 1993;13:702-711.
12.   Krauss RM. Low density lipoprotein subclasses and risk of coronary heart disease.
        Curr Opin Lipidol 1991;2:248-252.
13.   Austin MA, King MC, Vranigan KM, et al. Atherogenic lipoprotein phenotype. A
        proposed genetic marker for coronary heart disease risk. Circulation 1990;82:495-
        506.
14.   Zambon A, Austin MA, Brown BG, Hokanson JE, Brunzell JD. Effect of hepatic
        lipase on LDL in normal men and those with coronary artery disease. Arterioscler
        Thromb 1993;13:147-153.
15.   Griffin BA, Caslake MJ, Yip B, et al. Rapid isolation of low density lipoprotein
        subfractions from plasma by density gradient ultracentrifugation. Atherosclerosis
        1990;83:59-67.
16.   Superko HR, Krauss RM. Differential effects of nicotinic acid on subjects with
        different LDL subclass patterns. Atherosclerosis 1992;95:69-76.
17.   Gaw A, Packard CJ, Murray EF, et al. Effects of simvastatin on apoB metabolism
        and LDL subfraction distribution. Arterioscler Thromb 1993;13:170-189.
18.   Griffin BA, Freeman DJ, Tait GW, et al. Role of plasma triglyceride in the
        regulation of plasma low density lipoprotein (LDL) subfractions: Relative
        contribution of small, dense LDL to coronary heart disease risk. Atherosclerosis
        1994;106:241-253.

FIBRATES: MODES OF ACTION

Alberico L. Catapano
Institute of Pharmacological Science and
Centro per lo Studio, la Prevenzione e
la Terapia delle Vasculopatie Aterosclerotiche
University of Milan
Milan
ITALY

Summary

Fibrates are a class of hypolipidemic drugs that effectively reduce plasma triglyceride and cholesterol levels, but also increase HDL cholesterol. In recent years the attention of pharmacologists and clinicians to fibrates has been renewed, especially in the light of the results of prospective studies and of the multifaceted action on plasma lipids as well as on factors modulating the thrombotic homeostasis in blood. The mechanisms of actions underlying these effects are discussed in this brief article.

Introduction

Fibrates are a class of hypolipidemic compounds that effectively reduce plasma triglyceride and cholesterol levels and in many instances increase plasma high density lipoprotein levels (for a review see [1]).

The parent compound, clofibrate, was discovered during the screening of aryloxyacetic acid derivatives and was licensed for human use in 1962. Since then second- and third-generation compounds have been developed with higher potency and fewer side effects. Among them are bezafibrate, ciprofibrate, etrofibrate, fenofibrate, and gemfibrozil (see Figure 1).

Although there are some differences in the mode of action of these drugs it is generally agreed that the results observed with one compound are, in principle, applicable to the others.

In this short review attention is devoted to the action of fibrates on specific steps of lipid and lipoprotein metabolism. Individual differences among drugs will be discussed. The final part of this review will briefly address the action of fibrates on factors modulating thrombotic homeostasis in the blood.

A.M. Gotto et al. (eds.), Multiple Risk Factors in Cardiovascular Disease, 295-306.

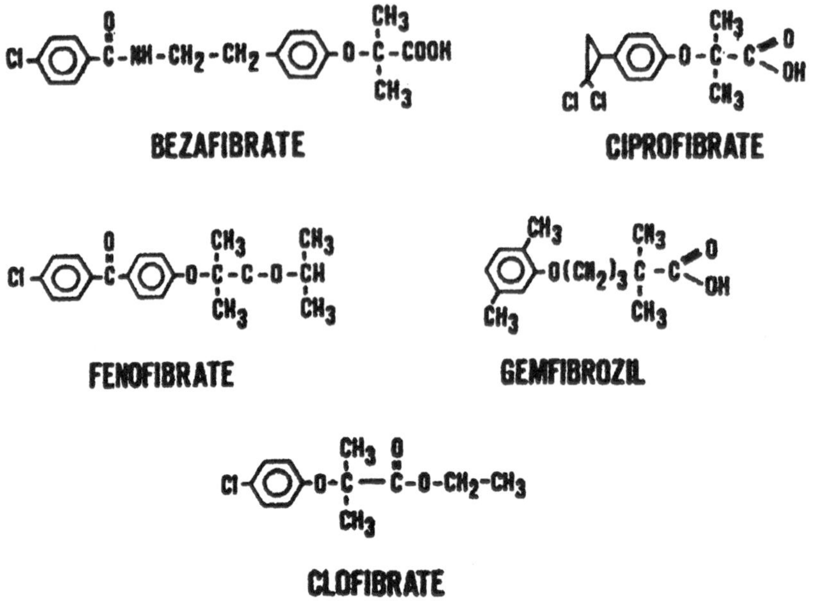

Figure 1. Chemical structures of the major available fibrates.

Mode of Action

EFFECTS ON PLASMA TRIGLYCERIDES

Synthesis. The reduction of plasma triglycerides (TG) which follows fibrate therapy may depend upon either decreased production, increased catabolism, or a combination of the two mechanisms.

Availability of fatty acids has a strong influence on the rate of TG and very low density lipoprotein (VLDL) production by the liver, *in vitro* and *in vivo* [2-4] and can probably control the secretion of apo B containing lipoproteins from the liver. Clofibrate as well as other fibrates lower fasting levels of free fatty acids (FFA) in man and blunt the adrenalin-induced release from adipose tissue [5-7]. These effects result in a decreased supply of FFA to the liver in the fasting state. Furthermore fibrates inhibit the liver acetyl CoA-carboxylase, the rate-limiting enzyme in the synthesis of fatty acids [8-10]. These effects combined should result in a reduced production of TG after fibrate treatment. Indeed *in vitro* and *in vivo* data in animals and man have confirmed this finding.

A second mechanism by which fibrates may interfere with plasma triglycerides production is by reducing lipid absorption and/or chylomicron formation. Several data, including studies on the postprandial phase suggest that this is the case (see section of postprandial lipedemia). Although these findings are of paramount relevance in understanding the mechanism of action of fibrates, only a few studies have directly addressed this point and many more are required to fully understand the relevance of this mechanism to the overall hypotriglyceridemic effect of fibrates.

Catabolism. There is now general agreement that a major effect of fibrates on plasma triglycerides is to promote their catabolism. A number of studies have shown that treatment with these drugs increases the utilization of TG-rich lipoprotein by peripheral tissues by increasing the activity of lipoprotein lipase in skeletal muscle and/or adipose tissue [11-14]. Some fibrates, but not all, also increase the hepatic lipase activity [11-13]. This latter effect should result in a more rapid conversion of HDL_2 to HDL_3, the former being a subpopulation of the HDL that is believed to promote the release of cholesterol from HDL to the liver [15-16]. The effect of fibrates on lipoprotein lipase also explains the paradoxical increase of low density lipoprotein (LDL) cholesterol in hypertriglyceridemic patients after fibrate therapy [17,18]. In several forms of hypertriglyceridemia, LDL are enriched with TG; in these subjects, therefore, the LDL cholesterol is lower than expected, compared with LDL protein (apo B) [19,20]. Normalization of the TG-rich lipoprotein catabolism restores the normal LDL composition, thus increasing LDL cholesterol in subjects with high plasma triglycerides and low LDL cholesterol [17,18]. This increase of LDL cholesterol is not seen in hypercholesterolemic subjects treated with fibrates, and is in agreement with the concept that fibrates restore a normal composition in lipoproteins enriched with triglycerides. Recently, LDL subclasses have been described that might bear relevance to the cardiovascular risk of a subject: "small" LDLs are believed to be more "atherogenic" than "large" LDLs [21]. Fibrates appear to interfere with this pattern in a favorable way (i.e. by reducing the small LDL) [22]. More studies, however, are required for a more detailed understanding of the clinical relevance of this observation.

EFFECTS ON CHOLESTEROL

Synthesis and Esterification. Although the hypocholesterolemic activity of clofibrate and its analogues is less dramatic than its effect on plasma triglycerides, it is a constant finding in animal models and certain forms of human hyperlipidemia [1,22].

Several authors have suggested an effect of clofibrate and analogues on cholesterol synthesis. This is true *in vitro*, although at very high doses [23,24], and *in vivo* in several animal species [25,26]. In man, however, the situation many differ; determination of mevalonate, an indicator of the total body cholesterol synthesis, shows no effect of fibrates on this parameter in man [27,28]. Probably inhibition of cholesterol synthesis, if present *in vivo*, plays a minor role in determining the hypocholesterolemic action of fibrates.

Recently bezafibrate has been reported to inhibit ACAT in rats [29,30]. This finding could explain, at least in part, the cholesterol lowering activity of fibrates in man. Further this could be related to the efficacy of some fibrates in promoting cholesterol efflux from sterol laden cells. In fact ACAT inhibition, by slowing down cholesterol esterification, could make more sterol available for removal by appropriate acceptors (i.e. HDL).

Catabolism and Excretion. Fibrates are known to promote excretion of cholesterol in the bile, thereby increasing biliary saturation with cholesterol and predisposing to gallstone formation [31-34]. This effect, rather than the suppression of cholesterol synthesis, may be viewed as responsible for an increased expression of LDL receptors (LDL-R) in the liver. In fact an increase of LDL-R expression has been demonstrated *in vivo* in hypercholesterolemic man after fibrate treatment: Shepherd et al. showed an increased receptor-mediated catabolism of LDL following treatment with bezafibrate, etofibrate, and fenofibrate, with no changes of nonreceptor mediated catabolism of LDL [35,36]. Studies *in vitro* are not available to show a direct effect of fibrates on LDL receptor expression, but if biliary cholesterol elimination is the driving force, these studies are not likely to be positive unless appropriate models are used. Cholesterol 7 α hydroxylase is the key enzyme in promoting bile acid synthesis; fibrates have apparently little effect on it, although at very high doses in rats [26,37,38], a slight reduction was demonstrated.

LDL RECEPTOR EXPRESSION AND LDL CATABOLISM

As mentioned above, fibrates appear *in vivo* to induce the LDL receptor expression [36,36]. To date we cannot identify the mechanism by which this effect occurs. One explanation (i.e. increased cholesterol elimination) has been discussed. Another possible explanation results from a series of very elegant studies by Eisenberg and co-workers [39] on the effects of bezafibrate (and therefore probably of other TG-lowering drugs) on LDL composition and catabolism *in vitro*. The authors showed that in hypertryceridemia LDL are enriched with triglycerides. This abnormality results in at least two metabolic derangements: 1) LDLs interact poorly with their receptors, owing to an altered conformation of apolipoprotein B-100, the ligand for the LDL receptor, on these lipoproteins [39]; and 2) less cholesterol per particle is delivered to the cell, thus hampering, in part, the control of endogenous sterol synthesis [39]. These metabolic derangements are fully corrected after bezafibrate treatment [22,40,41].

If these data bear any relation to the *in vivo* situation, an increased LDL receptor-mediated catabolism should be detected after treatment with fibrates. These observations are of paramount clinical relevance, and also contribute to a "unified" view of the action of fibrates on cholesterol and LDL metabolism. This observation, however, does not explain the increased receptor-mediated catabolism that can also be detected n type IIa patients after treatment with fibrates [35]. Clearly the effect of fibrates on LDL subfractions should be studied in more detail.

EFFECTS ON HDL

Fibrates increase HDL cholesterol levels [24,42-46]. This is a reproducible effect in hyper-triglyceridemic patients and is likely, at least in part, to be related to the increased catabolism of VLDL following fibrate treatment.

The low HDL cholesterol levels in hypertryceridemia (HTG) result from an increase of TG in HDLs as well as from a reduced number of lipoprotein particles [46]. Fibrates restore the composition of HDLs; however, some fibrates may also act by increasing HDL synthesis. Gemfibrozil and fenofibrate, for instance, increase apo A-I production rate [47]; this effect combined with the effect on TG catabolism, may explain the greater efficacy of gemfibrozil compared with other drugs in increasing HDL levels in man [48]. The mechanism of action by which the increase of apo A-I production occurs is not known. Also it is not clear whether apo A-I is derived from the intestine or from the liver, although the former possibility is the most likely, owing to the effect of fibrates on postprandial lipoproteins [49].

EFFECTS ON APOLIPOPROTEINS

The effects of fibrates on plasma apolipoprotein levels are consistent with the effect of these drugs on plasma lipids. Apolipoprotein B is decreased, while apo A-I is increased by fibrates [50-52]. Apolipoprotein E is also decreased, especially in type III subjects [53]. Finally, the C-II/CIII ratio in VLDL is decreased after treatment with fibrates [54]. Whether this reflects the increase of lipoprotein lipase activity or favors the action of this enzyme on TG-rich lipoproteins is unknown. Apo C-III slows down the hepatic catabolism of VLDL remnants [55] and in transgenic mice the level of expression of this apoprotein correlates very well with plasma TG (i.e. the higher the apo C-III plasma levels, the higher the plasma TG) [56].

EFFECTS ON LIPOPROTEIN COMPOSITION

As mentioned above, fibrates have profound effects on lipoprotein composition and structural abnormalities especially in patients with hypertriglyceridemia. Correction of these abnormalities is also associated with correction of abnormal cell metabolism of LDL isolated from the plasma of hypertriglyceridemic subjects before therapy is instituted (see section on LDL receptors and LDL catabolism). Moreover, binding, internalization, and degradation of VLDL isolated from plasma of hypertriglyceridemic subjects is appreciably higher than that of normal VLDL, and these abnormal lipoproteins also deliver cholesterol to the cell via a nonreceptor-mediated pathway. These two abnormalities are reversed toward normal upon fibrate treatment [40-42]. Fibrates also affect the distribution of lipoprotein subclasses [57,58].

EFFECTS OF FIBRATES ON POSTPRANDIAL LIPEMIA

Many subjects fasted for only a few hours during the day because of the time required for the intestinal absorption and removal from plasma of intestinally derived lipoproteins. Zilversmit [59] first proposed that the postprandial lipoproteins may be atherogenic via a direct action on endothelial cells, thus setting a stage for further research in the involvement of intestinal lipoproteins in atherogenesis. Further evidence have stressed this concept. It is now generally accepted that high postprandial response to a fat load may indeed represent a "negative" finding [60,61].

Fibrates, in general, effectively reduce postprandial lipemia in hypertriglyceridemic subjects [62-64]. The mechanism of action by which fibrates exert this action is not fully understood. Probably both reduced lipid absorption and/or incorporation into lipoproteins as well as increased catabolism of chylomicron and intestinal VLDL play a role.

Recent studies take advantage of the fact that intestinal lipoproteins transport vitamin A to the liver. Therefore plasma levels of vitamin A after a fat-rich meal containing this vitamin are good estimates of the plasma levels of intestinal lipoproteins [65]. Fibrates reduce very effectively the plasma levels of vitamin A during the postprandial lipemia [63].

However little is available on the "quality" of postprandial lipoproteins after hypolipidemic drug treatment. Studies aimed at determining whether these lipoproteins stimulate lipid accumulation in macrophage or are detrimental to cultured endothelial cells are urgently needed. These studies may help in explaining, at least in part, the effectiveness of fibrates as antiatherosclerotic compounds.

FIBRATES AND LDL STRUCTURE

As mentioned above, hypertriglyceridemia results in profound changes in the composition of lipoprotein classes. These changes also alter the conformation of apolipoprotein B at the surface of LDL resulting in a reduced interaction of the lipoprotein with the LDL receptor [39,41]. The altered apolipoprotein conformation is easily demonstrated by using monoclonal antibodies raised against apo B [42]. Some of these antibodies, especially those whose epitopes lie near the putative LDL-binding domain, recognize hypertriglyceridemic LDL with lower affinity. Lowering of plasma TG restores immunoreactivity [42]. It is clear that fibrates, probably via their lowering of plasma TG, also interfere with LDL catabolism and cellular cholesterol homeostasis. Whether this is of relevance to the phenomenon of atherosclerosis is not known; however, these observations have opened a new avenue of research in understanding the mechanism of action of fibrates at their cellular level.

FIBRATES AND Lp(a)

Lp(a) is a plasma lipoprotein that is present in most if not all individuals. This lipoprotein results from the linkage of one apo (a) molecule to LDL. Plasma levels of Lp(a) are directly related to the risk of coronary artery disease [66], are quite stable, and are difficult to modify, either by dietary or pharmacological approaches. More recently it has been reported that bezafibrate may lower Lp(a) plasma levels [67]. These findings are certainly of interest, although these studies need to be confirmed and extended to other fibrates.

FIBRATES AND FIBRINOGEN

Plasma levels of fibrinogen are an independent risk factor of coronary artery disease [68,69]. This finding probably relates to the role of fibrinogen in clot formation, thus predisposing to vascular stenosis. Reduction of fibrinogen plasma levels may therefore result in a protective effort in terms of number of coronary events.

Clofibrate was reported to reduce fibrinogen first [70]; bezafibrate and fenofibrate also possess this effect [71], being more efficacious in hyperfibrinogenemic subjects. These decreases of fibrinogen may relate to the effect to the drugs on plasma lipids; some preliminary data on fibrinogen synthesis demonstrate that synthesis is reduced by bezafibrate *in vitro* [72].

Conclusions

Fibrates are characterized by a multifaceted action on plasma lipid and lipoproteins. The relative contribution of each of the mechanisms indicated above is certainly difficult to determine *in vivo* in man, and may furthermore have a different relevance depending upon the type of patient.

Nevertheless this class of drugs acts on several of the known lipidic and some nonlipidic risk factors for atherosclerosis and thereby is of interest in the approach to the patient at risk for atherosclerosis.

Acknowledgements

This work was supported in part by MPI (Publication n. 941480). The author thanks Miss Maddalena Marazzini for typing the manuscript.

References

1. Sirtori CR, Franceschini G. Effect of fibrates on serum lipids and atherosclerosis. Pharmac Ther 1988;37:167-191.
2. Kissebah AH, Alfarsi S, Adams PW, Seed M, Folkard J, Wynn V. Transport kinetics of plasma-free fatty acid, very low density lipoprotein triglycerides and apoprotein in patients with endogenous hypertriglyceridemia. Effects of 2,2-dimethyl, 5(2,5-xylyloxy) valeric acid therapy. Atherosclerosis 1976;24:199-218.
3. Wong SH, Fisher EA, Marsh JB. Effects of eicosapentaenoic and docosahexaenoic acids on apoprotein B mRNA and secretion of very low density lipoprotein in HepG2 cells. Arteriosclerosis 1989;9:836-841.
4. Nestel PJ, Connor WE, Reardon MF, Connor S, Wong S, Boston R. Suppression by diets rich in fish oil of very low density lipoprotein production in man. J Clin Invest 1984;74:82-89.
5. Kissebah AH, Adams PW, Harrigan P, Wynn V. The mechanism of action of clofibrate and tetranicotinoylfructose (bradilan) on the kinetics of plasma free fatty acid and triglyceride transport in type IV and type V hypertriglyceridaemia. Europ J Clin Invest 1974;4:163-174.
6. Carlson LA. Effect of gemfibrozil in vitro on fat-mobilizing lipolysis in human adipose tissue. Proc Roy Soc Med 1976;69:101-103.
7. Bierman EL, Brunzell JD, Bagdade JD, Lerner RL, Hazzard WR, Porte D Jr. On the mechanism of action of atromid-S on triglyceride transport in man. Trans Assoc

Am Physicians Phila 1970;83:211-220.

8.   Stegmeier K, Stork H, Lenz H, Leuschner F, Liede V. Pharmacology and mode of action of bezafibrate in animals. In: Greten H, Lang PD, Schettler G, editors. Lipoproteins and coronary heart disease. New York :Gerhard Witzstrock Publishing House, 1980:76-82.

9.   Maragoudakis ME, Hankin H, Wasvary JM. On the mode of action of lipid-lowering agents. J Biol Chem 1972;247:342-347.

10. Maragandakis ME, Hankin H. On the mode of action of lipid lowering agents. V. Kinetics of the inhibition in vitro of rat acetyl CoA carboxylase. J Biochem 1971;246:348-354.

11. Greten H, Laible V, Zipperle G, Augustin J. Comparison of assay methods for selective measurement of plasma lipase. Atherosclerosis 1977;26:563-572.

12. Nikkilä EA, Huttunen JK, Ehnholm C. Effect of clofibrate on post-heparin plasma triglyceride lipase activities in patients with hypertriglyceridemia. Metabolism 1977; 26:279-186

13. Vessby B, Lithell H, Ledermann H. Elevated lipoprotein lipase activity in skeletal muscle tissue during treatment of hypertriglyceridemic patients with bezafibrate. Atherosclerosis 1982;44:113-118.

14. Lithell H, Boberg J, Hellsing K, Lunquist G, Vessby B. Increase of the lipoprotein lipase activity in human skeletal muscle during clofibrate administration. Eur J Clin Invest 1978;8:67-76.

15. Heller F, Harvengt C. Effects of clofibrate, bezafibrate, fenofibrate and probucol on plasma lipolytic enzymes in normolipaemic subjects. Europ J Clin Pharmacol 1983;25:57-63.

16. Goldberg AP, Applebaum-Bowden DM, Bierman EL, et al. Increase in lipoprotein lipase during clofibrate treatment of hypertriglyceridemia in patients on hemodialysis. N Engl J Med 1979;301:1073-1076.

17. Carlson LA, Olsson AG, Ballantyne D. On the rise in low density and high density lipoproteins in response to treatment of hypertriglyceridemia in type IV and type V hyperlipoproteinemias. Atherosclerosis 1977;26:603-609.

18. Shepherd J, Packard CJ. An overview of the effects of p-chlorophenoxyisobutyric acid derivatives on lipoprotein metabolism. In: Pharmacological control of hyperlipidaemia. Barcelona:JR Prous Science Publishers, 1986:135-144.

19. Rabkin SW, Hayden M, Frohlich J. Comparison of gemfibrozil and clofibrate on serum lipids in familial combined hyperlipidemia. A randomized placebo-controlled double blind crossover trial. Atherosclerosis 1988;73:233-240.

20. Crouse JR Grundy SM. Effect of colestipol, clofibrate and placebo on plasma lipoproteins of patients with hypercholesterolemia. Metabolism 1981;30:123-128.

21. Austin MA, Breslow JL, Hennekens CH, Buring JE, Willet WC, Krauss RM. Low density lipoprotein subclass patterns and risk of myocardial infarction. JAMA 1988; 260:1917-1921.

22. Eisenberg S, Gavish D, Kleinman Y. Bezafibrate. In: Pharmacological control of hyperlipidaemia. Barcelona:JR Prous Science Publishers, 1986:145-169.

23.   Berndt J, Gaumert R, Still J. Mode of action of the lipid-lowering agents clofibrate and BM 15075, on cholesterol biosynthesis in rat liver. Atherosclerosis 1978; 30:147-152.

24.   Newton RS, Krause BR. Mechanisms of action in gemfibrozil: Comparison of studies in the rat to clinical efficacy. In: Pharmacological control of hyperlipidaemia. Barcelona:JR Prous Science Publishers, 1986:171-186.

25.   Schneider AG, Ditschuneit HH, Stange EF, Ditschuneit H. Regulation of 3-hydroxy-methylglutaryl-coenzyme. A reductase in freshly isolated human mononuclear cells by fenofibrate. In:Carlson LA, Olsson AG, editors. Treatment of hyperlipoproteinemia. New York:Raven Press, 1984;181-184.

26.   Fantappiè S, Maggi FM, Cancellieri M, Bosisio E, Malavasi B, Catapano AL. Effect of bezafibrate on plasma lipid in strain of genetically hypercholesterolemic RICO rats. Pharmacol Res 1989;21:109-110.

27.   Beil FU, Schrameyer-Wernecke A, Biesiegel U, Greten H. Lovastatin versus bezafibrate in the treatment of primary hypercholesterolemia. Effects on lipoproteins and cholesterol synthesis. In: Abstract Book of X International Symposium on Drugs Affecting Lipid Metabolism; 1989 Nov 8-11; Houston, 1989; 54.

28.   Galli Kienle M, Del Puppo M, Cighetti G, Arca M, D'alò G, Galli G. Effects of long-term pravastatin therapy on whole body cholesterol synthesis in hyper-cholesterolemic patients. In: Abstract Book of X International Symposium on Drugs Affecting Lipid Metabolism; 1989 Nov 8-11; Houston, 1989; 59.

29.   Bosisio E, Catapano AL, Cighetti G, Paoletti R. Effect of bezafibrate on liver enzymes and lipoproteins in animal experiments. In: Greten H, Lang PD, Schettler G, editors. Lipoproteins and coronary heart disease. New York:Gerhard Witzstrock Publishing House, 1980:86-91.

30.   Ståhlberg D, Angelin B, Einarsson K. Effects of treatment with clofibrate, bezafibrate, and ciporfibrate on the metabolism of cholesterol in rat liver microsomes. J Lipid Res 30;953-958.

31.   Palmer RH. Effects of fibric acid derivatives on biliary lipid composition. Amer J Med 1987;83:37-43.

32.   Leiss O, Meyer-Krahmer K, Von Bergmann K. Biliary lipid secretion in patients with heterozygous familial hypercholesterolemia and combined hyperlipidemia. Influence of bezafibrate and fenofibrate. J Lipid Res 1986;27:713-723.

33.   Schlierf G, Chwat M, Feueborn E, et al. Biliary and plasma lipids-lowering chemotherapy. Atherosclerosis 1980;36:323-329.

34.   Kesaniemi YA, Grundy SM. Influence of gemfibrozil and clofibrate on metabolism of cholesterol and plasma triglycerides in man. JAMA 1984;251:2241-2246.

35.   Stewart JM, Packard CJ, Lorimer AR, Boag DE, Shepherd J. Effects of bezafibrate on receptor-mediated and receptor-independent low density lipoprotein catabolism in type II hyperlipoproteinaemic subjects. Atherosclerosis 1982;44:355-365.

36.   Series JJ, Caslake MJ, Kilday C, Cruickshank A, Demant T, Packard CJ, Shepherd J. Influence of etofibrate on low density lipoprotein metabolism. Atherosclerosis,

1988;69:233-239.

37.   Ståhlberg D, Reihnér E, Ewerth S, Einarsson K, Angelin B. Effects of bezafibrate on hepatic cholesterol metabolism. Eur J Clin Pharmacol 1991;40:S33-S36.

38.   Cohen BI, Raicht RF, Shefer S, Mosbach EH. Effects of clofibrate on sterol metabolism in the rat. Biochim Biophys Acta 1974;369:79-85.

39.   Kleinman Y, Eisenberg S, Oschry Y, Gavish D, Stein O, Stein Y. Defective metabolism of hypertriglyceridemic low density lipoprotein in cultured human skin fibroblasts. Normalization with bezafibrate therapy. Clin Invest 1985;75:1796-1803.

40.   Gavish D, Oschry Y, Fainaru M, Eisenberg S. Change in very low-, low-, and high-density lipoproteins during lipid lowering (bezafibrate) therapy: Studies in type IIA and type IIB hyperlipoproteinaemia. Eur J Clin Invest 1986;16:61-68.

41.   Kleinman Y, Schonfeld G, Gavish D, Oschry Y, Eisenberg S. Hypolipidemic therapy modulates expression of apolipoprotein B epitopes on low density lipoproteins. Studies in mild to moderate hypertriglyceridemic patients. J Lipid Res 1987;28:540-548.

42.   Witztum JL. Current approaches to drug therapy for the hypercholesterolemic patient. Circulation 1989;80:1101-1114.

43.   Fears R. Drug treatment of hyperlipidaemia. Drugs of Today 1984;20:257-294.

44.   Blane GF, Bogaievsky Y, Bonnefous F. Fenofibrate: Influence on circulating lipids and sideeffects in medium- and long-term clinical use. In: Pharmacological Control of Hyperlipidaemia. Barcelona:JR Prous Science Publishers, 1986:187-216.

45.   Rouffy J, Chanu B, Bakir R, Djian F, Goy-Loeper. Comparative evaluation of the effects of ciprofibrate and fenofibrate on lipids, lipoproteins and apoproteins A and B. Atherosclerosis 1985;54:273-281.

46.   Sorisky A, Ooi TC, Simo IE, Meuffels M, Hindmarsh JT, Nair R. Change in composition of high density lipoprotein during gemfibrozil therapy. Atherosclerosis 1987;67:181-189.

47.   Saku K, Gartside PS, Hynd BA, Kashyap ML. Mechanism of action of gemfibrozil on lipoprotein metabolism. J Clin Invest 1985;75:1702-1712.

48.   Kaukola S, Manninen V, Malkonen M, Enholm C. Gemfibrozil in the treatment of dyslipidemias in the middle-aged survivors of acute myocardial infarction. Acta Med Scand 1981:209:69-73.

49.   Cattin L, Da Col PG, Feruglio FS. Effects of gemfibrozil on serum triglycerides after an oral fat load in hyperlipidemic patients: A double-blind, placebo, crossover study. Advances in Therapy 1989;6:16-25.

50.   Vessby E, Lithell H, Hellsing K, et al. Effects of bezafibrate on the serum lipoprotein lipid and apolipoprotein composition of the plasma lipid esters. Atherosclerosis 1980;37:257-269.

51.   Nestel PJ, Hunt D, Wahlquist MS. Clofibrate raises plasma apoprotein AI and HDL-cholesterol concentrations. Atherosclerosis 1980;37:625-629.

52.   Olsson AG, Carlson LA, Erikson V, Helmius G, Hemmingsson A, Ruhn G. Regression of computer estimated femoral atherosclerosis after pronounced serum lipid lowering in patients with asymptomatic hyperlipidemia. Lancet 1982;ii:1311.

53. Patsch JR, Yeshurun D, Jackson R, Gotto A. Effects of clofibrate, nicotinic acid and diets on the plasma lipoproteins of a subject with type III hyperlipoproteinemia. Am J Med 1977;63:1001-1009.

54. Franceschini G, Sirtori M, Gianfranceschi G, Frosi G, Montanari G, Sirtori CR. Reversible increase of the apo CII/apo CIII-1 ratio in the very low density lipoproteins after procetofen treatment in hypertriglyceridemic patients. Artery 1985;12:363-381.

55. Windler E, Havel RJ. Inhibitory effects of C apolipoproteins from rats and humans on the uptake of triglyceride-rich lipoproteins and their remnants by the perfused rat liver. J. Lipid Research 1985;26:556-565.

56. Ito Y, Azrolan N, O'Connel A, Walsh A, Breslow JL. Hypertriglyceridemia as a result of human apo CIII gene expression in transgenic mice. Science 1990;249:790-793.

57. Moulin P, Bourdillon MC, De Parscau L, Perrot L, Ponsin G, Berthezene F. High density lipoprotein alternations induced by bezafibrate in healthy male volunteers. Atherosclerosis 1987;67:17-22.

58. Schwandt P, Weisweiler P. Effect of bezafibrate on the high density lipoprotein subfractions. HDL-2 and HDL-3 in primary hyperlipoproteinemia. Artery 1980;7:464-470.

59. Zilversmit DB. Atherogenesis: A post-prandial phenomenon. Circulation 1979;60:473-485.

60. Havel RJ. Role of triglyceride-rich lipoproteins in progression of atherosclerosis. Circulation 1990;81:694-696.

61. Patsch JR, Prasad S, Gotto AM, Bengtsson-Olivecrona G. Postprandial lipemia. A key for the conversion of HDL_2 and HDL_3 by hepatic lipase. J Clin Invest 1984;74:2011-2023.

62. Simpson HS, Williamson CM, Olivecrona T, et al. Postprandial lipemia, fenofibrate and coronary artery disease. Atherosclerosis 1990;85:193-202.

63. Weintraub MS, Eisenberg S, Breslow JL. Different patterns of postprandial lipoprotein metabolism in normal type IIa, type III and type IV hyperlipoproteinemic individuals. J Clin Invest 1987;79:1110-1119.

64. Oster P, Schlierf G, Land PD, Mordasini R, Vollmar J. Diurnal lipid and lipoprotein profiles with bezafibrate and clofibrate in healthy volunteers. Pharmatherapeutica 1985;4:267-277.

65. Ross AC, Zilversmith DB. Chylomicron remnant cholesteryl esters as the major constituent of very low density lipoprotein in plasma of cholesterol fed rabbits. J Lipid Res 1977;18:169-181.

66. Utermann G. The mysteries of lipoprotein(a). Science 1989;246:904-910.

67. Schwartzkopff W, Bimmermann A. Hyperlipoproteinamie type IIa, IIb und IV. Munch Med Wschr 1988;130:422-428.

68. Moller L, Kristensen TS. Plasma fibrinogen and ischemic heart disease risk factors. Arteriosclerosis and thrombosis 1991;11:344-350.

69. Meade TW, North WRS, Chakrabarti T, Stirling Y, Haines AP, Thompson SG.

Haemostatic function and cardiovascular death: Early results of a prospective study. Lancet 1980;1:1050-1054.

70.   Dormandy JA, Gutteridge JMC, Hoare E, Dormandy TL. Effect of clofibrate on blood viscosity in intermittent claudication. Br Med J 1974;4:259-262.

71.   Almér LO, Kjellström T. The fibrinolytic system and coagulation during bezafibrate treatment of hypertriglyceridemia. Atherosclerosis 1986;61:81-85.

72.   Catapano AL. Unpublished observations

FENOFIBRATE: A SAFETY EVALUATION OF A LARGE GERMAN PATIENT POPULATION

Klaus U. Kirchgässler
Research and Development
Fournier Pharma GmbH
Justus-von-Liebig-Strasse 16
D-66280 Sulzbach
GERMANY

Introduction

Fenofibrate, a fibric acid derivative of the second generation, was introduced into medical practice in 1975 for the treatment of dyslipidemia. Since then, its efficacy and safety profile has been well established. More recently, the micronized form of fenofibrate was introduced in several countries including the Federal Republic of Germany. The 200 mg dose of this new formulation is bioequivalent to 300 mg standard fenofibrate and allows convenient once daily dosing [1].

In the context of the introduction of fenofibrate 200 micronized into the German market, a drug monitoring program was set up to obtain data on tolerability and efficacy in a large sample of patients with various types of dyslipidemia. In this paper, safety data of more than 7,000 patients are presented and compared with data on standard fenofibrate. Furthermore, efficacy data of more than 3,200 patients from this program will be briefly described.

Material and methods

PATIENTS

The drug monitoring program under discussion here was conducted in approximately 2,000 private practices in Germany (mainly general practioners and doctors of internal medicine). Patients with hyperlipidemias type IIa, IIb, or IV were treated with 200 mg of micronized fenofibrate once daily for twelve weeks. Patients were supposed to have an LDL cholesterol level above or equal 160 mg/dl and/or total triglyceride levels above 250 mg/dl in order to participate in the program.

Patients were not supposed to participate in the program if they suffered from

307

A.M. Gotto et al. (eds.), Multiple Risk Factors in Cardiovascular Disease, 307-314.
© *1995 Kluwer Academic Publishers and Fondazione Giovanni Lorenzini.*

diseases that are known contraindications to treatment with fenofibrate such as chronic renal failure, nephrotic syndrome, acute or chronic hepatitis, liver insufficiency, or pancreatitis. All types of concomitant medications were allowed with the exception of other lipid lowering agents.

LABORATORY MEASUREMENTS

Blood samples were supposed to be taken at the beginning of the observation period as well as after 6 and 12 weeks of treatment. The measurements of total cholesterol, total triglycerides, and HDL cholesterol were carried out by local laboratory facilities. LDL cholesterol values were calculated using the Friedewald formula [2]. Blood sampling for safety laboratory measures were performed at the discretion of the participating physicians at baseline, after 6 weeks, and at the end of the observation period.

QUESTIONNAIRE

A standardized questionnaire was used to assess safety and tolerability at each visit. Patients were systematically questioned for adverse events at all visits. At the end of the observation period, the overall tolerability was classified by the investigators using a scale ranking from "very good" to "unsatisfactory."

STATISTICAL ANALYSIS

All data were analyzed and are presented descriptively. Adverse events were both listed as reported and classified using the COSTART code. The statistical evaluation was performed by BIODAT Gesellschaft für Biometrie und Statistik mbH, Berlin, FRG.

Results

PATIENTS

In total, 7,235 patients of the planned 10,000 patients (72%) participated in the drug monitoring program and are available for analysis of the tolerability of fenofibrate 200 micronized. Currently, demographic data are available only for 3,818 patients, and 3,724 patients were included in the analysis of efficacy. The most important demographic data are listed in Table 1:

Table 1. Demographic data.

	Total	Male	Female
Age	56 ± 10.9 yrs	54 ± 10.1 yrs	59 ± 11.2 yrs
Height	171 ± 8.5 cm	176 ± 6.5 cm	165 ± 5.9 cm
Weight	79 ± 12.6 kg	84 ± 11.8 kg	73 ± 10.3 kg

According to the results of lipid level measurements, the patients were classified into the different types of dyslipidemia as follows (Table 2):

Table 2. Classification of patients into different types of dyslipidemia (total n = 3,724 with missing data in n=757).

	Miss.	Type of Dyslipidemia					
		Type IIa		Type IIb		Type IV	
Total	757	1194	40.2%	777	26.2%	996	33.6%

With regard to treatment, 1,006 (27.3%) had no previous treatment of dyslipidemia, 1,570 (42.6%) were previously treated with diet only, 229 (6.2%) already had received lipid lowering medication and 883 (23.9%) reported a history of both, medication and diet. For almost all patients risk factors and/or concomitant diseases were documented at baseline which are given in Figure 1:

Figure 1. Frequency of risk factors.

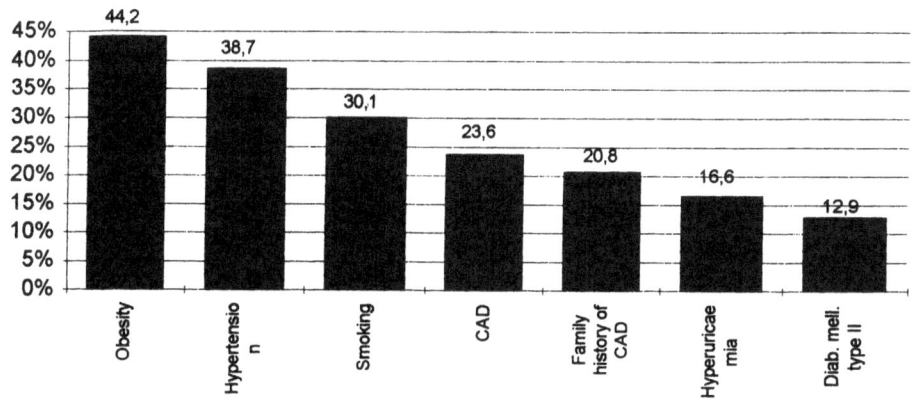

TOLERABILITY

In general, the trial medication was very well tolerated. At the end of the program, overall tolerability was rated as follows (Table 3):

Table 3. Ratings of overall tolerability at the final visit.

Miss.	Ratings of Tolerability							Total
	Very Good		Good		Moderate		Unsatisfactory	(100%)
161	2209	62.6%	1224	34.7%	62	1.8%	31	0.9%	3526

In total, 289 of 7,235 patients (4.0%) reported 335 adverse events. The affected organ systems and the number of adverse events (AE) for each organ system is listed in Table 4:

Table 4. Adverse events according to organ system.

Organ system (Costart classification)	Number of events	Frequency	
		% of pts.	% of AEs
Digestive system	145	2.0	43.2
Skin and appendages	53	0.7	15.8
Nervous system	34	0.5	10.1
Body as a whole	34	0.5	10.1
Cardiovascular system	23	0.3	6.9
Muscoskeletal system	11	0.15	3.2
Urogenital system	9	0.12	2.7
Metabolic and nutritional disorders	8	0.11	2.4
Respiratory system	7	0.10	2.1
Endocrine system	5	0.07	1.5
Special senses	3	0.04	0.9
Hemic and lymphatic system	2	0.03	0.6
Personality disorder	1	0.01	0.3

In 28 patients (0.4% of the entire population, and 8.4% of the patients with adverse events), a total of 34 adverse events (10.1% of all adverse events) were classified as serious adverse events according to the internationally accepted definition, that is an adverse event, which is fatal, life-threatening, disabling, or which results in in-patient hospitalization or prolongation of hospitalization. In addition, congenital anomalies and occurrence of malignancy are always considered serious adverse events.

The serious adverse events according to this definition which occurred during the two drug monitoring programs are listed in the Table 5:

Table 5. Serious adverse events.

Pt.No.	Adverse event	Outcome	Causal relationship (as reported)
0060/3	cerebral infarction	irreversible damage	improbable
0064/2	tendosynovitis (op)	recovered	improbable
	carcinoma of the prostate	ongoing	improbable
0097/1	Coronary artery disease (CABG)	recovered	improbable
0104/3	urolithiasis	recovered	not documented
	hydronephrosis	recovered	not documented
	convulsion	recovered	not documented
0117/4	Pulmonary embolism	died	improbable
0137/3	goiter (op.)	not documented	improbable
0155/1	carcinoma of the bladder	not documented	improbable
0162/4	thyroid adenoma	not documented	improbable
0273/2	severe angina (hospitalization)	recovered	improbable
0425/3	carcinoma of the liver	ongoing	improbable
0461/5	inguinal hernia (hospitalization)	recovered	improbable
0504/4	carcinoma of the colon	not documented	not documented
0516/2	necrotizing pancreatitis	irreversible damage	improbable
0538/2	cholelithiasis	recovered	probable
0546/5	necrosis of the large toe	irreversible damage	improbable
0592/1	cerebral infarction	died	improbable
0717/5	cholecystitis (op.)	not documented	improbable
0776/2	PTCA	recovered	improbable
0784/5	diabetes mellitus (hospitalization)	not documented	not documented
0787/5	cerebral ischemia	not completely	improbable
	tachyarrhythmia absoluta	recovered	
0832/3	hernia operation (hospitalization)	recovered	improbable
0866/5	inguinal hernia (hospitalization)	recovered	not documented
0984/1	diabetes mellitus	ongoing	improbable
1025/1	jaundice	recovered	possible
1029/2	bone fracture (hospitalization)	recovered	improbable
1159/3	myocardial infarction	recovered	improbable
1294/3	myocardial infarction	died	improbable
1463/2	cholelithiasis	recovered	possible
	pneumonia	recovered	improbable
1538/3	cerebral infarction	irreversible damage	improbable
1584/3	bronchitis (hospitalization)	recovered	improbable
1613/1	skull fracture	not documented	not documented
	subarachnoidal hemorrhage		

With respect to laboratory abnormalities, an increase in γ-GT was reported in 6 patients, and an increase in CPK in two cases. In one of these, micronized fenofibrate had to be discontinued in the presence of muscle pain. This finding of a very low incidence of laboratory abnormalities, however, cannot and should not be directly compared to findings from clinical trials, as not all physicians performed safety laboratory measurements on a regular basis during the drug monitoring program.

In total, 297 patients (4.1%) dropped out from the drug monitoring program. In 137 patients (1.9%), an adverse event was given as the reason for drop out regardless of whether or not the adverse event was thought to be related to treatment with micronized fenofibrate.

What do these results mean in the context of other results both with standard and micronized fenofibrate? The comparison with the data both for short- and long-term trials cumulated gathered by Blane et al. in 1986 [3] with standard fenofibrate is shown in Table 6. For micronized fenofibrate, the data from a recently terminated Belgian phase IV trial will be, in the near future, the best data base for a comparison with the present results.

Table 6. Global incidence of adverse events with standard and micronized fenofibrate

| | Standard fenofibrate | | Micronized fenofibrate |
| | Blane et al. 1986 | | German drug monitoring |
	Short term	Long term	Short term
Global incidence	6.3%	11.3%	4.0%
Discontinuation of treatment	3.5%	0.2%	1.9%

Looking at the relative distribution of the types of adverse events, the data presented are also comparable to previously generated data. This is especially true for the predominance of mild and transient gastrointestinal disturbances which account for almost 50% of all adverse events in various data bases. In addition, the German drug monitoring program revealed no previously unknown adverse events which were related to the treatment with fenofibrate.

EFFICACY

A summary of the effects of micronized fenofibrate on various lipid parameters in the first drug monitoring program (data from the second phase not yet being available) is given in Figure 2 (all values means with exception of HDL cholesterol where the median is given):

Figure 2. Relative changes in lipid parameters at 12 weeks compared to baseline for the entire patient population.

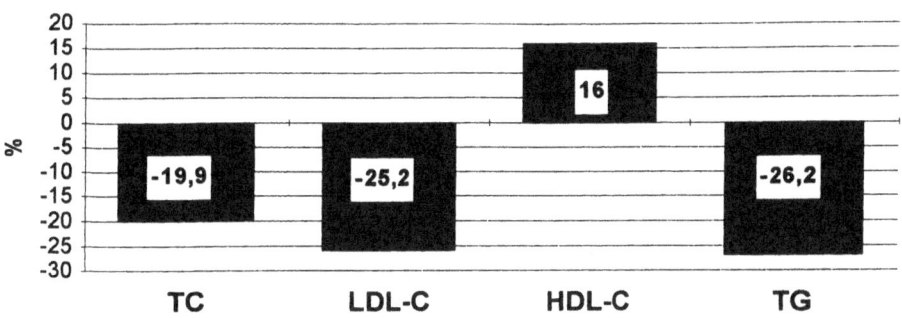

The effect of micronized fenofibrate was more pronounced when baseline levels were high as shown for LDL cholesterol in Figure 3:

Figure 3. Reduction in mean LDL cholesterol depending on baseline values in the entire patient population.

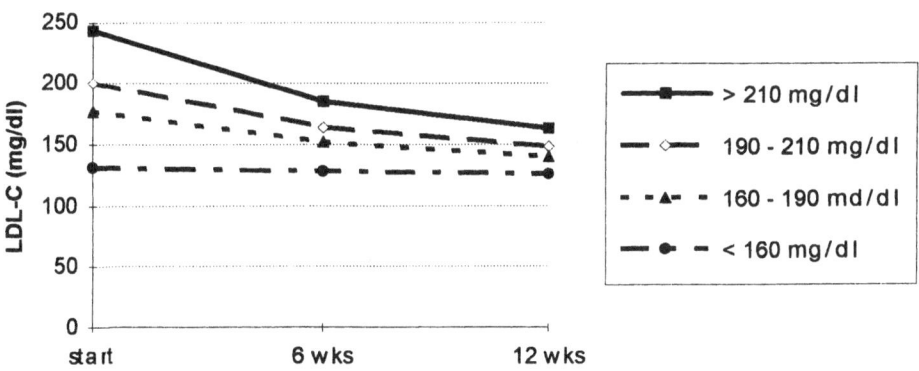

In summary, these data confirm the known profile of fenofibrate as a potent cholesterol and triglyceride lowering drug which also leads to substantial increase in HDL cholesterol. Its beneficial effects on the cardiovascular risk profile are further demonstrated by a reduction of the LDL/HDL quotient from 5.3 to 3.3 within the 12-week treatment period.

Conclusion

In this large drug monitoring program, the tolerability and efficacy of micronized fenofibrate was assessed in more than 7,000 patients. The micronized formulation was found to be efficacious in all major types of dyslipidemia; furthermore, the data presented here confirm the excellent tolerability profile of micronized fenofibrate.

References

1.   Guichard JP, Levy-Prades Sauron R. A comparison of the bioavailability of standard or micronized formulations of fenofibrate. Curr Therap Res Clin Exp 1993;54:610-14.
2.   Friedewald WT, Levy RI, Frederickson DS. Estimation of the concentration of low-density lipoprotein cholesterol in plasma without use of the preparative ultracentrifuge. Clin Chem 1972;18:499-502
3.   Blane GF, Bogaievsky Y, Bonnefous F. Fenofibrate: influence on circulating lipids and side effects in medium and long-term clinical use. In: Pharmacological control of hyperlipidemia. JR Prous Science Publ. S.A., 1986;187-216.

PLASMA CHOLESTEROL AND TOTAL MORTALITY

R. Paoletti and A. Poli
Institute of Pharmacological Sciences
University of Milan
20133 Milan
ITALY

The association between increased levels of plasma cholesterol, specifically LDL cholesterol, and the incidence of coronary heart disease (CHD) morbidity and mortality has been demonstrated in a number of epidemiological studies in the last thirty years [1,2,3]. Since CHD in industrialized countries accounts for about half of the deaths observed, an association between plasma cholesterol and total mortality should also be demonstrable, unless an inverse association between plasma cholesterol levels and noncardiovascular mortality exists. In fact, observational studies with long follow-up show that subjects with increased levels of plasma cholesterol are at higher risk of death for all causes (total mortality) [4,5].

In the Framingham cohort, for example, this observation is particularly evident [5]. If the cohort itself is stratified in quartiles according to plasma cholesterol levels at the first examination and the performance in the following thirty years is considered, it is easily appreciated that in the first fifteen years of follow-up the total mortality of the four groups with different plasma cholesterol levels does not significantly differ from one another. However in the following fifteen years, the total death rate of the four groups differentiates, the highest being observed in the patients with plasma cholesterol greater than 260 mg/dl, and lowest in the patients with plasma cholesterol less than 180 mg/dl. All these differences are particularly evident at the thirty-year follow-up, when they are statistically different from one another.

Similar results are observed in other cohorts when the follow-up is long enough. In the Belgian Bank study [6], for example, the total mortality of patients with plasma cholesterol higher and lower than 260 mg/dl differentiates after about 15 years of follow-up. In the 25 -year follow-up, patients with plasma cholesterol over 260 mg/dl have a crude rate of death for all causes about 15% greater than those with plasma cholesterol lower than 260 mg/dl.

Similar results are observed in the same study when the relationship between cigarette smoking and total death is considered. If nonsmokers and current smokers are compared, no significant difference in total death rate is observed in the first ten years of

A.M. Gotto et al. (eds.), Multiple Risk Factors in Cardiovascular Disease, 315-319.

follow-up; however, at the end of the 25-year period, a difference between current smokers and never-smokers appears, and is of the same amplitude of that observed for subjects with low or high plasma cholesterol.

If the results of the published studies, including the very large cohort of the patients screened for the Multiple Factors Intervention Trial (MRFIT), are pooled and analyzed, apparently different pictures can be obtained when death-rates are presented as relative risks or absolute risks [7]. When relative risks are considered, and the risk of individuals with plasma cholesterol between 160 and 199 is set at 1, it can be seen that after six years of follow-up the risk of CHD death is doubled in subjects with levels of plasma cholesterol around 240 mg/dl, and is reduced about 25% in individuals with plasma cholesterol ≤ 160 mg/dl.

On the other hand, patients with plasma cholesterol of 160 mg/dl or lower present a significantly high relative risk of intracranial hemorrhage (relative risk = 2.25) and a high relative risk of death for suicides, or for lung or gastrointestinal cancer. Lung and gastrointestinal cancer risk, on the other hand, is slightly reduced below the basal relative risk of 1 in patients with plasma cholesterol exceeding 240 mg/dl.

But when absolute risks are considered, the number of CHD deaths exceeds so greatly the other causes of death, that the overall picture becomes completely different. Increasing levels of plasma cholesterol are associated with an increasing risk of all-cause death, because the increasing risk of CHD, associated with high cholesterol levels, is not at all balanced by the small reductions observed in the lung and digestive tract cancer incidence, and in intracranial hemorrhage, associated with the same elevated cholesterol levels.

Problems arise in trying to interpret the observation of an increased rate of cancer deaths in patients with low levels of plasma cholesterol. A possible explanation could be that low blood cholesterol is causally involved in the generation of neoplasm, or that preclinical cancers decrease the level of plasma cholesterol .

Data from the Honolulu Heart Program Study support this latter view [8]. If the subjects in this study are classified into quintiles of serum cholesterol at enrollment, and followed up with time, one can observe that the excess death rate for cancer, observed in the first quintile (patients with lowest plasma cholesterol), disappears when patients with some disease involvement ("confounded group") are eliminated from the data analysis. If only patients in good health at enrollment ("healthy group") are considered, in fact, the total death rate does not change passing from the first to the third quintile, but rises when the fourth and the fifth quintile are considered. The only pathological conditions which clearly increase in incidence when plasma cholesterol decreases, seem to be subarachnoid hemorrhage or intracranial hemorrhage.

In the MRFIT screening follow-up study, Iso and colleagues [9] have shown that the relative risk of this condition decreases by some 50%, passing from plasma cholesterol lower than 160 mg/dl to plasma cholesterol higher than 280 mg/dl. On the other hand nonhemorrhagic stroke, with relative risk increasing from 1 to 2.5 in the same cholesterol range, follows an opposite pattern. The risk of total stroke, as a result of these different relationships, is essentially unaffected by plasma cholesterol concentration.

In conclusion, data from observational epidemiological studies support the view that increased levels of total cholesterol are associated with a higher risk of CHD mortality; in long enough follow-up studies this increases in the risk transfers into the total mortality risk. The apparent higher risk of cancer, which was observed for low plasma cholesterol levels, is likely to be explained by the effect of cancer on cholesterol and not by an effect of low plasma cholesterol on cancerogenesis; the only condition which is actually increased at low plasma cholesterol, intracranial or subarachnoid hemorrhage, has a total incidence in the population that is too low to affect the total mortality rate.

A completely different aspect of the relationship between plasma cholesterol and total mortality emerges from patients enrolled in cholesterol lowering trials. In these trials, such as the Lipid Research Clinics Coronary Primary Prevention Trial (LRC-CPTT) and the Helsinki Heart Study (HHS), the reduced incidence of coronary heart disease morbidity and mortality has been observed in patients treated with cholestyramine or gemfibrozil respectively, while no difference in the total death rate has appeared between treated and control patients.

For this reason it has been suggested that hypocholesterolemic drugs could negatively affect the noncardiovascular mortality, without leading to any significant result on the total mortality incidence in treated patients [10,11]. Specifically, some authors have described an increasing incidence of suicides, homicides, accidents, and violent deaths in patients treated with hypolipidemic drugs as compared to controls [12]. But a careful analysis of the data of the two major trials performed, and their follow-up, allows this interpretation to be ruled out.

First of all one should consider that plasma cholesterol levels in patients enrolled in hypocholesterolemic trials are reduced, using diet and drugs, to levels which can still be considered high. In the LRC-CPTT patients with plasma cholesterol of about 280 mg/dl were brought to plasma cholesterol levels of 250 mg/dl using cholestyramine; a similar reduction (10%) was observed in the HHS, in patients with plasma cholesterol levels of about 260-280 mg/dl at enrollment [13,14]. The on-trial plasma cholesterol of patients assuming active drugs in these studies, as a consequence of this consideration, falls in a range that in general public is not associated with an increase of any kind of noncardiovascular mortality.

However let us analyze in more detail the results of these two trials. The twelve-year follow-up of the LRC-CPTT trial shows that the incidence of cardiovascular and coronary deaths during and after the end of the trial is always lower in patients who received active treatment during the trial itself [15]. The advantage of cholestyramine-treated patients over control patients was greatest at the end of the trial, was maintained for about 4.5 years after the end of the trial itself, and was slightly reduced after a further 1.5 years of follow-up. It is noteworthy that drug administration was stopped at the end of the trial by the large majority of participants.

During the whole twelve-year period, no significant cancer incidence difference was observed in the two groups; the total (all-causes) death rate, which seemed unaffected by the active treatment at the formal completion of the trial (at six years), was indeed reduced, although not significantly, during both the trial and the follow-up after the trial end. The general picture of the data clearly indicates that patients treated with cholestyramine feared better than those treated with placebo.

In the Helsinki Heart Study, a small increase in deaths from accident, suicides, and homicides was observed in the treated group as compared with the control group, when patients were analyzed on an "intention-to-treat" basis. But when one analyzes the individual cases, a different picture emerges [16]. Patients who committed suicide or who died in accidents were in most cases no longer taking the active drug, and some of them had actually never taken the drug itself, even if they had been enrolled in the treatment group and not in the control group. If we consider only patients actually using the drug at the time of death, no significant difference emerges in the death rate for violent causes in the two treatment groups.

Also in interventional studies, a long follow-up is likely to be needed to show that hypolipidemic treatment affects total mortality. In the Program of Surgical Control of Hyperlipidemia (POSCH), the total death rate, not significantly improved at the formal end of the trial, ameliorated at the eleven-year follow-up evaluation [17].

In the Niacin branch of the Coronary Drug Project, performed on patients already affected by a myocardial infarction, a clear and significant benefit for patients treated with the active drug, compared to those administered a placebo, and of statistically high significance (P=0.0012), appeared after 6 years of follow-up, being of good evidence at the sixteenth year of observation [18].

A similar scene emerges from a recent meta-analysis on this topic by Holme [19]. The author shows that to obtain a reduction in CHD morbidity and mortality, a large-enough reduction in the plasma cholesterol level must be obtained. If only studies in which this diminution was greater than 10% are considered, the cholesterol reduction also positively affects the total death rate of the treated patients [19].

The expected publication of the 4S study, a secondary prevention trial designed to test the effect of an HMGCoA reductase inhibitor on the total survival [20], will soon add relevant information to the discussion on this controversial topic. In the meanwhile, the discussion on the effect of hypocholesterolemic drugs on total mortality cannot justify a change in attitude of physicians and cardiologists toward plasma cholesterol and its reduction. The effect of these drugs on CHD incidence and on the evolution of the disease are in fact clear enough to warrant treatment in high risk hypercholesterolemic patients.

References

1.   Hoes AW, Grobbe DE, Valkenburg HA, et al. Cardiovascular risk and all-cause mortality; a 12 year follow-up study in the Netherlands. Eur J Epidemiol 1993;9: 285-292.
2.   Law MR, Wald NJ, Wu T, et al. Systematic underestimation of association between serum cholesterol concentration and ischaemic heart disease in observational studies: Data from the BUPA study. Br Med J 1994;308:363-366.
3.   Castelli WP, Garrison RJ, Wilson PWF, et al. Incidence of coronary heart disease and lipoprotein cholesterol levels. J Am Med Assoc 1986;256:2835-2838.

4.   Klag MJ, Ford DE, Mead LA, et al. Serum cholesterol in young men and subsequent cardiovascular disease. N Engl J Med 1993;328:313-318.
5.   Anderson KM, Castelli WP, Levy D. Cholesterol and mortality: 30 years follow-up from the Framingham Study. J Am Med Assoc 1987;257:2176-2180.
6.   Kornitzer M, Dramaix M, Beroit I, et al. Twenty-five-year mortality follow-up in the Belgian bank study. Cardiology 1993;82:153-171.
7.   Jacobs D, Blackburn H, Higgins M, et al. Report of the conference on low blood cholesterol: mortality associations. Circulation 1992;86:1046-1060.
8.   Iribarren C, Dwyer JH, Burchfield CM, et al. Can the U-shaped relationship between mortality and serum cholesterol be explained by confounding? Circulation 1993;87 (Suppl.2):7.
9   Iso H, Jacobs DR, Wentworth D, et al. Serum cholesterol levels and six-year mortality from stroke in 350,977 men screened for the multiple risk factor intervention trial. N Engl J Med 1989;320:904-910.
10. Oliver MF. Doubts about preventing coronary heart disease. Br Med J 1992;304:393-394.
11. Smith GD, Pekkanen J. Should there be a moratorium on the use of cholesterol lowering drugs? Br Med J 1992;304:431-434.
12. Strandberg TE, Salomaa VV, Naukkarinen VA, et al: Long-term mortality after 5-year multifactorial primary prevention of cardiovascular diseases in middle-aged men. J Am Med Assoc 1991;266:1225-1229.
13. The Lipid Research Clinics. Coronary Primary Prevention Trial. Results 1. Reduction in incidence of coronary heart disease. J Am Med Assoc 1984;251:351-374.
14. Frick MH, Elo O, Haapa K, et al. Helsinki heart study:Primary prevention trial with gemfibrozil in middle-aged men with dyslipidemia. N Engl J Med 1987;317:1237-1245.
15. The Lipid Research Clinics. Coronary Primary Prevention Trial: Results of 6 years of post-trial follow-up. Arch Intern Med 1992;152:1399-1410.
16. Wysowski DK, Gross TP. Deaths due to accidents and violence in two recent trials of cholesterol-lowering drugs. Arch Intern Med 1990;150:2169-2172.
17. Buckwald H, Varco RL, Matts JP, et al. Effect of partial ileal bypass surgery on mortality and morbidity from coronary heart disease in patients with hyper-cholesterolemia. N Engl J Med 1990;323:946-955.
18. Canner PL, Berge KG, Wenger NK, et al. Fifteen year mortality in coronary drug project patients: long-term benefit with niacin. J Am Coll Cardiol 1986;8:1245-1255.
19. Holme I. Relation of coronary heart disease incidence and total mortality to plasma cholesterol reduction in randomized trials: Use of meta-analysis. Br Heart J 1993;69 (Suppl.1):S42-S47.
20. The Scandinavian Simvastatin Survival Study Group. Design and baseline results of the Scandinavian Simvastatin Survival Study of patients with stable angina and/or previous myocardial infarction. Am J Cardiol 1993;71:393-400.

CHOLESTEROL-LOWERING CORONARY ANGIOGRAPHY TRIALS: AN OVERVIEW

Laurence J. Hirsch
Merck Research Laboratories
Rahway, New Jersey 07065
USA

Introduction

Beginning with the Cholesterol-Lowering Atherosclerosis Study (CLAS) trial in 1987, there have been 10 randomized, controlled trials that tested the effects of aggressive cholesterol lowering (low density lipoprotein cholesterol [LDL-C] decrease >10%) on coronary atherosclerosis. Interventions have included combined pharmacological therapy and/or lifestyle changes, ileal bypass surgery, and either cholestyramine or HMG-CoA reductase inhibitors as lipid-lowering monotherapies, in addition to low-fat diets. Both visual reading of films by blinded panels of expert angiographers and computerized quantitative coronary angiography (QCA) have been used. The primary arteriographic endpoint in 9 studies showed less average progression of lesions in active treatment patients, with $p < 0.05$ in 8 trials. Analyses also showed a decrease in the proportions of patients with definite disease progression, and an increase in patients with regression, in nearly all studies. However, the numbers of lesions showing marked change, either worsening or improvement, is rather small. The degree of LDL-C lowering observed in different studies is significantly correlated with change in percent diameter stenosis, and with proportions of patients with both progression and regression of disease. Although between-group differences in absolute lumen diameter changes are small, clinical coronary events have generally been reduced, significantly in three trials, suggesting other possible benefits of cholesterol lowering (plaque stabilization, improved endothelial function, etc.). In three trials using lovastatin (either monotherapy or with colestipol), progression of coronary lesions was significantly associated with clinical coronary events, and in three other trials angiographic worsening of disease strongly predicted subsequent clinical events. These findings support the concept that lowering LDL-C slows the progression of coronary atherosclerotic lesions, which in turn is related to reductions in clinical coronary events. Ongoing clinical endpoint trials will ultimately address the effect of intensive cholesterol reduction on coronary heart disease (CHD) morbidity and mortality.

A.M. Gotto et al. (eds.), Multiple Risk Factors in Cardiovascular Disease, 321-333.
© *1995 Kluwer Academic Publishers and Fondazione Giovanni Lorenzini.*

Background

The relationship between elevations of total cholesterol (TC) and LDL-C, and of low levels of high density lipoprotein cholesterol (HDL-C) to the incidence of CHD is well established [1,2]. Primary and secondary prevention trials have demonstrated that by lowering serum cholesterol, particularly LDL-C, combined coronary events (cardiac death and nonfatal myocardial infarction (MI)) may be reduced [3-5]. Although meta-analyses suggest significant benefits on CHD mortality as well [6], definitive data from properly designed intervention trials are lacking at this time. A number of such trials (reviewed in [7]) are now underway, the majority using HMG-CoA reductase inhibitors such as the Scandinavian Simvastatin Survival Study (4S) [8]. Nevertheless, such studies generally require the randomization and treatment of several thousand patients for periods of five or more years, at costs of tens of millions of dollars.

An alternative approach to evaluate the effect of cholesterol lowering on coronary atherosclerosis is by assessment of arteriographic change over time. Recent advances in imaging technology and standardization of cardiac catheterization procedures to improve the precision of lesion measurements [9] have enabled the conduct of coronary antiatheroma trials that can detect differences in atherosclerotic lesions between much smaller treatment groups over shorter periods of time. Such studies are the only way to directly assess potential mechanisms whereby cholesterol lowering affects the underlying pathological condition, i.e. coronary atherosclerosis, that leads to CHD morbidity and mortality. Thus effects on lesion progression, stabilization, and regression may be differentiated by angiographic endpoint trials.

The studies reviewed here were included if they were prospective, randomized and controlled, with defined arteriographic endpoints and validated assessment procedures, and if significant LDL-C lowering in the treatment group (defined as a decrease from baseline >10%) was achieved. In all cases the individuals analyzing the study angiograms were blinded to patient treatment assignment. The first such study was CLAS [10]; 9 other trials have subsequently either been published [11-18] or presented in abstract form [19]. One other trial, PLAC-1, has recently been presented, but the data are preliminary and so are not included here [20]. With the exception of the Program on the Surgical Control of the Hyperlipidemias (POSCH) [12], no study was designed to show a reduction in cardiac morbidity or mortality. This review is not a formal meta-analysis of the clinical outcomes in these trials; nevertheless certain findings regarding relationships between changes in LDL-C or HDL-C and coronary lesion progression/regression, and between lesion progression and clinical CHD events are highlighted. Other recent articles also summarize angiographic and clinical endpoint data from coronary regression trials [21-23].

Trial Descriptions

Visual scoring of individual lesion and of overall angiographic change by panels of expert angiographers, using the methods developed by Blankenhorn and coworkers [24], was employed in CLAS, POSCH, and the Monitored Atherosclerosis Regression Study (MARS)

[10,12,16]. Fully computerized QCA [11,15-19] and "hybrid" computer assisted QCA (human lesion tracing followed by digitization and computerized analysis) [13,14] were used in the other studies. MARS is the only coronary regression trial that prospectively used both QCA (primary method) and visual evaluation of coronary arteriograms. In CLAS the primary approach was by panel, but a QCA analysis in a subset of the original patients has subsequently been published [25]. In all trials (except POSCH), angiographic evidence of coronary atherosclerosis was an entry criterion, and all patients (except controls in the St. Thomas' Atherosclerosis Regression Study [STARS]) received counselling for low fat, low cholesterol diets. Brief descriptions of each study follow.

1) CLAS [10]: The Cholesterol-Lowering Atherosclerosis Study compared diet with niacin and colestipol for 2 years in 188 nonsmoking males post coronary artery bypass graft (CABG) with baseline TC 4.81-9.10 mmol/L; angiographic follow-up was obtained in 162 subjects.

2) LHT [11]: The Lifestyle Heart Trial compared the effects of a low-fat vegetarian diet, stress management and moderate exercise training, and smoking cessation to usual care in 48 patients for 1 year; follow-up QCA was performed in 41 subjects.

3) POSCH [12]: The Program on the Surgical Control of the Hyperlipidemias randomized 838 patients who survived a first myocardial infarction with TC > 5.69 mmol/L to either partial ileal bypass or usual medical care. Follow-up to 9.7 years (with repeat angiography at 3, 5, 7, and 10 years) has been reported; 634 patients had 5-year angiograms evaluated.

4) FATS [13]: The Familial Atherosclerosis Treatment Study compared a moderate approach to lipid lowering (diet ± colestipol) to either niacin and colestipol, or lovastatin and colestipol, in 146 men with apolipoprotein B ≥ 125 mg/dl and a family history of coronary artery disease; 120 subjects had follow-up QCA at 2.5 years.

5) SCOR [14]: The Specialized Center of Research (U. California, San Francisco) study randomized 97 patients with heterozygous familial hypercholesterolemia to either usual care or that plus colestipol, niacin, and in some cases, lovastatin for 2.2 years; 72 (41 female) completed the trial.

6) STARS [15]: The St. Thomas' Atherosclerosis Regression Study compared usual care versus either dietary counseling or diet plus cholestyramine in 90 men with angina or prior MI, and TC > 6.0 mmol/L; 74 patients completed the 3.2 year study.

7) MARS [16]: The Monitored Atherosclerosis Regression Study randomized 270 men and women with TC 4.92-7.64 mmol/L to diet and either placebo or lovastatin, 40 mg twice daily for 2 years; 247 patients had angiographic evaluation by the panel method, and 220 by QCA.

8) CCAIT [17]: The Canadian Coronary Atherosclerosis Intervention Trial compared diet and either placebo or lovastatin 20 to 80 mg/day (to lower LDL-C < 3.4 mmol/L) in 331 patients with TC 5.7-7.8 mmol/L for 2 years; 299 had QCA follow-up.

9) SCRIP [18]: The Stanford Coronary Risk Intervention Project compared usual care and individualized, combined programs including diet, exercise, weight loss, smoking cessation, and medications to reduce LDL-C < 2.84 mmol/L, and increase HDL-C > 1.42 mmol/L, in 300 patients over 4 years; 246 had follow-up QCA.

10) HARP [19, and Pasternack R, personal communication]: The Harvard Atherosclerosis Reversibility Project randomized 91 patients with TC 4.7-6.5 mmol/L and TC/HDL ratio ≥ 4 to diet and either placebo or stepped care with pravastatin, niacin, cholestyramine, and gemfibrozil for 2.5 years, to reduce TC < 4.1 mmol/L and LDL/HDL ≤ 2.0; 79 had follow-up QCA.

Results

LIPIDS

As shown in Table 1, the active treatment groups in all studies sustained significant reductions in LDL-C. TC and, when measured, apolipoprotein B were also significantly lowered in these patients (not shown). Changes in HDL-C, however, were much more variable, with some treatment groups (particularly those receiving high-dose niacin) showing increases of ≥ 25% [10,13,14], and others no change or even slight decreases [11,15]. Triglyceride responses in active treatment groups were also variable across these trials, ranging from reductions of about 20 to 30% [10,13-16,18] to no change or slight increases [11,12,15].

ANGIOGRAPHIC FINDINGS

The primary angiographic endpoints in the studies differ, in part depending on the method(s) of analysis. For visual film reading, the panelists reviewed individual lesions for change, but assigned a single number ranging from 0 to 3, the global change score (GCS), to indicate the overall panel consensus as to the degree of angiographic change, 0 representing no change, and 3, extreme change [10,24]. This was the primary angiographic endpoint in CLAS and POSCH, and a secondary endpoint in MARS. For the QCA studies, both relative (percent diameter stenosis, or %S) and absolute (minimum or mean lumen diameter, in mm) measures of lumen narrowing may be calculated, usually on a per-patient basis. Because %S has been reported for all QCA studies, it is summarized in Table 1. It is clear that with one exception (HARP, the study with the lowest baseline TC and LDL-C levels), the rate of coronary arterial narrowing due to atherosclerosis is slowed with aggressive reductions of LDL-C. The differences are significant between treatment and control groups except for HARP, SCRIP, and MARS (in MARS for change in %S by the panel method, p < 0.001). It is worth noting that in SCRIP, the primary endpoint was change in minimum lumen diameter, which was significantly slowed by the multifactorial treatment regimen [18]; and in STARS, mean lumen diameter, the primary endpoint, showed even greater treatment efficacy than did change in %S [15]. In MARS, GCS was also significantly reduced (improved) with lovastatin treatment (p=0.002) [16].

Spearman correlation coefficients were calculated for mean changes in LDL-C and HDL-C, each against mean change in %S, using the within-group changes observed in each of the regression trials. Use of such coefficients may be questioned because the observations are not independent; that is, changes observed for the two or three treatment groups within each trial cannot be considered to be independent of each other. Nevertheless the coefficients can be used to roughly assess the relationship between lipid changes and angiographic effects. As shown in Figure 1, mean change in %S is strongly correlated with changes in LDL-C (r=0.72, p=0.0003). In other words, the greater the decrease in LDL-C, the less the degree of worsening of %S, and the greater the chance of net improvement (regression), as assessed by QCA. A similar correlation was found between changes in %S and TC, but there was no significant correlation with HDL-C changes (r=-0.16, p=NS).

Table 1. Changes in lipids and percent diameter stenosis in coronary antiatheroma studies.

Study	Lipid Responses (%)				Change in Percent Diameter Stenosis (%)		
	Control Groups		Treatment Groups		Control Groups	Treatment Groups	p-value
	LDL-C	HDL-C	LDL-C	HDL-C			
CLAS	-5	+2	-43	+37	+1.6	-1.8	0.002
Lifestyle	-6	-3	-37	-3	+3.4	-2.2	0.001
POSCH	-5	-1	-42	+5	NA		
FATS (N+C)			-32	+43		-0.9	<0.005
	-7	+4			+2.1		
(L+C)			-46	+15		-0.7	<0.02
SCOR	-11	-1	-39	+25	+0.8	-1.5	0.039
STARS (Diet)			-16	0		-1.1	NS*
	-3	-1			+5.8		
(Diet + Chol)			-36	-4		-1.9	<0.01
MARS	-1	+2	-38	+9	+2.2	+1.6	NS
MARS (panel)					+4.0	+1.3	<0.001
CCAIT	-2	+3	-29	+7	+2.9	+1.7	0.039†
SCRIP	-4	+5	-23	+12	+2.8	+2.0	NS**
HARP	+3	0	-38	+13	+2.4	+2.1	NS

See text for descriptions and full names of studies. N=niacin; C=colestipol; L=lovastatin; Diet=low-fat diet; Chol=cholestyramine; LDL-C and HDL-C=low-density and high-density lipoprotein cholesterol; NA=not applicable; NS=not significant. For change in percent diameter stenosis (%S), a positive (+) value indicates progression or worsening; a negative (-) value indicates regression or improvement. All %S results are by QCA, except for the panel results noted for MARS. Lifestyle and HARP use lesion-based methods for statistical comparison; all other trials are per-patient averages. *p=0.06 for change in mean lumen diameter, study primary endpoint; †p=0.01 for change in minimum lumen diameter, study primary endpoint; **p=0.02 for change in minimum lumen diameter, study primary endpoint, expressed over 4-year duration of study.

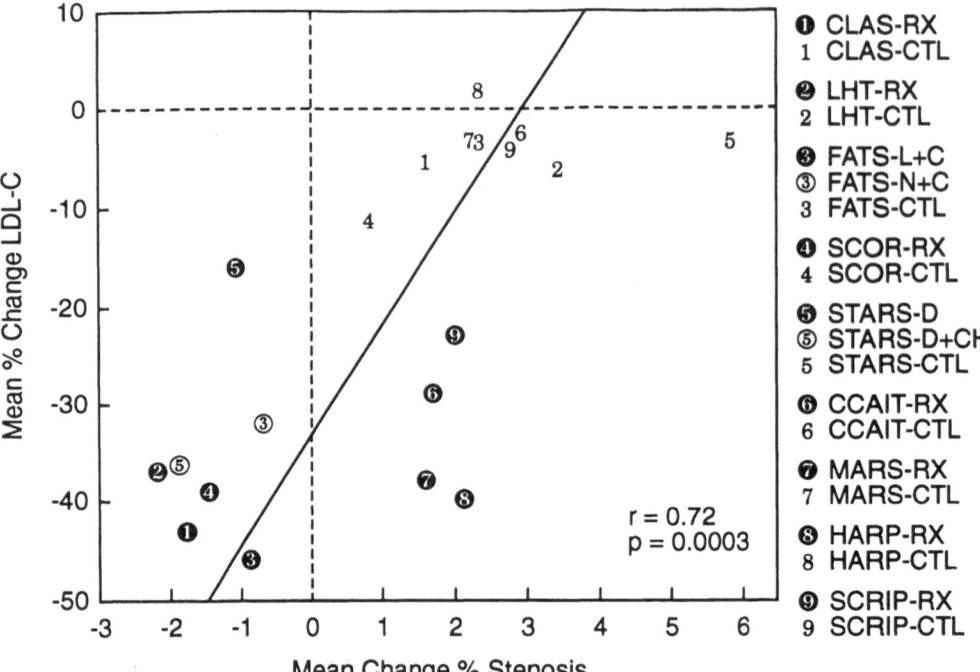

Figure 1. Correlation of within-group change from baseline in LDL-C and mean change in percent diameter stenosis, in nine coronary regression trials. The Spearman correlation coefficient is highly significant. Closed numbers (❶,③) represent active treatment groups (RX); open numbers (3) represent control groups (CTL). L=lovastatin; N=niacin; C=colestipol; D=diet; CH=cholestyramine.

Categorical Analyses. The above QCA analyses are performed on changes in lumen diameter parameters as continuous variables, usually on a per-patient basis. The precision of the methods allows detection of small differences between groups as statistically significant. However, it is usual to assign a threshold degree of lesion or segment diameter change (generally a value 2 or 3 times the standard deviation of repeated measures variability) beyond which the change is considered definite [26]. A potentially more clinically meaningful outcome is to then define patients as progressors if at least one lesion worsens beyond the threshold, and no lesions improve by a similar amount; patients may be considered regressors if the converse happens. Table 2 summarizes these data from all of the trials, and it is again clear that aggressive cholesterol lowering decreases the proportion of patients with disease progression (by nearly 50%, on average), and increases the proportion with disease regression (by 2.5-fold, on average). As with mean change in %S,

LDL-C change correlated significantly with both types of categorical change (data not shown).

Table 2. Proportions of patients with angiographic progression or regression, and with clinical coronary heart disease (CHD) events, in coronary antiatheroma studies.

Study	Patients With Progression (%)		Patients With Regression (%)		CHD Events	
	Control	Treatment	Control	Treatment	Control Patients (%)	Treatment Patients (%)
CLAS	61	39	4	16	18(19)	15(16)
Lifestyle	NA	NA	NA	NA	1	0
POSCH (5 yrs)	65	37	5	13	125(30)	82(20)*
FATS (N+C)		25		39		2(4)**
	46		11		10(19)	
(L+C)		21		32		3(7)**
SCOR	41	13	20	33	1	0
STARS (Diet)		15		38		3(11)†
	46		4		10(36)	
(Diet + Chol)		12		33		1(4)†
MARS	41	29	12	23	31(23)	22(16)
MARS (panel)	65	47	11	23		
CCAIT	50	33	7	10	21(13)	17(10)
SCRIP	50	50	10	20	35(23)	20(14)‡
HARP	38	33	15	13	10(21)	6(14)

See text for descriptions and full names of studies. N=niacin; C=colestipol; L=lovastatin; Diet=low-fat diet; Chol=cholestyramine. CHD events are variably defined, and include cardiac death, nonfatal myocardial infarction, unstable angina, and either coronary bypass surgery or angioplasty. STARS includes cerebrovascular accidents; FATS includes peripheral revascularization procedures; HARP includes congestive heart failure.
*p < 0.001 (combined cardiac death and nonfatal MI); **p=0.03 (N+C), p=0.08 (L+C), overall p=0.01; †p < 0.05 (diet), p < 0.01 (diet+chol); ‡p=0.07.

CLINICAL EVENTS

None of these studies, except POSCH, was designed to look at clinical endpoints, and even POSCH was inadequately powered for detection of decreased all-cause mortality, the primary endpoint. Nevertheless, CHD events have been reported in all studies, and these data are summarized in Table 2. It must be remembered that specific criteria for event classification vary between studies, and different studies do not report the exact same events. Keeping these points in mind, there are consistently positive effects of cholesterol lowering on the incidence of clinical CHD events in these studies, with reported decreases of up to 70-80%. In 3 trials (POSCH, FATS, and STARS), the event reductions are significant [12,13,15], and in SCRIP, nearly so [18]. Nevertheless, the small number of events in most of these trials preclude drawing definitive conclusions on the clinical benefits of aggressive lipid lowering in this population of patients.

Angiographic Change and CHD Events. An important question is whether angiographic progression is associated with the incidence of clinical CHD events. Data from the two lovastatin monotherapy trials, MARS and CCAIT, as well as from FATS support such a relationship. In CCAIT, all patients considered to be progressors were significantly more likely to have a clinical CHD event as were patients who were not. Conversely, more patients with at least one cardiac event were considered progressors as were patients without an event. Similarly in MARS, the distribution of GCS was shifted toward significantly more disease progression in those patients who sustained a clinical CHD event than in those who did not (manuscript in preparation). Data from FATS also demonstrate a clear relationship between lesion deterioration and acute clinical events. In this study, using a multivariate model to estimate change in %S in proximal coronary artery segments, patients in the highest tercile of estimated change (i.e. those with the most progression) had a 9-fold risk of a clinical event, compared to those in the lowest tercile (p < 0.002) [13].

Angiographic Progression as a Predictor of Clinical Events. Data from the POSCH, CLAS, and nicardipine intervention trials all provide strong evidence that not only are angiographic progression and CHD events related, but that the former is predictive of the latter. In POSCH, progression of coronary disease by GCS in 695 patients at 3 years was correlated with subsequent clinical events from 3 to 10 years [27]. Specifically, the combined outcome of CHD mortality or nonfatal MI (p=0.04, ileal bypass group, and p < 0.0001, control group), as well as coronary- and all-cause mortality (p=0.003, and p=0.01, respectively, both groups) were all twice as common in those patients who were progressors at 3 years as in those who were not. Similar findings have recently been presented from the 10 year follow-up of CLAS patients [28]. In the nicardipine study [29], progression of disease (defined as a worsening ≥ 15%S by QCA in at least one lesion) was found in 141 of 335 patients after 2 years. During a mean follow-up of 44 +/- 10 months, patients with progression at 2 years were 7.3 times as likely to have suffered a cardiac death (p < 0.001), and 2.3 times as likely to have had a nonfatal MI or cardiac death (p=0.009).

PLAQUE STABILIZATION WITH CHOLESTEROL LOWERING

The strength of the relationship between angiographic disease progression and clinical coronary heart disease events is impressive, particularly given the relatively small absolute differences in %S between treatment groups in the various studies, as shown in Table 1. Several of the coronary antiatheroma studies have found that relatively few lesions (in the range of 10%) show definite progression (or regression) [13,17], implying that a minority of lesions progress sufficiently to account for acute clinical CHD events (death, MI, unstable angina). A detailed discussion is beyond the scope of this overview, but work by Davies and colleagues [30,31], Fuster et al. [32], and more recently Brown et al. [21] strongly suggests that there is indeed a relatively small number of "culprit" lesions that account for clinical CHD events. Such lesions number no more than 10-20% of all coronary lesions, and are characterized by several features: usually mild-to-moderate stenosis severity, a large extracellular lipid core, a weakened fibrous cap with decreased collagen content and smooth muscle cells, and increased numbers of macrophages. These lesions are often shaped eccentrically at bend or branch points in the coronary arteries. These factors predispose these lesions to rupture or fissure, exposing the highly thrombogenic core contents to the circulation, resulting in intramural (plaque) hemorrhage, and mural, or worse, occlusive intraluminal thrombus.

Brown has suggested that intensive lipid lowering therapies stabilize such plaques [21]. Such effects may therefore result in small average angiographic changes, but lead to seemingly disproportionate reductions in clinical CHD events [33]. In FATS, Brown has analyzed 13 coronary events that occurred among the 146 patients. The events were associated with a "culprit" lesion (in the appropriate distribution of worsening ischemia) that had markedly progressed in severity from baseline measurement to that at the time of the event. In the control patients, 8 of 9 cardiac events arose from 414 lesions that were less than 70%S at baseline. Conversely, only 1 of 683 similar lesions in the two intensively treated groups precipitated a clinical event (p < 0.004), implying a stabilizing effect on the pool of potential culprit plaques [21]. Other beneficial effects of cholesterol lowering have also been suggested, including healing of the coronary endothelium and restoration of normal coronary vascular reactivity [34,35], and reductions in prothrombotic tendencies, including the augmented platelet adhesiveness seen in hypercholesterolemia [36]. Further work is needed to better understand what role aggressive lowering of cholesterol may have on these possible risks for acute cardiac events.

Summary

The coronary angiographic trials reviewed show consistent beneficial effects of intensive cholesterol lowering to slow the average progression of coronary atherosclerosis, whether assessed visually or by QCA. Patient-based analyses clearly demonstrate decreased progression, and increased regression of disease. Reductions in LDL-C correlate strongly with these angiographic outcomes. Absolute differences in lumen diameter measures between control and active treatment groups tend to be small, yet most studies show positive trends in clinical coronary event reductions; in three trials the differences are significant. These findings, in concert with histopathological and angiographic studies, suggest the existence of a small group of "culprit" lesions with large extracellular lipid cores and weakened fibrous caps that are prone to fissure or rupture, leading to intramural or plaque hemorrhage, with mural and possibly intraluminal thrombus formation; clinically these present as acute myocardial infarction, unstable angina, and cardiac death. Arteriographic disease progression, in turn, increases the risk of clinical CHD events. The data suggest that lowering LDL-C promotes plaque stabilization, which reduces the likelihood of acute cardiac events.

Acknowledgments

The performance of the statistical correlation analyses by Dr. Deborah Shapiro, and the efforts of Mss. Maria Kanellos and Donna Walters in the preparation of this manuscript are greatly, and gratefully, appreciated.

Note Added Post-Symposium

The results of the HARP, MAAS, and 4S studies were all published shortly after presentation of these analyses at the symposium [37-39]. The MAAS trial demonstrated that simvastatin slows the progression of coronary atherosclerosis, including reductions of new lesions and new occlusions, as assessed by QCA [38]. The 4S trial has convincingly shown that aggressive lowering of serum cholesterol and LDL-C with simvastatin reduces total mortality 30% (by preventing CHD deaths) with no adverse effects on non-CHD morbidity or mortality, in patients with a history of MI or unstable angina [39].

References

1.   LaRosa JC, Hunninghake D, Bush D, et al. Special report: The cholesterol facts. A summary of the evidence relating dietary fats, serum cholesterol, and coronary heart disease. A joint statement by the American Heart Association and the National Heart, Lung, and Blood Institute. Circulation 1990;81:1721-1733.

2.   Pekkanen J, Linn S, Heiss G, et al. Ten-year mortality from cardiovascular disease in relation to cholesterol level among men with and without pre-existing cardiovascular disease. N Engl J Med 1990;322:1700-1707.

3.   Rossouw JE, Lewis B, Rifkind BM. The value of lowering cholesterol after myocardial infarction. N Engl J Med 1990;323:1112-1119.

4.   Lipid Research Clinics Program. Lipid Research Clinics Coronary Primary Prevention Trial results. I. Reduction of coronary heart disease. JAMA 1984;251: 365-374.

5.   Frick MH, Elo O, Haapak E, et al. Helsinki Heart Study: Primary prevention trial with gemfibrozil in middle-aged men with dyslipidemia. N Engl J Med 1987;317: 1237-1245.

6.   Law MR, Wald, NJ Thompson SG. By how much and how quickly does reduction in serum cholesterol concentration lower risk of ischemic heart disease? BMJ 1994; 308:367-372.

7.   Mellies MJ. Ongoing and planned clinical trials for atherosclerosis prevention and regression. Curr Opin Invest Drugs 1993;2:529-539.

8.   Scandinavian Simvastatin Survival Study Group. Design and baseline results of the Scandinavian Simvastatin Survival Study of patients with unstable angina or previous myocardial infarction. Amer J Cardiol 1993;71:393-400.

9. Reiber JHC, Serruys PW, Kooijman CJ, et. al. Assessment of short-, medium-, and long-term variations in arterial dimensions from computer-assisted quantitation of coronary cineangiograms. Circulation 1985;71:280-288.
10. Blankenhorn DH, Nessim SA, Johnson RL, et al. Beneficial effects of combined colestipol-niacin therapy on coronary atherosclerosis and coronary venous bypass grafts. JAMA 1987;257:3233-3240.
11. Ornish D, Brown SE, Scherwitz LW, et al. Can lifestyle changes reverse coronary heart disease? The Lifestyle Heart Trial. Lancet 1990;336:129-133.
12. Buchwald H, Varco RL, Matts JP, et al. Effect of partial ileal bypass surgery on mortality and morbidity from coronary heart disease in patients with hyper-cholesterolemia. Report of the Program on the Surgical Control of the Hyper-lipidemias (POSCH). New Engl J Med 1990;323:946-955.
13. Brown G, Albers JJ, Fisher LD, et al. Regression of coronary artery disease as a result of intensive lipid-lowering therapy in men with high levels of apolipoprotein B. New Engl J Med 1990;323:1289-1298
14. Kane JP, Malloy MJ, Ports TA, Phillips NR, Diehl JC, Havel RJ. Regression of coronary atherosclerosis during treatment of familial hypercholesterolemia with combined drug regimens. JAMA 1990;264:3007-3012.
15. Watts GF, Lewis B, Brunt JNH, et al. Effects on coronary artery disease of lipid-lowering diet, or diet plus cholestyramine, in the St. Thomas' Atherosclerosis Regression Study (STARS). Lancet 1992;339:563-569.
16. Blankenhorn DH, Azen SP, Kramsch DM, et al. Coronary angiographic changes with lovastatin therapy. The Monitored Atherosclerosis Regression Study (MARS). Ann Int Med 1993;11:969-976.
17. Waters D, Higginson L, Gallstone P, et al. Effects of monotherapy with an HMG-CoA reductase inhibitor on the progression of coronary atherosclerosis as assessed by serial quantitative arteriography. The Canadian Coronary Atherosclerosis Intervention Trial. Circulation 1993;89:959-968.
18. Haskell WL, Alderman EL, Fair JM, et al. Effects of intensive multiple risk factor reduction on coronary atherosclerosis and clinical cardiac events in men and women with coronary artery disease. The Stanford Coronary Risk Intervention Project (SCRIP). Circulation 1993;89:975-990.
19. Sacks FM, Pasternak RC, Gibson CM, Rosner B, Stone PH for the HARP Group. The effect on coronary artery stenosis of intensive pharmacologic step therapy to improve LDL and HDL in patients with normal plasma lipid levels. Circulation 1992;86(Suppl.I):I-743.
20. Pitt B, Mancini GBJ, Ellis SG, Rosman HS, McGovern ME for the PLAC I Investigators. Pravastatin Limitation of Atherosclerosis in the Coronary Arteries (PLAC I). J Amer Coll Cardiol 1994:ii-131A.
21. Brown BG, Zhao XQ, Sacco DE, Albers JJ. Lipid lowering and plaque regression. New insights into prevention of plaque disruption and clinical events in coronary disease. Circulation 1993;87:1781-1791.

22.   Vos J, de Feyter PJ, Simoons ML, Tijssen JGP and Deckers JW. Retardation and arrest of progression or regression of coronary artery disease: A review. Prog Cardiovasc Dis 1993;35:435-454.

23.   Blankenhorn DH, Hodis HN. Arterial imaging and atherosclerosis reversal. Arterioscler Thromb 1994;14:177-192.

24.   Azen SP, Cashin-Hemphill L, Pogoda J, et al. Evaluation of human panelists in assessing coronary atherosclerosis. Arterioscler Thromb 1991;11:385-394.

25.   Blankenhorn DH, Selzer RH, Mack WJ, et al. Evaluation of colestipol/niacin therapy with computer-derived coronary end point measures. A comparison of different measures of treatment effect. Circulation 1992;86:1701-1709.

26.   Brown BG, Hillger LA, Lewis C, et al. A maximum confidence approach for measuring progression and regression of coronary artery disease in clinical trials. Circulation 1993;87(Suppl.II):II-66-II-73.

27.   Buchwald H, Matts J, Fitch L, et al. for the Program on the Surgical Control of the Hyperlipidemias (POSCH) Group. Changes in sequential coronary arteriograms and subsequent coronary events. JAMA 1992;268:1429-1433.

28.   Cashin-Hemphill L, Mack W, LaBree L, et al. Coronary progression predicts future cardiac events. Circulation 1993;88(4):I-363.

29.   Waters D, Craven T, Lesperance J. Prognostic significance of progression of coronary atherosclerosis. Circulation 1993;87:1067-1075.

30.   Davies MJ. A macro and micro view of coronary vascular insult in ischemic heart disease. Circulation 1990;82(3):II-38-II-46.

31.   Richardson P, Davies MJ, Born GVR. Influence of plaque configuration and stress distribution on fissuring of coronary atherosclerotic plaques. Lancet 1989;ii:941-944.

32.   Fuster V, Badimon L, Badimon JJ, Chesebro JH. The pathogenesis of coronary artery disease and acute coronary syndromes. N Engl J Med 1992;326:242-250, 310-318.

33.   Applegate, RJ, Herrington DM, Little WC. Coronary angiography: More than meets the eye. Circulation 1993;87:1399-1401.

34.   Treasure CB, Talleyu JD, Stillabower ME, and the Lovastatin Restenosis Trial Study Group. Coronary endothelial responses are improved with aggressive lipid lowering therapy in patients with coronary atherosclerosis. Circulation 1993;88(4):I-368.

35.   Egashira K, Hirooka Y, Kai H, et al. Reduction in serum cholesterol with pravastatin improves endothelium-dependent coronary vasomotion in patients with hypercholesterolemia. Circulation 1994;89:2519-2524.

36.   Kaul S, Waack BJ, Padgett RC, Brooks RM, Heistad DD. Altered vascular responses to platelets from hypercholesterolemic humans. Circ Res 1993;72:737-743.

37.   Sacks FM, Pasternack RC, Gibson CM, Rosner B, Stone PH for the Harvard Atherosclerosis Reversibility Project (HARP) Group. Effect on coronary atherosclerosis of decrease in plasma cholesterol concentrations in

normocholesterolaemic patients. Lancet 1994;344:1182-1186.

38. MAAS Investigators. Effect of simvastatin on coronary atheroma: the Multicentre Anti-Atheroma Study (MAAS). Lancet 1994;344:633-638.

39. Scandinavian Simvastatin Survival Study Group. Randomized trial of cholesterol lowering in 4444 patients with coronary heart disease: the Scandinavian Simvastatin Survival Study (4S). Lancet 1994;344:1383-1389.

TREATMENT OF HYPERLIPIDEMIA IN SPECIFIC TYPES OF PATIENTS: THE ELDERLY, WOMEN, AND PATIENTS WITH CORONARY ARTERY DISEASE

D. Roger Illingworth
Division of Endocrinology
Diabetes and Clinical Nutrition
Department of Medicine
Oregon Health Sciences University
Portland, Oregon 97201
USA

Introduction

The well-recognized association between hypercholesterolemia and an increased risk of premature coronary artery disease, together with angiographic evidence that treatment of patients identified to have hypercholesterolemia attributable to increased concentrations of low density lipoproteins (LDL), leading to regression, slowed progression, and a substantial reduction in the number of cardiovascular events, prompted the development of guidelines for evaluation and treatment of hypercholesterolemia in Europe and the USA [1-3]. These guidelines suggest that in a given patient with hypercholesterolemia the concentration of LDL cholesterol at which diet and potentially drug therapy should be recommended depends on the presence or absence of coronary artery disease, the presence or absence of other risk factors, and the age and sex of the patient. The present paper discusses approaches to the treatment of hypercholesterolemia in three specific patient populations: older individuals (age > 65 years); women; and patients with established coronary artery disease.

Hyperlipidemia in Older Patients

The evaluation and potential treatment of older patients identified to have hypercholesterolemia should proceed along a logical sequence which should include establishing the lipoprotein phenotype, evaluating the patient for potential secondary causes of hypercholesterolemia, close examination of the patient for physical stigmata of genetic dyslipidemias as well as subclinical evidence of vascular disease (e.g. the presence of carotid or femoral bruits), and evaluating the patient's family history, presence or absence of other cardiovascular risk factors, and the potential role of other concurrent medications as contributing factors in the causation of hyperlipidemia. Hypothyroidism represents a

335

A.M. Gotto et al. (eds.), Multiple Risk Factors in Cardiovascular Disease, 335-339.
© 1995 Kluwer Academic Publishers and Fondazione Giovanni Lorenzini.

common and potentially treatable secondary cause of hypercholesterolemia in older patients. Hypothyroidism was present in 6% of patients screened for the Cholesterol Reduction in Senior People (CRISP) study which evaluated the safety and efficacy of lovastatin in patients with hypercholesterolemia who were over 65 years of age [4]. In this patient population hypothyroidism was the most common secondary cause of hypercholesterolemia. A thyroid-stimulating hormone (TSH) determination should be included in the evaluation of every patient identified to have hypercholesterolemia regardless of whether or not the patient has clinical stigmata suggestive of hypothyroidism. Studies have demonstrated that although the relative risk of coronary heart disease as a function of increasing plasma concentrations of total and LDL cholesterol becomes lower with advancing age, the absolute or attributable risk becomes greater. This is well illustrated by the studies of Rubin et al [5] who followed 2,746 men, initially aged 60-79, for a period of 10.1 years and assessed cardiovascular mortality as a function of cholesterol concentration. Although the relative risk varied from 1.4 to 1.7 between the lower and upper quintile of cholesterol concentrations in men ranging in age between 60-64 years and 75-79 years, the excess risk from coronary artery disease between the lower and upper quintiles of cholesterol concentration rose from 2.2 in the men aged 60-64 to 11.3 in the men aged 75-79. These results justify treatment of hypercholesterolemia in selected older male patients with no other life-limiting disorders who are functionally active with a view to reducing their excess risk from cardiovascular disease. If dietary therapy proves inadequate, HMG CoA reductase inhibitors may be the preferred therapy for older patients with hypercholesterolemia in whom the incidence of clinical side effects associated with bile acid sequestrants and nicotinic acid may be unacceptable. Recent studies [4,6] have assessed the efficacy of lovastatin in older patients with primary hypercholesterolemia. In the EXCEL Study [6] slightly greater reductions in the plasma concentrations of LDL cholesterol were observed in older men and women treated with lovastatin at doses ranging from 20-80 mg/day. Similar results were observed in the CRISP Pilot Study [4]. In both studies the clinical side-effect profile of lovastatin was similar to that observed in younger patients [6]. Although several reports have indicated that the frequency of drug-associated side effects is 20-35% higher in older patients as compared to their younger counterparts, this may be in large part due to the high frequency of polypharmacy in older patients, a higher frequency of patient error, and variations in patient compliance as well as slowed drug metabolism of systemically acting agents in this patient population [7]. In the opinion of the author, it is important to individualize therapy and assess in each patient the benefit:risk ratio of treatment in the primary prevention of cardiovascular disease.

Hyperlipidemia in Women

Cardiovascular disease remains the number one cause of death in women and the primary prevention of premature coronary artery disease is appropriate in selected female patients with multiple risk factors or those with genetic disorders of lipoprotein metabolism, particularly heterozygous familial hypercholesterolemia. In premenopausal women with hypercholesterolemia it is important to define the causal etiology of this disorder, exclude potential exacerbating secondary factors and evaluate the patient for the presence or absence of other cardiovascular risk factors or subclinical evidence of atherosclerosis. Dietary therapy should be recommended for adult female patients with LDL concentrations which exceed 160 mg/dl and drug therapy should be considered in patients in whom the LDL concentrations exceed 190-220 mg/dl on maximal dietary therapy. Drug therapy is most appropriate in premenopausal women with heterozygous familial hypercholesterolemia, particularly those with a strongly positive family history of premature coronary artery disease, those with other known cardiovascular risk factors or patients with increased plasma concentrations of Lp(a).

Similar considerations should be applied to the evaluation and treatment of postmenopausal women with primary hypercholesterolemia for whom the goal of therapy is the primary prevention of coronary artery disease. In this population, however, estrogen replacement therapy should be regarded as an integral part of treatment in those women who do not have a contraindication to the use of estrogens, either alone in women who have undergone a hysterectomy or, estrogen plus progesterone therapy in women who have not undergone a hysterectomy [8].

As illustrated in Table 1 the hypolipidemic effects of lovastatin appear slightly greater in female as compared to male patients with heterozygous familial hypercholesterolemia. The percent reduction in LDL is greatest in postmenopausal women who are not receiving estrogen replacement therapy. However, the overall magnitude of reduction in LDL cholesterol concentrations is greatest in postmenopausal women who are treated sequentially with diet, oral estrogen therapy, and drug therapy, as compared to diet plus drug therapy with the omission of estrogen replacement therapy.

Table 1.   Response to lovastatin therapy (40 mg/day) in male and female patients with heterozygous familial hypercholesterolemia.

		Percent Change	
	N	LDL-Chol	HDL-Chol
Males	69	-30 ± 13	+12 ± 18
Females	82	-34 ± 13*	+13 ± 23
Cycling	40	-32 ± 13ns	+15 ± 28
Post-menopausal	24	-38 ± 12**	+13 ± 16
PM + Estrogen	15	-31 ± 11	+11 ± 21

Values shown are the percent change in plasma lipid concentrations + S.D.

*= $p < .05$ for differences between males and females
**= $p < .002$ for differences between males and females by one-way anova
N= number of patients, PM = postmenopausal, ns = not significant

Treatment of Patients with Coronary Heart Disease

Available evidence justifies an aggressive approach to treatment of hypercholesterolemia in male and female patients with known coronary artery disease in whom an optimal goal of therapy is an LDL cholesterol concentration of < 100-130 mg/dl [1-3]. In the opinion of the author, the National Cholesterol Education Program (NCEP) Guidelines, which are the most aggressive in terms of therapy goals, are supported by the angiographic studies and should be regarded as optimal targets of therapy for those patients with known coronary artery disease. These guidelines are appropriate in both male and female patients and should also be applied to older patients with coronary artery disease who do not have other life-limiting illnesses and in whom therapy is likely to improve the quality of life and reduce the risk of subsequent cardiovascular procedures or death. The NCEP Panel has recommended HMG CoA reductase inhibitors, bile acid sequestrants, and nicotinic acid as the drugs of first choice for the treatment of primary hypercholesterolemia and, of these three classes of agents, the HMG CoA reductase inhibitors are the most effective. However, even at maximal doses, simvastatin, the most effective of the currently available HMG CoA reductase inhibitors, reduces LDL concentrations by up to 45% which, in patients with more severe degrees of hypercholesterolemia who concurrently have coronary heart disease, still leaves the patient with significant hypercholesterolemia. The percent reduction in LDL cholesterol concentrations to achieve target values as defined by the NCEP Panel is illustrated in Table 2. From this table it is apparent that in patients with LDL concentrations exceeding 190-240 mg/dl, combination drug therapy is likely to be necessary if optimal goals are to be obtained. In patients with more severe degrees of hypercholesterolemia, other measures including the use of LDL apheresis may be appropriate.

Table 2. NCEP II Guidelines [1]; % reduction needed to meet LDL-C goals.

Base LDL-C (mg/dl)	< 160 mg/dl	2 RF/DM < 130 mg/dl	CAD < 100 mg/dl
190 -240	16 to 33%	32 to 46%	47 to 58%
160 - 190	N/A	19 to 32%	38 to 47%
130 - 160	N/A	N/A	23 to 38%

LDL-C, low density lipoprotein cholesterol; RF, risk factors; DM, diabetes; CAD, coronary artery disease; N/A, not applicable

References

1.   The Expert Panel. Summary of the second report of the National Cholesterol Education Program Expert Panel on Detection, Evaluation and Treatment of High

Blood Cholesterol in Adults. JAMA 1993;269:3015-3023.

2.   European Atherosclerosis Society. Prevention of coronary heart disease - scientific background and new clinical guidelines. Nutrition Metabolism Cardiovascular Diseases 1992;2:113-156.

3.   Betteridge DJ, Dodson PM, Durrington BN, et al. Management of hyperlipidemia. Guidelines of the British Hyperlipidemia Association. Postgrad Med J 1993;69:359-369.

4.   LaRosa JC, Applingate W, Crouse JR, III, et al. Cholesterol-lowering in the elderly. Results of the Cholesterol Reduction in Seniors Program (CRISP) Pilot Study. Arch Intern Med 1994;154:529-539.

5.   Rubin SM, Sidney S, Black DM, et al. High blood cholesterol in elderly men and the excess risk for coronary heart disease. Ann Intern Med 1990;113:916-920.

6.   Shear CL, Franklin FA, Stinnett S, et al. Expanded clinical evaluation of lovastatin (EXCEL) - study results. Effect of patient characteristics on lovastatin-induced changes in plasma concentrations of lipids and lipoproteins. Circulation 1992;85:1293-1303.

7.   LaRosa JC. Dyslipoproteinemia in women and the elderly. Med Clinics Nth America 1994;78:163-180.

8.   Belchetz PE. Hormonal treatment of postmenopausal women. N Engl J Med 1994;330:1062-1071.

AN ITALIAN MULTICENTER STUDY ON EFFICACY AND TOLERABILITY OF SIMVASTATIN IN MALE PATIENTS WITH ESSENTIAL HYPERTENSION AND PRIMARY HYPERCHOLESTEROLEMIA

Antonio Salvetti, Gianfranco Argenio, and Giampaolo Bernini
Cattedra di Medicina Interna, 1a Clinica Medica
on the behalf of participating Centers of IMSS
University of Pisa
Pisa
ITALY

Summary

Hypertension and hypercholesterolemia frequently coexist and may require concomitant drug treatment. Avalaible data suggested that simvastatin is able to improve the lipid profile in hypercholesterolemic hypertensive patients without changing the antihypertensive effect of the pharmacological therapy.

A recent Italian Multicenter Study with Simvastatin (IMSS) has adressed the effects of this drug on the lipid profile and blood pressure of 122 male hypercholesterolemic essential hypertensive patients, whose blood pressure was stably controlled by drug treatment. Simvastatin, given at the titrated dose from 10 to 40 mg o.d. (mean dosage 21.9 mg) for 48 weeks, significantly reduced total cholesterol (-31%), LDL-cholesterol (-44%), and triglycerides (-13%) and significantly increased HDL-cholesterol (+11%). At the end of the study 92.8% and 93.7% of patients reached the end points of total cholesterol < 200 mg/dl and of LDL-cholesterol < 130 mg/dl respectively. Blood pressure did not show any significant change and subgroup analysis showed that the effect of simvastatin was unaffected by the kind of antihypertensive treatment and vice versa. The incidence of subjective side effects was 0.8%, that of adverse biochemical drug-related effects was 5.7%, and the drop-out rate due to adverse biochemical effects, 1.6%.

In conclusion, the IMSS showed that simvastatin is an effective and well-tolerated drug for improving the lipid profile in male hypercholesterolemic hypertensive patients. Moreover, simvastatin did not interfere with the blood pressure lowering effect of commonly used antihypertensive drugs.

A.M. Gotto et al. (eds.), Multiple Risk Factors in Cardiovascular Disease, 341-347.
© *1995 Kluwer Academic Publishers and Fondazione Giovanni Lorenzini.*

Introduction

Epidemiological data have clearly shown that coexistence of several risk factors increases the likelihood of developing atherosclerotic vascular disease. Since hypertension, male sex, and hypercholesterolemia are well-known cardiovascular risk factors, it seems rational to reduce increased serum cholesterol levels in hypertensive males, a goal which can be achieved by drug treatment when appropriate dietary intervention is ineffective.

Experimental [1,2] and clinical [1] data have shown that LDL-cholesterol can modify vascular reactivity, and recently it has been reported that LDL-cholesterol reduction induced by statin treatment lowered diastolic blood pressure in untreated hypercholes-terolemic essential hypertensive patients [3]. However, it has also been reported that in WKY and SHR rats lovastatin increased *in vivo* blood pressure and impaired endothelium-dependent and -independent vasodilation *in vitro* [4]. Therefore, the possibility may exist that simvastatin can influence blood pressure in two opposite ways.

Simvastatin, a 3-hydroxy-3-methylglutaryl Coenzyme A (HMG-CoA) reductase inhibitor, is a well-proven cholesterol lowering drug both in familial and nonfamilial hypercholesterolemic patients [5]. To our knowledge, only two studies have evaluated the effects of simvastatin on lipids and blood pressure of stably treated hypercholesterolemic essential hypertensive patients, and results obtained show that this drug significantly lowered total cholesterol and improved lipid profile without changing blood pressure [6,7]. However, in these two placebo-controlled studies the effects of simvastatin were assessed in a relatively small number of patients treated for a relatively short period.

Therefore, we decided to evaluate the efficacy and tolerability of simvastatin in essential hypertensive males with primary hypercholesterolemia in a larger population and for a longer treatment period. In addition, investigation also focused on assessing whether this drug can modify blood pressure in these hypertensive patients, whose blood pressure was stably and well controlled by commonly used antihypertensive drugs.

Material and Methods

Subjects: One-hundred-twenty-two essential hypertensive males (age: 42.6 + 8.3 years, range 18-65 yrs, body mass index < 27 Kg/m2) with primary hypercholesterolemia were selected, in 13 Italian Medical Centers, after giving informed consent, according to the following criteria.

- Serum total cholesterol > 240 mg/dl and calculated (by Friedwald's formula) LDL-cholesterol > 160 mg/dl at the end of a 6-month period of hypolipidemic drug wash-out and of low cholesterol (cholesterol intake < 300 mg/day) diet.
- Blood pressure stably controlled (diastolic blood pressure < 95mmHg at four consecutive measurements at 4-week intervals) by active drug treatment during the same 6-month observation period.

Trial plan: According to a sequential open-trial design, patients, while continuing antihypertensive drug treatment at a constant schedule and the low cholesterol diet, received simvastatin, with dosage titration over a 12-week period in order to achieve the target point of total cholesterol < 200 mg/dl and of calculated LDL-cholesterol < 130 mg/dl. All patients started by taking 10 mg simvastatin once daily with their evening meal for a 4-week period and the dose was eventually increased to 20 mg up to 40 mg every 4 weeks. Thereafter, the dosage of simvastatin which achieved target points was given up to 48 weeks.

At week 0, 4, 8, 12, 24, 36, and 48 blood samples were collected for determination of total cholesterol, HDL-cholesterol, triglycerides, white blood cell count (WBC), red blood cell count (RBC), hemoglobin, hematocrit, alanine aminotransferase (ALT), aspartate aminotransferase (AST), gamma glutamyltransferase (GGT), creatinine phosphokinase (CPK), alkaline phosphatase, creatinine, and glucose.

At the same time blood pressure was measured by mercury sphygmomanometer in the same arm and by the same observer three times, with patients seated in a comfortable chair for at least 15 minutes. The three values were then averaged. A complete clinical hystory was recorded to monitor possible side effects or adverse effects at the same intervals.

Lipid measurements: All 13 Medical Centers involved in the study applied standard methods. Serum total cholesterol and triglycerides were measured using the enzyme method. HDL-cholesterol was evaluated by the same enzyme method after precipitation with phosphotustic acid and magnesium chloride. LDL-cholesterol was calculated by Friedwald's formula.

Results

At the end of the titration phase 30 (24.6%) patients received 10 mg/day of simvastatin, 65 (53.3%) received 20 mg/day and 27 (22.1%) received 40 mg/day. In accordance with the trial plan, this dosage schedule was maintained until the end of the study. Mean dosage of simvastatin was 21.9 mg/day.

Twelve patients dropped out after the titration phase for the following reasons: 2 deaths (1 sudden death, 1 car accident), 1 protocol violator, 7 lost at follow-up and 2 for laboratory adverse effects. As shown in Table 1, both total and LDL-cholesterol were significantly (p < 0.0001) reduced. Total cholesterol was already reduced at the 4th week (-16%); it reached the target point (< 200 mg/dl) at the 12th week (-29%) and maintained similar values at the 48th week (-31%). LDL-cholesterol declined at the 4th week (-22%), was further reduced at the 12th week (-41%) below target point (< 130 mg/dl) and showed similar values at the 48th week (-44%). At the end of the study 92.8% and 93.7% of patients showed values of total cholesterol < 200 mg/dl and of LDL-cholesterol below 130 mg/dl, respectively. Triglycerides significantly (p < 0.05) decreased at the 4th week (-9%) and were further (-14%, p < 0.01) reduced at the 8th week and remained so up to the 48th week (-13%). HDL-cholesterol started to rise from the 4th week (+6%, n.s.), reaching the maximum increment at the 12th week (+12%, p < 0.005), and remained at similar values at the end of the study (+11%).

Subgroup analysis of patients receiving different antihypertensive drugs alone or in combination (Table 2) showed that the effect of simvastatin on total cholesterol was unaffected by the kind of antihypertensive treatment.

Table 1. Absolute values of total (TC), LDL (LDL-C), and HDL (HDL-C) cholesterol, of triglycerides (TG) and of systolic (SBP) and diastolic (DPB) blood pressure before (0) and during simvastatin treatment.

weeks	0	4	8	12	24	36	48
TC mg/dl	274.2 ± 2.0	230.9 ± 2.7*	206.3 ± 2.7*	195.8 ± 2.4*	191.2 ± 2.6*	187.4 ± 2.6*	190.3 ± 2.9*
LDL-C mg/dl	192.3 ± 2.5	149.5 ± 2.8*	125.7 ± 2.8*	114.0± 2.4*	110.9 ± 2.7*	107.3 ± 2.6*	108.5 ± 2.9*
TG mg/dl	187.5 ± 4.6	170.0 ± 4.3§	161.8 ± 4.1°	160.6 ± 6.4°	158.4 ± 5.7°	158.9 ± 5.9°	162.0 ± 5.9°
HDL-C mg/dl	44.4 ± 1.0	47.3 ± 1.0	48.5 ± 1.0°	49.6 ± 1.0"	49.1 ± 1.1§	48.7 ± 1.0§	49.2 ± 1.1§
SBP mmHg	146.1 ± 0.9	146.3 ± 0.9	146.0 ±0.9	144.3 ± 0.8	145.5 ± 1.1	144.8 ± 0.8	144.4 ± 0.8
DBP mmHg	86.3 ±0.4	86.4 ± 0.5	86.3 ± 0.5	85.9 ± 0.4	85.5 ± 0.5	85.6± 0.5	85.2 ± 0.5

§ p < 0.05; ° p < 0.01; " p <0.005; * p < 0.0001

Table 2. Effects of simvastatin treatment on total cholesterol (TC, mg/dl) levels in the various antihypertensive treatment subgroups.

Treatments Subgroups	Patients Number	TC Basal	TC at 48th Week	Percent Decrease	p
Ace-Inhibitors	39	292	198	-32.1%	NS
Ace-Inhibitors + Diuretics	18	275	196	-28.7%	NS
Ca-Antagonists	24	267	186	-30.3%	NS
Ca-Antagonists + Ace-Inihibitors	11	271	199	-26.5%	NS
β-Blockers, Diuretics or β-Blockers + Diuretics	15	263	190	-27.7%	NS
Other Associations	15	260	194	-25.3%	NS

Results are expressed as means.
NS: Not Significant versus the other treatment subgroups
Other Associations: Ca-Antagonists + β-Blockers, Ca-Antagonists + Diuretics, β-Blockers + Ace-Inhibitors

Systolic and diastolic blood pressure did not show any significant change under simvastatin treatment in the overall group (Table 1) as well as in the subgroups receiving different antihypertensive treatments. There were 4 clinical cardiovascular events (1 sudden death, 2 acute myocardial infarction, and 1 stroke) and 1 patient complained of gastralgia. Moreover, 9 adverse biochemical effects were observed: 3 increments in ALT or AST (2 drug related), 2 drug-related increments in GGT, 1 drug-related increment in alkaline phosphatase, and 3 increments in CPK (2 drug-related) without muscle symptoms. Two patients dropped out owing to adverse biochemical effects, 1 for CPK increment, and 1 for GGT increment. The other biochemical parameters did not show any significant change. Thus, the incidence of subjective side effects was 0.8%, that of adverse drug related biochemical effects 5.7%, and drop-out rate due to adverse biochemical effects 1.6%.

Discussion

Our data show that simvastatin, given at the dosage ranging from 10 to 40 mg once daily in hypercholesterolemic male hypertensive patients treated with antihypertensive drugs, was highly effective in lowering total and LDL-cholesterol. In addition, this drug also significantly reduced triglycerides and increased HDL-cholesterol, thus further improving lipid profile. In accordance with the trial plan, the great majority (> 90%) of patients reached the end points of total cholesterol < 200 mg/dl and of LDL-cholesterol < 130 mg/dl, so that their cardiovascular risk as related to lipid profile was normalized. This target was achieved with a mean dosage of 21.9 mg/day of simvastatin and in about 80% of patients with a dose ranging from 10 to 20 mg/day. This dosage schedule is similar to that employed in most studies on normotensive hypercholesterolemic patients [5,8,9] and in one study on hypercholesterolemic hypertensive patients under antihypertensive drug treatment [7], and lower than that used in another similar study [6]. The amount of total and LDL-cholesterol reduction in our study was similar to that found in two previous studies in which a relatively small number of hypercholesterolemic hypertensive patients under antihypertensive drug treatement received simvastatin for a relatively short period [6,7]. Thus, our data extend to a greater number of patients treated over a longer time period the finding that simvastatin is an efficient hypolipidemic drug in male hypertensive patients under antihypertensive drug treatment.

Interestingly, the lipid lowering effect of simvastatin was unaffected by the kind of antihypertensive treatment, a finding substantially confirming the results of a previous study [10], in which a large number of patients were treated with lovastatin. However, the limited number of patients in our subgroups did not allow definitive conclusions and more specifically it cannot be excluded that the effect of simvastatin may be more evident in patients receiving Ca-antagonists, as suggested by the above reported study with lovastatin [10].

In the present study, while simvastatin significantly reduced LDL-cholesterol, it did not change blood pressure in essential hypertensive patients, whose blood pressure values were stably reduced to the normotensive range by treatment with commonly used antihypertensive drugs. Although our data may be biased by lack of a placebo control group, they fit very well with the findings of two previous placebo-controlled studies [6,7], which showed that simvastatin did not change blood pressure in hypertensive patients treated with antihypertensive drugs.

It cannot be excluded that LDL-cholesterol reduction induced by statin treatment may reduce diastolic blood pressure in untreated hypertensive patients, as already reported

[3]. However, our data and those of previous studies [6,7] reasonably exclude the possibility that simvastatin could increase blood pressure at least in essential hypertensive patients under antihypertensive drug treatment.

In the present study subjective side effects occurred in less than 1% of patients, and overall incidence of drug-related adverse biochemical events was 5.7% with a 1.6% drop-out rate due to these biochemical abnormalities. These data, which are similar to those reported in normotensive [5,8,9,11] and hypertensive hypercholesterolemic patients [6,7] receiving simvastatin, confirm the favorable safety profile of this drug.

In conclusion, our data show that simvastatin is an effective and well- tolerated drug for treatment of hypercholesterolemia in male essential hypertensive patients and that this drug did not interfere with the blood pressure lowering effect of antihypertensive therapy.

Participating Centers

Cattedra di Medicina Interna, Clinica Medica 1, University of Pisa (Argenio GF, Bernini GP).
Divisione di Medicina, Ospedale Civile di Fidenza (Ambrosoli S).
Divisione di Nefrologia, Ospedale Civile di LIvorno (Baldari G).
Divisione di Medicina, Ospedale Civile di Castelnuovo Garfagnana (Bianchini A).
Divisione di Cardiologia, Ospedale Civile di Empoli (Bini A).
Divisione di Medicina 1, Ospedale Civile di Pontedera (Cagianelli A).
Divisione di Medicina, Ospedale Civile di Aosta (Cardellino G).
Divisione di Medicina 1, Ospedale Civile di Pistoia (Federighi G).
Centro Ipertensione, Ospedale Civile di La Spezia (Gandolfi E).
Divisione di Medicina, Ospedale Civile di Carrara (Innocenti P).
Divisione di Medicina, Ospedale Civile di Pistoia (Pettina' G).
Divisione di Medicina, Ospedale Civile di Pescia (Saba P).
Divisione di Medicina, Ospedale Civile di Fiesole (Toso M).

References

1.   Stewart DJ, Monge JC. Hyperlipidemia and endothelial dysfunction. Curr Op Lipidol 1993;4:319-24.
2.   Sachidinis A, Mengden T, Locher R, Brunner C, Vetter W. Novel cellular activities for low density lipoprotein in vascular smooth muscle cells. Hypertension 1990;15:704-11.
3.   Glorioso N, Troffa C, Tonolo G, et al. High circulating LDLs play a role in the maintenance of high blood pressure in essential hypertensive patients. Am J Hypertens 1993;6:17A.
4.   Roullet JB, Xue H, Pappu AS, Roullet C, Holcomb S, McCarron DA. Mevalonate availability and cardiovascular function. Proc Natl Acad Sci USA 1993; 90:11728-32.
5.   Todd PA, Goa KL. Simvastatin: A review of its pharmacological propierties and

therapeutic potential in hypercholesterolemia. Drugs 1990;40:583-607.

6. Morgan T, Anderson A, McDonald P, Hopper J, Macaskill G. Simvastatin in the treatment of hypercholesterolaemia in patients with essential hypertension. J Hypertens 1990;8(Suppl.1):S25-S32.

7. Farish E, MacDonald N-J, Barnes JF, Stark S, Reid JL. A double-blind twelve-week placebo-controlled study to assess the efficacy of Simvastatin in the treatment of hypercholesterolaemia in hypertensive patients. J Drug Dev 1990;3(Suppl. 1):259-63.

8. Ziegler O, Drouin P, Simvastatin-Fenofibrate Study Group. Safety, tolerability and efficacy of Simvastatin and Fenofibrate. A multicenter study. Cardiology 1990;77 (Suppl.4):50-57.

9. Molgaard J, Lundh BL, von Schenck H, Olsson AG. Long-term efficacy and safety of simvastatin alone and in combination therapy in treatment of hypercholesterolaemia. Atherosclerosis 1991;91:S21-S28.

10. Pool JL, Shear CL, Downton M, et al. Lovastatin and coadministered antihyper-tensive/cardiovascular agents. Hypertension 1992;19:242-48.

11. Bilheimer DW. Long-term clinical tolerance of lovastatin and simvastatin. Cardiology 1990;77(Suppl.4):58-65.

EFFECTS OF SIMVASTATIN TREATMENT ON THROMBOXANE (TX) BIOSYNTHESIS AND PLATELET FUNCTION IN TYPE II HYPER-CHOLESTEROLEMIA (HC)

Alberto Notarbartolo
Department of Internal Medicine
University of Palermo
Palermo
ITALY

Eicosanoids are derived from arachidonate and the resulting biologically active derivatives with paracrine function include prostaglandins (PGs), thromboxane (TX)A_2, and sulfidopeptide leukotrienes (LTs).

PGI_2 is the pivotal prostaglandin synthesized by arterial tissue particularly by endothelial cells. On the other hand, platelets synthesize TXA_2 which is a potent vasoconstrictor and platelet aggregator. Moncada and Vane [1] hypothesized that the balance of TXA_2 and PGI_2 maintained "vascular integrity" consistent with a good anticoagulant state. Their effects on platelets are mediated by c-AMP, increased by PGI_2, and reduced by TXA_2.

Hypercholesterolemia and Abnormal Platelet Function

A high incidence of atherosclerosis and thrombotic complications has been associated with type IIa hypercholesterolemia (HC) [2]. Because platelet "hyperreactivity" has been considered as being responsible or at least contributing to acute thromboembolic complications, such as myocardial infarction and ischemic stroke, several studies have assessed platelet function in type IIa hyperlipoproteinemia [3,4,5,6]. Increased sensitivity of platelets to the aggregatory effects of various agonists and higher production of arachidonic acid metabolites have been described in HC in association with increased activity of platelet phospholipases [7].

Washed platelets from type IIa hypercholesterolemic subjects incubated with exogenous arachidonate produce higher amounts of thromboxane (TXB_2) that correlate linearly with cholesterol levels. To verify the relevance of these capacity-related measurements to the actual rate of TXA_2 biosynthesis *in vivo*, we studied the urinary excretion of its major enzymatic metabolites in 46 patients with type IIa HC and 20 age-matched controls [8]. The excretion rate of 11-dehydro-TXB_2 was significantly ($p < 0.001$)

A.M. Gotto et al. (eds.), Multiple Risk Factors in Cardiovascular Disease, 349-352.
© 1995 *Kluwer Academic Publishers and Fondazione Giovanni Lorenzini.*

higher in patients (68.7 ± 35.1 ng/hr, mean ± SD) than in controls (22.4 ± 9.4 ng/h), with metabolite excretion > 2 SD of the normal mean in 74% of the patients. Moreover, a statistically significant correlation (r=0.673, p < 0.001, n=66) was found between 11-dehydro-TXB$_2$ excretion and total plasma cholesterol.

In conclusion TXA$_2$ biosynthesis is enhanced in the majority of patients with type IIa HC; this may be, at least in part, a consequence of abnormal cholesterol levels, as suggested by the correlation between the two. Low-dose aspirin can largely suppress increased metabolite excretion, thus suggesting that it reflects TXA$_2$-dependent platelet activation *in vivo*.

Effect of Treatment on TXA$_2$ and PGI$_2$ Biosynthesis and Platelet Sensitivity to Aggregating Agents in Type IIa Hypercholesterolemia

K. Schrör and colleagues have studied the effect of lowering LDL cholesterol in familial hypercholesterolemia (FH) heterozygous patients on platelet function, TX formation, and platelet sensitivity against iloprost, a stable prostacyclin mimetic [9]. Seven FH were treated with cholestyramine (12 g/day) for 8-11 months and were compared with 8 untreated FH and 11 healthy controls, obtaining a 21% reduction of plasma cholesterol; levels of immunoreactive TXB$_2$ in collagen-stimulated platelets were not different from the untreated FH. However, cholestyramine treatment normalized the platelet reactivity of FH against iloprost. It is possible to suggest that if deposition of cholesterol in cellular components of vessel wall is a primary event in atherosclerosis, any reduction in its deposition, might be considered beneficial.

The same authors reported in *Eicosanoids* in 1989, together with a 25% decrease of total cholesterol, a 50% decrease of TXB$_2$ level in platelet-rich plasma after stimulation with adenosine diphosphate in 12 FH patients treated for 8 months with simvastatin (20-40 mg/day), an HMGCoA reductase inhibitor analogue of lovastatin, compared with 10 controls and 10 untreated FH patients. The new and exciting finding presented in this study is that long-term treatment with S, not only normalizes platelet reactivity against PGI$_2$, as previously shown with cholestyramine, but also reduces platelet hyperreactivity [10].

At the same time as the Schrör report, we published in *Atherosclerosis* in 1989 similar results, regarding the effect of simvastatin on platelet aggregation and TXA$_2$ synthesis *ex vivo* [11].

We investigated TXA$_2$ biosynthesis *in vivo* in 24 patients with type IIa HC, randomized to receive in a double-blind fashion simvastatin (20 mg/day) or placebo for 3 months. Total blood cholesterol was significantly (p < 0.001) reduced by simvastatin: 283 ± 27 mg/dl (mean ± SD, n=12) at baseline, 220 ± 34 at 1 month and 205 ± 26 at 3 months. The 11-dehydro-TXB$_2$ excretion was also significantly (p < 0.001) reduced: 62 ± 20 ng/h at week 4; placebo-treated patients did not show any significant changes in either blood cholesterol (294 ± 50 at baseline, 291 ± 54 at 1 month and 295 ± 46 at 3 months) or U-11-dehydro-TXB$_2$ (71 ± 26, 70 ± 32 and 72 ± 26, respectively). The reduction in U-11-dehydro-TXB$_2$ associated with simvastatin was correlated with the reduction in blood cholesterol (r=0.80; p < 0.0001), LDL-cholesterol (r=0.79; p < 0.0001), and Apo B (r=0.75;

$p < 0.0001$) levels. Platelets from patients with type IIa HC required significantly ($p < 0.005$) more collagen and ADP to aggregate and synthesized less TXB_2 in response to both agonists after simvastatin therapy. Bleeding time, platelet sensitivity to iloprost, blood Lp(a) and HDL cholesterol levels were not significantly affected by drug therapy. We conclude that enhanced TXA_2 biosynthesis in type IIa HC is at least in part dependent on abnormal cholesterol levels and/or other simvastatin-sensitive mechanisms affecting platelet function.

It is not easy to explain the observed different results with the two hypocholesterolemic treatments (cholestyramine and simvastatin). It may be suggested that with cholestyramine a better vasomotility is achieved with a decrease of cholesterol content of vessel wall cellular component, while with simvastatin not only is the sensitivity of platelets to PGI_2 normalized but also the cholesterol/phospholipid ratio with a consequently reduced TXA_2 synthesis. These different findings could be due to the pharmacologic mechanism of cholestyramine and simvastatin. Cholestyramine acts by binding the bile acids in the intestinal lumen with a decrease of circulating LDL and enhanced uptake of LDL by liver receptors; there is also an increased liver production of VLDL. Simvastatin increases the liver LDL and VLDL remnants uptake via Apo B-E receptors and also diminishes the LDL and VLDL cholesterol hepatic synthesis. An hypothesis to be verified could be that the sharp and more evident decrease of LDL cholesterol obtained after simvastatin treatment is able to reduce megakaryocytes cholesterol content.

Conclusions

In coronary atherosclerosis elevated levels of LDL and TXA_2 platelet biosynthesis may induce coronary spasm and/or acute thrombosis. Simvastatin, an analogue of lovastatin, reduces both LDL and TXA_2. The Familial Atherosclerosis Treatment Study (FATS) showed that drug combinations which predominantly lowered LDL (colestipol and lovastatin) or raised HDL (nicotinic acid and cholestyramine) were effective in arresting progression, inducing regression of coronary artery disease and decreasing coronary events [12]. In postcoronary angioplasty patients treated for 6 months with lovastatin in one study restenosis was significantly less frequent than in untreated patients [13].

Some argue that achievement of clinical benefits with HC treatment within a short period of time can be ascribed to changes in coronary flow reserve possibly related to improved endothelial function. In New Zealand white rabbits with acute HC the impaired endothelium-dependent relaxation is significantly attenuated by treatment with lovastatin.

Finally it may be suggested that whatever the molecular mechanism of action of simvastatin (and not necessarily other lipid lowering maneuvers) in modulating platelet TXA_2 biosynthesis, these effects may contribute to the overall impact of the drug on thrombotic risk.

Acknowledgements

I wish to thank Giovanni Davì, M.D. (Haematology and Thrombosis Laboratory, Head, Chieti and Palermo University); Carlo Patrono, M.D. (Pharmacology Department, Head,

University of Chieti); and Maurizio Averna, M.D. (Lipid Core Laboratory, Head, University of Palermo). We are also grateful for the technical assistance of Gisella Marino, Ph. D.; Isabella Catalano, M.D.; Antonella Ganci, M.D.; Angela Rao Camemi, Ph. D.; Carlo Barbagallo, M.D.; Carlo Giammarresi, M.D.; and Francesco La Placa, M.D.

References

1.   Moncada S, Vane JR. Arachidonic acid metabolites and the interactions between platelets and blood vessels walls. NEJM 1979;300:1142-47.
2.   Ross R. The pathogenesis of atherosclerosis. In: Braunwald E, editor. Heart disease. Philadelphia: WB Saunders Co. 1988:1135-52.
3.   Gotto AM Jr, Farmer JA. Risk factors for coronary artery disease. In: Braunwald E, editor. Heart disease. Philadelphia: WB Saunders Co. 1988:1153-90.
4.   Strano A, Davì G, Averna M, et al. Platelet sensitivity to prostacyclin and thromboxane production in hyperlipidemic patients. Throm Haemost 1982;77:18-21.
5.   Tremoli E, Folco G, Agradi E, Galli C. Platelet thromboxane and serum cholesterol. Lancet 1979;1:107-8.
6.   Prisco D, Rogasi PG, Paniccia R, et al. Altered lipid composition and thromboxane A_2 formation in platelets from patients affected by IIa hyperlipoproteinemia. Thromb Res 1988; 50:593-604.
7.   Kramer RM, Jakubowski JA, Vaillancourt R, Deykin D. Effect of membrane cholesterol on phospholipid metabolism in thrombin-stimulated platelets. J Biol Chem 1982;257:6844-49.
8.   Davì G, Averna M, Catalano I, et al. Increased thromboxane biosynthesis in type IIa hyper-cholesterolemia. Circulation 1992;85:1792-98.
9.   Lobel P, Steinhagen-Thiessen E, Schrör K. Cholestyramine treatment of type IIa hypercholesterolemia normalizes platelet reactivity against prostacyclin. Eur J Clin Invest 1988;18:256-60.
10.   Schrör K, Steinhagen-Thiessen E, Lobel P. Simvastatin reduces platelet thromboxane formation and restores normal platelet sensitivity against prostacyclin in type IIa hypercholesterolemia. Eicosanoids 1989;2:39-45.
11.   Davì G, Averna M, Novo S, et al.. Effects of synvolin on platelet aggregation and thromboxane B_2 synthesis in type IIa hypercholesterolemic patients. Atherosclerosis 1989;79:79-83.
12.   Brown G, Albers JJ, Lloyd DF, et al. Regression of coronary artery disease as a result of intensive lipid lowering therapy in men with high levels of apolipoprotein B. NEJM 1990;323:1289-98.
13.   Sahni R, Maniet AR, Voci G, Banka VS. Prevention of restenosis by lovastatin after successful coronary angioplasty. Am Heart J 1991;121:77-85.

RISK FACTOR INTERACTIONS INVOLVING PRESSOR AGENTS

Gustav V.R. Born and Luis E. Cardona-Sanclemente
The William Harvey Research Institute
St. Bartholomew's Hospital Medical College
Charterhouse Square
London EC1M 6BQ
UNITED KINGDOM

The risk of coronary and cerebral events is increased more than additively by hypertension in conjunction with high plasma low density lipoprotein (LDL) and fibrinogen. This could be accounted for by our *in vivo* experiments showing that LDL and fibrinogen uptake into arterial walls is accelerated by the pressor agents noradrenaline, adrenaline, angiotensin II, and the nitric oxide inhibitor L-NAME concomitantly with moderate rises in blood pressure. Angiotensin II increased uptake when blood pressure increased only transiently; and uptake was not increased in otherwise comparable spontaneously hypertensive rats. Nevertheless, these findings may provide a rationale for drug combinations.

Introduction

The first indication of atherosclerosis is the accumulation of lipid in the intima of susceptible arteries. These initial lesions, classified by the World Health Organization as Stage 1 of atherosclerosis, are known as "fatty streaks." Characteristically the lesions consist of a pool of lipid material in the intima beneath apparently intact endothelium. The lipid is predominantly derived from LDL of the plasma with contributions, so far quantitatively uncertain, from other lipoproteins including Lp(a). The lesions also contain fibrinogen and fibrin in considerable amounts [1].

Plasma LDL passes through arterial endothelium by transcytosis, apparently within the plasmalemmal vesicles that are characteristic of endothelial cells [2,3] and identical with pinosomes in which lipoprotein particles were first demonstrated by autoradiography [4]. The predominant rate-determining factor of the arterial uptake of LDL is its concentration in the plasma [5-7]. In looking for other possible rate determinants we demonstrated that in anesthetized rabbits the process is accelerated by noradrenaline or adrenaline at their pathophysiological concentrations in the blood [8-10]. Amongst the immediate questions arising were (i) whether such an effect is demonstrable also with other potentially atherogenic plasma proteins, e.g. fibrinogen; and (ii) whether the effect might be connected

A.M. Gotto et al. (eds.), Multiple Risk Factors in Cardiovascular Disease, 353-357.
© *1995 Kluwer Academic Publishers and Fondazione Giovanni Lorenzini.*

with the hypertensive action of catecholamines. Hypertension is established as a risk factor for coronary heart disease as well as for stroke [11,12]. Similar experiments with another pressor agent, viz. angiotensin II, showed that it also increased the uptake of LDL as well as of fibrinogen by aortic walls in conscious, unrestrained rats. Extending our previous findings, adrenaline also increased the uptake of both proteins (Cardona-Sanclemente and Born, submitted for publication).

In these experiments adrenaline or angiotensin II infused by implanted minipump for six days significantly increased aortic wall radioactivities derived from rat and human LDL or human fibrinogen which had been circulating for 24 hours. The proteins were labelled with radioiodine attached to tyramine cellobiose, so that the aortic wall radioactivities predominately represented the amounts of LDL or fibrinogen degradation products trapped in the tissues during the 24-hour period [13]. This labelling technique excluded the possibility that the increased radioactivities were due to decreased elimination of the proteins, but gave no measure of LDL and fibrinogen present in the artery walls which had not been metabolized.

In the first series of experiments the minipumps were implanted under the skin of the neck and connected by cannula to alternate carotid arteries, in order to make the experiments to this extent similar to previous experiments with anesthetized rabbits in which catecholamines were infused into alternate carotids [8,10]. In later rat experiments the procedure was simplified by implanting the minipumps as before but not connecting them to the arteries, so that the agents were infused into the subcutaneous tissues of the neck. With both of these infusion arrangements, adrenaline or angiotensin II increased the radioactivities in the aortic walls.

Infusions of adrenaline or angiotensin II had no significant effect on the rates of clearance or LDL or fibrinogen from the plasma. Therefore, the increased uptakes caused by the agents could not be attributed to an effect on the concentrations of the labelled proteins in the circulating blood.

At the concentrations at which they were infused, both adrenaline and angiotensin II increased the blood pressure progressively from control values around 105 to about 130 mm Hg. Compared to saline-infused control rats, in which the diastolic blood pressure gradually decreased, the increase with adrenaline became significant after 3 days and with angiotensin II after 5 days.

These results would be compatible with the conclusion that the increased uptake of LDL or fibrinogen by aortic walls caused by noradrenaline, adrenaline, or angiotensin II is mediated by a common mechanism involving their pressor effects. This conclusion would appear to be supported by our recent finding that administration of N^Gnitro-L-arginine methyl ester (L-NAME) to conscious, unrestrained, normotensive rats increased the uptake of LDL and fibrinogen by the walls of the aorta (Cardona-Sanclemente and Born, accepted for publication). L-NAME inhibits the formation of the potent vasodilator substance nitric oxide (NO) from L-arginine by endothelial cells [14] and causes a progressive rise in blood pressure [15]. Thus the increased uptake of the atherogenic plasma proteins by aortic walls was again associated with moderate hypertension. In this respect, therefore, our findings with L-NAME resemble those previously obtained with the other pressor agents noradrenaline, adrenaline, and angiotensin II. Indeed, this previously observed association of uptake and blood pressure increases was a major reason for determining the effect of L-NAME as yet another means of raising blood pressure.

At first sight, therefore, the latest results would support some direct connection between the two effects. Such a connection would also plausibly emerge from observations showing that the labelling of vascular endothelial cell vesicles with ferritin is increased with increasing intralumenal pressure [16]. However, some of our own findings are inconsistent with such a conclusion. Thus, angiotensin II infused at a concentration sufficiently low as to cause only a very small and temporary rise in blood pressure still produced highly significant increases in LDL and fibrinogen uptake [17]. Even more striking was the absence of any increase in uptake in age-matched spontaneously hypertensive rats (SHR) in which the blood pressure was higher than that produced by any of the administered pressor agents, although still well within the range occurring in clinical hypertension [17]. For this there are, of course, several possible explanations. SHR begin to be hypertensive soon after birth, so that three-month-old animals may have developed some kind of adaptation to the mechanism(s) responsible for the uptake increases produced by administered pressor agents after five or six days. The development of an adaptive process in these rats is also suggested by the fact that nether angiotensin II nor L-NAME increased the uptake of LDL or fibrinogen in SHR. Alternatively, although both control and spontaneously hypertensive rats were Wistars, there may have been genetic factors to account for the difference.

Considering our experimental findings in relation to human atherosclerotic disease, there is striking epidemiological evidence that the risk of both coronary heart disease and stroke is increased more than additively when both LDL or fibrinogen and systolic or diastolic blood pressure are high [18,19]. If our work should after all point to some mechanistic connection between blood pressure and the accumulation of atherogenic plasma proteins in arterial walls they would provide, at least in principle, an explanation of these epidemiological facts.

Acknowledgement

We wish to thank the Garfield Weston Foundation and the British Heart Foundation for generous support.

References

1.   Smith EB, Crosbie L. Fibrinogen and fibrin in atherogenesis. In: Ernst E, Koenig W, Lowe GDO, Mead TW, editors. Fibrinogen: A "new" cardiovascular risk factor. Vienna:Blackwell, 1992;4-10.
2.   Vasile E, Simionescu M, Simionescu N. Visualization of the binding, endocytosis, and transcytosis of low-density lipoproteins in the arterial endothelium in situ. J Cell Biol 1983;96:1677-1689.
3.   Simionescu N, Vasile E, Lupu F, Popescu G, Simionescu M. Prelesional events in

atherogenesis: Accumulation of extracellular cholesterol-rich liposomes in the arterial intima and cardiac values of the hyperlipidaemic rabbit. Am J Path 1986;123:109-125.

4.   Stein O, Stein Y, Eisenberg S. A radiographic study of the transport of I-labelled serum lipoproteins in rat aorta. Cell Tissue Res 1973;138:223-232.

5.   Nagelkerke JF, Havekes L, Van Hinsbergh VWM, Van Berkel TJC. *In vivo* and *in vitro* catabolism of native and biologically modified LDL. FEBS Lett 1984;171:149-153.

6.   Goldstein JL, Brown MS. The low-density lipoprotein pathway and its relation to atherosclerosis. Ann Rev Biochem 1977;46:897-930.

7.   Brown MS, Goldstein JL. A receptor-mediated pathway for cholesterol homeostasis. Science 1986;232:34-47.

8.   Shafi S, Cusack NJ, Born GVR. Increased uptake of methylated low density lipoprotein induced by noradrenaline in carotid arteries of anaesthetized rabbits. Proc Royal Soc Lond 1989;235:289-298.

9.   Cardona-Sanclemente LE, Görög P, Born GVR. Increased uptake of low-density lipoproteins induced by adrenaline in the aortae of unrestrained rats. J Physiol 1992;452:56P.

10.   Cardona-Sanclemente LE, Born GVR. Adrenaline increases the uptake of low density lipoproteins in carotid arteries of rabbits. Atherosclerosis 1992;96:215-218.

11.   Collins R, Peto R, MacMahon S, et al. Blood pressure, stroke, and coronary heart disease: Part 2, Short-term reductions in blood pressure: Overview of randomised drug trials in their epidemiological context. Lancet 1990;335:827-838.

12.   MRC Working Party. Medical Research Council trial of treatment of hypertension in older adults: Principal results. BMJ 1992;304:405-412.

13.   Pittmann RC, Carew TE, Glass CK, Green SR, Taylor CA, Attie AD. A radioiodinated, intracellularly trapped ligand for determining the sites of plasma protein degradation *in vivo*. Biochem J 1983;212:791-800.

14.   Moncada S, Radomski MW, Palmer RMJ. Endothelium-derived relaxing factor. Biochem Pharmacol 1988;37:2495-2501.

15.   Rees DD, Palmer RMJ, Schulz R, Hodson HF, Moncada S. Characterization of three inhibitors or endothelial nitric oxide synthase *in vitro* and *in vivo*. Br J Pharmacol 1990;101:746-752.

16.   Moffitt H, Clough G, Michel CC. Effects of intraluminal pressures on the labelling of endothelial cell vesicles with native ferritin. Int J Microcirculation: Clin Exp 1992;11:90.

17.   Cardona-Sanclemente LE, Medina R, Born GVR. Effect of increasing concentrations of angiotensin II infused into unrestrained conscious rats on LDL and fibrinogen uptake by aorta. Br J Pharmacol 1994;111:22.

18.   Wilhelmsen L, Svardsudd K, Korsan-Bengtsen K, Larsson B, Welin L, Tibblin G. Fibrinogen as a risk factor for stroke and myocardial infarction. New Engl J Med 1984;311:501-505.

19.   Heinrich J, Balleisen L, Sculte H, Assmann G, Van de Loo J. Fibrinogen and Factor

VII in the prediction of coronary risk. Results from the PROCAM study in healthy men. Atherosclero Thromb 1994;14:54-59.

HEMODYNAMIC AND ADRENERGIC EFFECTS OF CIGARETTE SMOKING

Guido Grassi, Antonio Lanfranchi, Sabrina Vailati, Gino Seravalle, Bianca M. Cattaneo, and Giuseppe Mancia
Cattedra di Medicina Interna I
Ospedale S. Gerardo dei Tintori
Monza
and
Centro Fisiologia Clinica e Ipertensione
Università di Milano
Milan
ITALY

Introduction

Epidemiological and clinical studies carried out over the past thirty years have unequivocally shown that the cardiovascular risks of smoking are widespread and severe; they include peripheral and coronary atherosclerosis, angina pectoris, and sudden death [1-3]. The pathophysiological mechanisms responsible for the adverse clinical consequences of cigarette smoking are complex and heterogeneous. There is unequivocal evidence, however, that smoking induces: 1) marked alterations in plasma lipid profile, characterized by a reduction in HDL cholesterol levels and by an increase in free fatty acids [4], 2) unfavorable effects on the hemostatic function, with an increase in platelet aggregation and in plasma fibrinogen levels [5,6], and 3) structural and functional abnormalities of the endothelium, directly induced by nicotine and other several thousands of compounds of tobacco combustion [6].

Along with these well-documented metabolic and cardiovascular alterations, there is also clearcut evidence that smoking induces profound alterations in systemic and regional hemodynamics. This paper will review recent data collected by our group on the effects of cigarette smoking on blood pressure and on the functional properties of large arteries. It will also examine the adrenergic mechanisms involved in the pressor effects of smoking.

Pressor Effects of Cigarette Smoking

A number of epidemiological studies performed in the past have reported that blood pressure levels are lower in smokers than in nonsmokers [2,7]. This finding is in contrast

A.M. Gotto et al. (eds), Multiple Risk Factors in Cardiovascular Disease, 359-364.
© 1995 *Kluwer Academic Publishers and Fondazione Giovanni Lorenzini.*

with the evidence that smoking a cigarette induces an acute and marked pressor response, which is accompanied by an increase in heart rate and in peripheral vascular resistance [8-11].

There are several hypotheses advanced for explaining the contrasting hemodynamic effects of acute and chronic exposure to cigarette smoking. For example, it has been suggested that heavy smokers may have a lower body weight than nonsmokers and that this difference may account for the blood pressure differences reported in the two groups [2,7]. It has also been suggested, however, that a tolerance phoenomenon might prevent a persistent blood pressure elevation to occur during repeated cigarette smoking [12]. To test this hypothesis, in a study recently performed by our group [13], we examined in 10 normotensive smokers (who refrained from smoking for the 24 hours preceding the study) the effects of repeated cigarette smoking (4 cigarettes in one hour) on systolic and diastolic blood pressure, measured beat-to-beat by means of the Finapres device, and on heart rate, assessed by a cardiotachometer triggered by the R-wave on an electrocardiographic lead. As expected, smoking the first cigarette caused a marked increase in systolic blood pressure ($+28.7 \pm 4.0$ mmHg, mean $\pm$ SEM), diastolic blood pressure ($+12.4 \pm 3.8$ mmHg) and heart rate ($+20.7 \pm 2.8$ beats/min), all these changes being highly statistically significant ($p < 0.01$).

The major and new finding of the study, however, was the evidence that similar peak blood pressure and heart rate values were observed for the other three cigarettes smoked. It should also be emphasized that in each instance the responses were so prolonged that blood pressure and heart rate values remained persistently elevated throughout the whole smoking period. Beat-to-beat computer analysis of the recorded values showed that, compared to the hour-long nonsmoking control period, the hourly increase in systolic and diastolic blood pressure amounted to $18.8 \pm 2.3\%$ and to $14.0 \pm 2.1\%$, respectively, while the hourly increase in heart rate amounted to $29.7 \pm 1.8\%$ ($p < 0.01$ for all changes). This first set of studies provides clearcut evidence that smoking elicits marked and long-lasting pressor and tachycardic responses.

Further evidence of the prolonged hemodynamic effects of cigarette smoking is provided by the results of a study [14], which we performed in 6 normotensive subjects by employing 8-hour noninvasive ambulatory blood pressure monitoring during day-time period in two different experimental sessions. One recording was performed with subjects not smoking and the other while they smoked two cigarettes per hour, i.e. a total of 16 cigarettes. Ambulatory blood pressure data, after being visually edited and stored on floppy disks, were analyzed by computer to obtain mean values for each hour and for the whole recording period. The standard deviations of the means were taken as indices of blood pressure (and heart rate) variability. The results of this study show that ambulatory blood pressure and heart rate values are higher during smoking than during the nonsmoking session. Indeed, for the whole day-time period, the increase in systolic and diastolic blood pressure induced by smoking amounted to 5.2 ± 1.7 mmHg and to 6.4 ± 1.1 mmHg respectively, while the heart rate increase was 8.0 ± 3.1 beats/min ($p < 0.01$ for all). Not only absolute blood pressure values, but also blood pressure variability was markedly affected by smoking. A 20% increase in the standard deviations of mean arterial pressure values was indeed found in the smoking as compared to the nonsmoking ambulatory blood pressure recording. Because the magnitude of blood pressure variability is directly related to end-organ damage [15], its increase during smoking may account for several of the cardiovascular complications associated with the smoking habits.

Taken together, these results demonstrate that 1) repeated cigarette smoking is always accompanied by a pressor response and 2) each response is so long-lasting as to increase blood pressure for a prolonged period of time. They also suggest that there is no short-term tolerance to the hemodynamic effects of smoking and that the lower blood pressure values reported in smokers probably depend on the fact that blood pressure measurements are usually taken after a more or less prolonged period of abstinence from smoking.

Adrenergic Mechanisms Involved in the Pressor Effect of Smoking

Several studies have provided evidence that the mechanisms responsible for the pressor and tachycardic responses induced by cigarette smoking have an adrenergic nature. It has been indeed shown that these hemodynamic effects 1) are markedly attenuated by alpha- and beta-adrenergic blockade [8,9,13] and 2) are associated with a marked and prolonged increase in plasma norepinephrine and epinephrine [8,9,16].

The results of these studies, however, do not allow us to clarify whether the adrenergic stimulation induced by smoking occurs at the level of the central nervous system or at a peripheral adrenergic nerve site. To better clarify this issue, we have recently performed a study [17] in which, along with several hemodynamic variables (blood pressure, heart rate, calf blood flow and vascular resistance), plasma catecholamine levels (high-performance liquid chromatography assay), and postganglionic muscle sympathetic nerve activity (microneurography from the peroneal nerve) were measured in 9 normotensive subjects before and during cigarette smoking. As outlined in previous papers [18-20] microneurographic assessment of sympathetic nerve activity allows direct and precise quantification of sympathetic tone in man, thus overcoming technical and biological limitations of plasma catecholamines as markers of adrenergic activity. By employing this technique, we were able to demonstrate that cigarette smoking, despite markedly and significantly increasing plasma norepinephrine ($+34.8 \pm 7.0\%$, $p < 0.05$) and plasma epinephrine ($+90.5 \pm 39.0\%$, $p < 0.01$), induced a clearcut reduction ($-31.8 \pm 5.1\%$, $p < 0.01$) in muscle sympathetic nerve activity.

This finding suggests that the adrenergic activation associated with smoking does not have a central origin, but rather depends on the effects of nicotine and other products of tobacco combustion at peripheral sympathetic nerve sites. These effects may 1) enhance catecholamine release from chromaffin tissues, 2) reduce the reuptake of the neurotransmitter from adrenergic nerve terminals, and finally 3) decrease the tissue clearance of these neurohumoral substances, by reducing blood flow supplying various cardiovascular districts (for example, skeletal muscle district).

By which mechanisms does smoking cause inhibition of sympathetic nerve traffic? In the same study, we provided evidence that this inhibition has a reflex nature, and specifically depends on an arterial baroreceptor stimulation brought about by the smoking-dependent blood pressure rise.

Finally, there is also evidence that smoking may adversely affect baroreflex control of cardiovascular system. We have indeed shown [17] that the degree of sympathetic inhibition triggered by cigarette smoking was markedly less (-54.1 ± 7.5%, p < 0.05) than that induced by stimulation of arterial baroreceptors brought about by intravenous infusion of phenylephrine [21].

Thus arterial baroreflex, i.e. one of the major homeostatic mechanisms involved in blood pressure control [21], is impaired by smoking. This impairment, in turn, may be responsible for the smoking-related pressor effects, which therefore do not only depend on peripheral vasoconstriction.

Effects of Smoking on the Functional Properties of Large Arteries

In dealing with the effects of cigarette smoking on the functional properties of large arteries, an important variable to be evaluated is represented by arterial compliance. As outlined in previous papers [22,23], arterial compliance is of primary importance for the optimal function of the cardiovascular system because 1) it buffers the increase in blood pressure induced by the ejection of blood from the heart, thereby reducing cardiac work and vessel trauma and 2) it allows, by recoiling, blood flow to continue during diastole.

Despite the well-known methodological problems in evaluating arterial compliance in man, the recent development of new ultrasonographic measuring devices has allowed to investigate this index of the viscoelastic arterial properties in a dynamic fashion, i.e. throughout the whole cardial cycle. Because arterial compliance values have been shown to markedly change from diastolic to systolic pressure, this new approach undoubtedly represents an important technical improvement.

By using this new technique, our group has recently examined whether smoking affects arterial compliance and thus interferes with the arterial ability to become more distensible under appropriate physiological circumstances [24]. To clarify this question, in 13 young normotensive subjects before and during cigarette smoking, arterial compliance was measured by a new A-mode ultrasonic echo-tracking device [25], capable of continuously providing (300 readings/sec) radial artery diameter and, along with blood pressure values (Finapres recording), arterial compliance.

Smoking induced a reduction in radial artery diameter and arterial compliance which became progressively greater from the first to the fifth minute of smoking and was maintained for several minutes following the smoking procedure. On the whole, the magnitude of this reduction amounted to 35.7 ± 4.8% for arterial diameter data and to 22.5 ± 4.2% for arterial compliance values (p < 0.01 for both).

Thus cigarette smoking not only increases blood pressure but also causes an impairment of the viscoelastic properties of large arteries.

Conclusions

Although several questions related to the cardiovascular effects of cigarette smoking remain to be clarified, it is clear that not only blood pressure but also the sympathetic nervous system and the functional properties of large arteries are adversely affected by smoking. These alterations may play an important physiopathological role in the development of several cardiovascular complications of smoking, including hypertension and atherosclerosis.

References

1.   Pooling Project Research Group: Relationship of blood pressure, serum cholesterol, smoking habit, relative weight and ECG abnormalities to incidence of major coronary events; final report of the Pooling Project. J Chron Dis 1978;31:201-306.
2.   Wilhelmsen L. Coronary heart disease: Epidemiology of smoking and intervention studies of smoking. Am Heart J 1988;115:242-249.
3.   Kannel WB, McGee DL, Castelli WP. Latest perspectives on cigarette smoking and cardiovascular disease: The Framingham Study. J Card Rehab 1984;4:267-277.
4.   Craig WY, Palomaki GE, Haddow JE. Cigarette smoking and serum lipid and lipoprotein concentrations: An analysis of published data. Br Med J 1989;298:784-788.
5.   Meade TW, Imeson J, Stirling Y. Effects of changes in smoking and other characteristics on clotting factors and the risk of ischaemic heart disease. Lancet 1987;ii:986-988.
6.   Nowak J, Murray JJ, Oates JA, et al. Biochemical evidence of a chronic abnormality in platelet and vascular function in healthy individuals who smoke cigarettes. Circulation 1987;76:6-14.
7.   Karvonen M, Orma E, Keys A, Fidanza S, Brozek J. Cigarette smoking, serum cholesterol, blood pressure and body fatness: Observation in Finland. Lancet 1959;i:492-496.
8.   Cryer PE, Haymond MW, Santiago JW, Shah SD. Norepinephrine and epinephrine release and adrenergic mediation of smoking associated hemodynamic and metabolic events. N Engl J Med 1976;295:573-577.
9.   Trap-Jensen J, Carlsen JE, Svendsen TL, Christensen NS. Cardiovascular and adrenergic effects of cigarette smoking during immediate non-selective beta-adrenergic blockade in humans. Eur J Clin Invest 1979;9:181-183.
10.   Tachmes L, Fernandez RJ, Sachner MA. Haemodynamic effects of smoking cigarette of high and low nicotine content. Chest 1978;74:243-246.
11.   Mancia G, Groppelli A, Casadei R, Omboni S, Mutti E, Parati G. Cardiovascular effects of smoking. Clin Exper Hypertens 1990;A12:917-929.
12.   Benowitz NL, Jacob III P, Jones RT, Rosenberg J. Interindividual variability in the metabolism and cardiovascular effects of nicotine in man. J Pharmacol Exper Ther 1982;221:368-372.

13. Groppelli A, Omboni S, Parati G, Mancia G. Blood pressure and heart rate response to repeated smoking before and after ß-blockade and selective α_1 inhibition. J Hypertens 1990;8(Suppl.5):S35-S40.

14. Groppelli A, Giorgi MA, Omboni S, Parati G, Mancia G. Persistent blood pressure increase induced by heavy smoking. J Hypertens 1992;10:495-499.

15. Frattola A, Parati G, Cuspidi C, Albini F, Mancia G. Prognostic value of 24-hour blood pressure variability. J Hypertens 1993;11:1133-1137.

16. Baer L, Radichevich I. Cigarette smoking in hypertensive patients. Am J Med 1965;78:564-568.

17. Grassi G, Seravalle G, Calhoun DA, et al. Mechanisms responsible for sympathetic activation by cigarette smoking in humans. Circulation 1994;90:248-253.

18. Wallin BG, Fagius J. Peripheral sympathetic neural activity in conscious humans. Ann Rev Physiol 1988;50:565-576.

19. Grassi G, Seravalle G, Calhoun DA, et al. Monitoring of sympathetic activity in man: Physiology and pharmacology. Eur Heart J 1992;13(Suppl.A):22-25.

20. Mancia G, Grassi G, Parati G, Daffonchio A. Evaluating sympathetic activity in human hypertension. J Hypertens 1993;11(Suppl.5):S13-S19.

21. Mancia G, Mark AL. Arterial baroreflex in humans. In: Shepherd JT, Abboud FM, editors. Handbook of Physiology, Section 2: The Cardiovascular System, vol III, part II. Bethesda: American Physiological Society, 1983:755-793.

22. O'Rourke MF. Arterial function in health and disease.Edinburgh: Churchill Livingstone, 1982:3-32, 53-93, 224-270.

23. Safar ME, Levy BI, Laurent S, London GM. Hypertension and the arterial system: clinical and therapeutic aspects. J Hypertens 1990;8(Suppl.7):S113-S119.

24. Giannattasio C, Mangoni AA, Stella ML, Carugo S, Grassi G, Mancia G. Acute effects of smoking on radial artery compliance in humans. J Hypertens 1994;12:691-696.

25. Tardy Y, Meister JJ, Perret F, Brunner HR, Arditi M. Non-invasive estimate of the mechanical properties of peripheral arteries from ultrasonic and photoplethysmographic measurements. Clin Phys Physiol Meas 1991;12:39-54.

SERUM URIC ACID AND 18-YEAR CARDIOVASCULAR MORTALITY IN THE CHICAGO HEART ASSOCIATION DETECTION PROJECT IN INDUSTRY

Alan R. Dyer, Rose Stamler, Jeremiah Stamler, Dan Garside
Department of Preventive Medicine
Northwestern University Medical School
Chicago, Illinois 60611
USA

This report examines associations of serum uric acid (SUA) with 18-year cardiovascular (CVD) mortality in men and women ages 30-49 and 50-69 from the Chicago Heart Association Detection Project in Industry. In Cox regression analyses, with adjustment only for age and ethnicity, serum uric acid was significantly related to CVD mortality in women 50-69 (relative risks [RR]=1.35 for SUA higher by 1 mg/dl, 95% confidence intervals [CI]=1.21 to 1.50) but not women 30-49. With adjustment for multiple additional variables, the RR in women 50-69 became 1.25 (CI=1.11 to 1.40). For these women, serum uric acid was more strongly related to mortality in those with asymptomatic hyperglycemia (casual glucose $\geq$ 145 mg/dl or one-hour post load plasma glucose $\geq$ 205 mg/dl) (RR=1.61) compared to normoglycemic women (RR=1.18), in smokers (RR=1.30) compared to nonsmokers (RR=1.21), and in hypertensives (RR=1.36) compared to nonhypertensives (RR=1.07). For men, the association was significant only in men 30-49 when adjusted for age and ethnicity (RR=1.13, CI=1.02 to 1.26). While the association in men 50-69 was not statistically significant (RR=1.07, CI=1.00 to 1.15), there was evidence of increased CVD mortality at the high and low ends of the serum uric acid distribution. For these men, RR for those with serum uric acid $\geq$ 7.8 mg/dl compared to those with lower levels was 1.52 (CI=1.15 to 2.01) with adjustment for age and ethnicity, and 1.33 (CI=1.00 to 1.76) with multiple adjustment. These results suggest that uric acid is more strongly related to CVD mortality in women than in men and that uric acid is an important independent risk factor for CVD mortality in postmenopausal women.

Methods

The Chicago Heart Association Detection Project in Industry has been described at length elsewhere [1-3]. Briefly, from November 1967 to January 1973, the Chicago Heart Association Detection Project in Industry screened 39,572 men and women ages 18 and older at 84 cooperating companies and organizations in the Chicago area. All employees

A.M. Gotto et al. (eds), Multiple Risk Factors in Cardiovascular Disease, 365-372.
© 1995 *Kluwer Academic Publishers and Fondazione Giovanni Lorenzini.*

in the labor forces of these firms were encouraged to participate, and a 55% volunteer rate was obtained. A self-administered questionnaire was used to collect demographic data, smoking history, and information, including current treatment, on previous medical diagnoses of hypertension and diabetes, and beginning in August 1970, of hyperuricemia and gout. Measurements included height, weight, and a single casual supine blood pressure. A resting electrocardiogram (ECG) was also obtained [4]. Venous blood samples were collected one hour following a 50 g oral glucose load, and analyzed for serum cholesterol and plasma glucose, and subsequently, beginning in March 1970, for serum uric acid. Uric acid levels were determined by Autoanalyzer [5] on approximately 28,000 of the 39,572 screenees.

All participants have been followed periodically for the determination of vital status; for men and women with uric acid measurements, average follow-up is 18 years. Cause of death was determined from the death certificate and coded according to the eighth revision of the International Classification of Diseases adapted for use in the United States (ICDA) [6]. Deaths from cardiovascular diseases (CVD) were those assigned to ICDA codes 390-458.

Men and women were excluded from these analyses if they were less than 30 or ≥ 70 years of age; had evidence of a myocardial infarction by ECG at entry; if they were missing data on serum uric acid or other variables; or if they were receiving drug treatment for high blood pressure or diabetes.

This report thus focuses on the associations between serum uric acid and 18-year CVD mortality in 4,579 women and 6,828 men ages 30-49 and 3,438 women and 3,342 men ages 50-69.

Results

Mean serum uric acid was higher with age in women but not in men (Table 1).

Table 1. Correlations of serum uric acid with other variables.

Variable	Women 30-49	Women 50-69	Men 30-49	Men 50-69
Age	0.10	0.09	0.00	-0.01
Systolic pressure	0.16	0.18	0.18	0.14
Diastolic pressure	0.16	0.17	0.20	0.16
Body mass index	0.33	0.32	0.33	0.26
Serum cholesterol	0.11	0.05	0.12	0.08
Cigarettes/day	-0.01	-0.01	-0.08	-0.06
Post load glucose	0.13	0.16	0.09	0.07
Heart rate	0.04	0.05	0.07	0.09
Years of education	-0.01	0.00	0.04	0.00

Among other variables considered in these analyses, uric acid was most strongly correlated with body mass index (kg/m^2), with correlations ranging from 0.26 to 0.33. Uric acid was also positively correlated with systolic and diastolic blood pressure, serum cholesterol, plasma glucose, and heart rate in men and women, and inversely with number of cigarettes smoked per day in men.

In Cox regression analyses [7], with adjustment for age and ethnicity (white versus nonwhite), serum uric acid was positively related to CVD mortality in all four subgroups, with RRs associated with a 1 mg/dl increase in serum uric acid ranging from 1.07 in men 50-69 to 1.35 in women 50-69 (Table 2). However, as indicated by the lower limits of the 95% CI, only the RRs for women 50-69 and men 30-49 differed significantly from 1.0. With further adjustment for systolic blood pressure, body mass index, serum cholesterol, heart rate, untreated diabetes, asymptomatic hyperglycemia (casual glucose $\geq$ 145 mg/dl or one-hour post load glucose $\geq$ 205 mg/dl), years of education, and major and minor ECG abnormalities (defined according to Pooling Project criteria) [8], only the RR in women 50-69 continued to differ significantly from 1.0. Cox regression coefficients in women 50-69 also differed significantly from those in men 50-69.

Table 2. Relative risks (RR) and 95% confidence intervals (CI) for associations of serum uric acid with cardiovascular mortality.

		Age, ethinicity adjusted		Multiple adjustment*	
Cohort	Deaths	RR[+]	95% CI	RR[+]	95% CI
Women 30-49	54	1.16	(0.93, 1.44)	1.03	(0.81, 1.32)
Women 50-69	186	1.35	(1.21, 1.50)	1.25	(1.11, 1.40)
Men 30-49	188	1.13	(1.02, 1.26)	1.06	(0.94, 1.19)
Men 50-69	449	1.07	(1.00, 1.15)	1.04	(0.96, 1.12)

*Age, ethnicity, systolic blood pressure, body mass index, heart rate, serum cholesterol, cigarettes/day, untreated diabetes, asymptomatic hyperglycemia, education, ECG abnormalities
[+]For serum uric acid higher by 1 mg/dl

The association of serum uric acid with 18-year CVD mortality was also examined in subgroups of women and men ages 50-69 with subgroups defined based on values for glucose, blood pressure, and smoking status. For women 50-69, the association was significantly stronger in those with asymptomatic hyperglycemia (casual glucose $\geq$ 145 mg/dl or one-hour post load plasma glucose $\geq$ 205 mg/dl) with a RR of 1.61 for serum uric acid higher by 1 mg/dl compared to those with normal glucose levels, with a RR of 1.18 (Table 3). The RR was also larger in smokers compared to nonsmokers, 1.30 versus 1.21, and in hypertensives (systolic blood pressure $\geq$ 150 mm Hg or diastolic blood pressure $\geq$ 95 mm Hg) compared to nonhypertensives, 1.36 versus 1.07, although the differences in these RRs were not statistically significant. Only the RR of 1.07 for nonhypertensives did not differ significantly from 1.0.

The risk of CVD mortality was also increased in men 50-69 with asymptomatic hyperglycemia, although the RR of 1.17 was substantially less than the RR of 1.61 observed in the hyperglycemic women 50-69 and was virtually identical to the RR in normoglycemic women (Table 3). None of the RRs for the other subgroups of men 50-69 differed significantly from 1.0, and with the exception of the RR for nonhypertensives, all were smaller than the corresponding RRs in women.

Table 3. Relative risks (RR) and 95% confidence intervals (CI) for associations of serum uric acid with CVD mortality in subgroups of women and men 50-69.

Subgroup	N	Deaths	RR*	95% CI
Women 50-69				
Hyperglycemia+	364	25	1.16	(1.26, 2.06)
Normoglycemia	3022	157	1.18	(1.03, 1.36)
Smokers	1087	86	1.30	(1.09, 1.56)
Nonsmokers	2351	100	1.21	(1.03, 1.42)
Hypertensives#	1240	106	1.36	(1.18, 1.58)
Nonhypertensives	2198	80	1.07	(0.88, 1.31)
Men 50-69				
Hyperglycemia+	498	91	1.17	(1.00, 1.37)
Normoglycemia	2775	343	1.00	(0.91, 1.09)
Smokers	1202	218	1.09	(0.97, 1.21)
Nonsmokers	2140	231	1.01	(0.91, 1.12)
Hypertensives#	1551	275	1.03	(0.94, 1.13)
Nonhypertensives	1791	174	1.07	(0.94, 1.22)

*For serum uric acid higher by 1 mg/dl with multiple adjustment
+Casual glucose $\geq$ 145 mg/dl or one-hour post load plasma glucose $\geq$ 205 mg/dl
#Systolic pressure $\geq$ 150 mm Hg or diastolic pressure $\geq$ 95 mm Hg

In men 50-69, while the association between serum uric acid and 18-year CVD mortality was not statistically significant in the Cox regression analyses, examination of CVD mortality by uric acid decile revealed a J-shaped relationship, with mortality higher in the first quintile compared to the second and third quintiles and a RR of 1.38 for the top decile ($\geq$ 7.8 mg/dl) compared to the lowest quintile (Table 4). There was no increase in risk for those with uric acid in the range of 7.2 to 7.7 mg/dl compared to men in the lowest quintile, although the CVD mortality rate for these men was greater than that for men in the middle three quintiles.

Table 4. Relative risks (RR) of CVD mortality in serum uric acid deciles in men and women 50-69.

	Men 50-69				Women 50-69		
Deciles	N	Deaths	RR*	Deciles	N	Deaths	RR*
1-2: <5.1	651	90	1.00	<3.9	629	21	1.00
3-4: 5.1-5.7	696	86	0.86	3.9-4.4	755	35	1.44
5-6: 5.8-6.3	655	71	0.74	4.5-4.9	691	32	1.37
7-8: 6.4-7.1	695	98	0.98	5.0-5.6	646	40	1.88
9: 7.2-7.7	335	47	1.01	5.7-6.2	368	21	1.61
10: >7.8	311	57	1.38	>6.3	349	37	2.99

*Adjusted for age and ethnicity by Cox regression

A similar analysis in women 50-69 showed increased risks of CVD mortality in all quintiles compared to the first, and for women in the highest decile (≥ 6.3 mg/dl) the RR compared to the lowest quintile was 2.99, a value much larger than that in men 50-69.

Because of the apparent increased risk of CVD mortality in the upper 10% of the serum uric acid distribution for men 50-69, the risks of CVD mortality were compared for those above and below the 90th percentile of the serum uric distribution for each of the four cohorts (Table 5). With adjustment only for age and ethnicity, the RRs for those in the upper

Table 5. Relative risks (RR) and 95% confidence intervals (CI) for CVD mortality for the highest serum uric acid decile in men and women.

	Age, ethnicity adjusted		Multiple adjustment*	
Cohort	RR+	95% CI	RR+	95% CI
Women 30-49	1.68	(0.85, 3.35)	1.17	(0.56, 2.43)
Women 50-69	2.06	(1.44, 2.96)	1.55	(1.06, 2.29)
Men 30-49	1.38	(0.90, 2.10)	1.12	(0.73, 1.73)
Men 50-69	1.52	(1.15, 2.01)	1.33	(1.00, 1.76)

*Age, ethnicity, systolic blood pressure, body mass index, heart rate, serum cholesterol, cigarettes/day, untreated diabetes, asymptomatic hyperglycemia, education, ECG abnormalities
+For the highest serum uric acid decile versus all others; cutpoints were 5.7 mg/dl for women 30-49, 6.3 mg/dl for women 50-69, and 7.8 for men

10% were 2.06 for women 50-69, 1.68 for women 30-49, 1.52 for men 50-69, and 1.38 for men 30-49. However, as indicated by the lower limits for the 95% confidence intervals, only the RRs for men and women 50-69 differed significantly from 1.0. With multiple adjustment, the RR for women 50-69 was reduced to 1.55, but continued to differ significantly from 1.0, while the RR for men 50-69 was reduced to 1.33 with a lower limit on the 95% confidence interval that included 1.0. The RR for women 30-49 was reduced to 1.17 with multiple adjustment, and that for men 30-49 to 1.12.

Analyses comparing the upper 10% of the serum uric acid distribution with the lower 90% were also conducted for the subgroups based on glucose levels, blood pressure, and smoking status (Table 6). For women 50-69, the RR of CVD mortality in the top 10% of the serum uric acid distribution was larger for women with hyperglycemia compared to normoglycemia, for smokers compared to nonsmokers, and for hypertensives compared to nonhypertensives, consistent with the results of the Cox regression analyses given in Table 3 above. The RRs for women with asymptomatic hyperglycemia, smokers, and hypertensives all differed significantly from 1.0, whereas the RRs for normoglycemic women, nonsmokers, and nonhypertensives did not.

For men 50-69, the RRs were also larger for men with asymptomatic hyperglycemia compared to men with normal glucose levels and for smokers compared to nonsmokers (Table 6). However, for men 50-69, in contrast to women 50-69, the RR was larger for nonhypertensives compared to hypertensives. Only the RR for smokers differed significantly from 1.0 and with the exception of the RR for nonhypertensives, all RRs were smaller than those in the comparable subgroup of women 50-69.

Table 6. Relative risks (RR) and 95% confidence intervals (CI) for CVD mortality for the highest serum uric acid decile in men and women ages 50-69.

Subgroup	Women 50-69		Men 50-69	
	RR*	95% CI	RR*	95% CI
Hyperglycemia	2.66	(1.07, 6.63)	1.35	(0.78, 2.32)
Normoglycemia	1.32	(0.84, 2.06)	1.21	(0.85, 1.72)
Smokers	1.90	(1.10, 3.31)	1.63	(1.08, 2.46)
Nonsmokers	1.26	(0.74, 2.15)	1.16	(0.78, 1.73)
Hypertensives	1.72	(1.07, 2.76)	1.25	(0.89, 1.75)
Nonhypertensives	1.30	(0.65, 2.59)	1.62	(0.95, 2.74)

*For the highest serum uric acid decile versus all others with multiple adjustment

Comment

We previously examined the association between serum uric acid and CVD mortality in white men and women ages 45-64 from the Chicago Heart Association Detection Project white men and women ages 45-64 from the Chicago Heart Association Detection Project in Industry based on shorter lengths of follow-up [2,3]. In analyses based on 11.5 years of follow-up, serum uric acid was found to be positively related to CVD mortality in women ages 55-64 [3]. The present report extends those findings by examining the association between serum uric acid and CVD mortality in all men and women ages 30-69 based on 18 years of follow-up and by examining the associations in men and women ages 50-69 in specific subgroups based on glucose level, blood pressure, and smoking status.

In the analyses reported here, serum uric acid was significantly and independently related to increased CVD mortality in women ages 50-69, but not in women 30-49, or men 30-49 or 50-69. The positive association in women 50-69 appeared to be stronger in women with asymptomatic hyperglycemia, in smokers, and in hypertensives.

In men, while serum uric acid was not independently related to increased CVD mortality in either age group, for men 50-69 there was some evidence of increased mortality in both the low and high ($\geq$ 7.8 mg/dl) ends of the distribution. There was also some evidence of a positive association between serum uric acid and CVD mortality in men 50-69 for those with asymptomatic hyperglycemia and in smokers in this age group for those with uric acid levels $\geq$ 7.8 mg/dl.

These results suggest that serum uric acid is more strongly related to CVD risk in women than in men and that serum uric acid is an important CVD risk factor in postmenopausal women.

Acknowledgements

The Chicago Heart Association Detection Project in Industry has been supported by the Chicago Heart Association, the American Heart Association, the Illinois Regional Medical Program, and by grant number HL21010 from the National Heart, Lung, and Blood Institute. For a listing of other organizations supporting this Project and the many individuals who planned and carried out the field work, see the acknowledgements in reference 3 below.

References

1.   Stamler J, Rhomberg P, Schoenberger JA, et al. Multivariate analysis of the relationship of seven variables to blood pressure: Findings of Chicago Heart Association Detection Project in Industry, 1967-1972. J Chron Dis 1975;28:527-48.

2.   Persky VW, Dyer AR, Idris-Soven E, et al. Uric acid: A risk factor for coronary heart disease? Circulation 1979;59:969-77.

3.   Levine W, Dyer AR, Shekelle RB, Schoenberger JA, Stamler J. Serum uric acid and 11.5-year mortality of middle-aged women: Findings of the Chicago Heart Association Detection Project in Industry. J Clin Epidemiol 1989;42:257-67.

4.   Cedres LB, Liu K, Stamler J, et al. Independent contribution of electrocardiographic abnormalities to risk of death from coronary heart disease,

cardiovascular disease and all causes -- findings of three Chicago epidemiologic studies. Circulation 1982;65:146-53.

5.   Hawk PB, Oser BL, Summerson WH. Practical physiological chemistry. 13th ed. New York: Blakiston, 1954: 564.

6.   US Department of Health, Education, and Welfare, National Center for Health Statistics. International Classification of Diseases (8th revision) adapted for use in the United States (ICDA), PHS Publication No. 1693. Washington, D.C.: U.S. Government Printing Office, 1967.

7.   Cox DR. Regression models and life tables. J R Stat Soc Ser B 1972;34:187-202.

8.   Pooling Project Research Group. Relationship of blood pressure, serum cholesterol, smoking habit, relative weight and ECG abnormalities to incidence of major coronary events: Final report of the pooling project. J Chron Dis 1978;31:201-306.

THE IMPACT OF HIGH-DENSITY LIPOPROTEIN CHOLESTEROL ON CARDIOVASCULAR RISK: THE BEZAFIBRATE INFARCTION PREVENTION (BIP) STUDY

Uri Goldbourt for the BIP Study Research Group.
The Henry N. Neufeld Cardiac Research Institute
Sheba Medical Center and the Institute of Physiological Hygiene
Edith Wolfson Medical Center
Holon
ISRAEL

An inverse relationship of low blood concentration of high-density lipoprotein cholesterol (HDL-C) to the risk of developing coronary heart disease (CHD) is well established [1]. In studies of progression of atherosclerosis, low initial levels of serum HDL cholesterol have also been associated with subsequent rapid progression of coronary arterial lesions. For example, in the Leiden Dietary Intervention Study, the smaller the proportion of cholesterol on HDL, the larger was the mean change of coronary arterial diameter [2]. Treatment of hyperlipidemic patients with drugs possessing a strong HDL elevating capacity, such as fibrates and nicotinic acid, has resulted in reduced rates of clinical CHD [3] or slowed lesion progression [4]. When large samples of patients with CHD are examined, low HDL-C is quite frequent. Among those patients with so-called "desirable" total cholesterol, below 200 mg/dl, HDL-C below 35 mg/dl is often found [5].

Nevertheless, the precise etiology behind the association between low HDL and increased CHD risk is unclear. Most likely, these levels are markers of complex changes in the metabolism of triglycerides and cholesterol. Unequivocal evidence that elevating HDL-C would be beneficial in terms of coronary event rate is not available. In 1990 and 1991, two relevant large-scale multicenter clinical trials were initiated. These trials aimed at examining the hypothesis that elevating so-called "isolated" low HDL-C and reducing triglycerides would bring about a long-term benefit in terms of cardiac incidence. One trial is the US Veteran Administration trial [HIT] (N=2500) coordinated in Minneapolis. The larger, and ahead timewise, in terms of follow-up duration, is the Bezafibrate Infarction Prevention (BIP) Study in 18 Israeli medical centers [6].

Population and Methods

The aim of the study is to determine whether the long-term administration of bezafibrate

A.M. Gotto et al. (eds), Multiple Risk Factors in Cardiovascular Disease, 373-378.
© *1995 Kluwer Academic Publishers and Fondazione Giovanni Lorenzini.*

retard (400 mg/day) to CHD patients whose total serum cholesterol is in the normal or slightly elevated range of 180 to 250 mg/dl, HDL-C $\leq$ 45 mg/dl, and triglycerides $\leq$ 300 mg/dl would lead to reduced rates of fatal and nonfatal coronary events attributable to an underlying atherosclerosis of the coronary arteries, as compared with placebo. Randomization to bezafibrate or placebo was restricted to males and females, aged 45-74, whose lipids were at the above ranges and whose calculated low density lipoprotein cholesterol (LDL-C) was below 180 mg/dl (aged below 50, < 160 mg/dl). Thus it is a study that examines the effect of bezafibrate in a population that would not be normally on a sweeping pharmaceutical therapy to reduce LDL cholesterol. The main criteria for exclusion [6] were myocardial infarction (MI) during the preceding six months, congestive heart failure, unstable angina, insulin-dependent diabetes, pacemakers, and severe peripheral or cerebrovascular disease. The primary endpoint is nonfatal MI, death within 28 days after an acute MI, or sudden death within 24 hours from the onset of symptoms. Patients are being followed up until January 1998, a mean follow-up period of 6.25 years. The rationale and design of the study have been described in detail [6].

The mean age of patients included in BIP was 60 years. Of these, 92% were men, primarily due to the tighter restriction of the upper bound of HDL cholesterol on women and age differences. A previous MI had occurred in 77%. The others suffered from angina, objectively supported by catheterization or noninvasive evidence.

Results

The first patient was screened on February 1990 and randomized on May 1990. The last patient was randomized on January 15, 1993. Presently, at four years of follow-up, an average 2.75 years of follow-up, 92% of planned medical visits have taken place and 81% are still on study medication. The percentage of persons who discontinued medication other than because of a critical event, approximates 10%. There is a great variation between the centers, with one center showing an excellent low rate of 2.5% whereas four centers have suffered a permanent withdrawal rate between 13 and 14%. Only a few dozen patients actually severed contact with the respective clinical center and do not show up for examination.

Table 1 shows event incidence in the study sample. Confirmed primary endpoints occurred in 193 patients (6.2%). Fifteen patients subsequently suffered a recurrent fatal or nonfatal MI. We are also counting additional cardiac events. Reported so far were the occurrence of unstable angina in 4.4% of patients, CABG operation in 6.5%, and PTCA in 4.1%. The death of 113 patients (3.6%) was reported and confirmed. Survival analysis (not shown) has indicated that the rate of primary endpoints has been somewhat slower than expected on the basis of the more conservative assumption. This may reflect a study participation effect beyond that projected and/or an expression of the continuing decline of CHD mortality in Israel.

While follow-up continues, interesting early results arise from a mortality ascertainment in the screenees. In contrast to the BIP sample proper, the screenees includes a large number of women with CHD, rendering possible the elucidation of factors associated with their prognosis.

Table 1. Study Progression. Follow-up to June 1994.

	N	%
Primary Endpoints		
Fatal or Nonfatal MI	156	5.0
Sudden Death	37	1.2
Secondary Endpoints		
Coronary Artery Bypass-Graft (CABG)	202	6.5
Percutaneous Transluminal Coronary		
Angioplasty (PTCA)	127	4.1
Unstable Angina	137	4.4
Total Mortality	113	3.6

We were able to match 14,458 screened patients (including the study participants) with the national mortality registry. Table 2 shows the reported underlying causes of death for 642 of the 682 identified deaths through September 1993. Note that deaths attributable to CHD account for around one-half of deaths. The limitation of death certificate coding notwithstanding, we believe that in an era of rapidly decreasing case fatality and possibly decreasing incidence, an increasing portion of CHD patient mortality will be caused by competing causes, and thus the importance of all-cause mortality will become paramount.

Table 2. Mortality Among 14,458 BIP Screenees. May 1990-September 1993 (N=642).

	Men		Women	
	N	%	N	%
Coronary Heart Disease	271	(53)	59	(47)
Cancer	69	(13)	12	(10)
Noncoronary Heart Disease	57	(11)	7	(6)
Stroke	20	(4)	11	(9)
Injury	15	(3)	2	(2)
Other	84	(16)	35	(28)
Total	516	(100)	12	(100)

Co-morbid condition in these CHD patients carried a strong association with their fate over the ensuing 2.25 years. These conditions are strongly associated with subsequent mortality. Diabetes has an overwhelming effect on mortality in women. A more than doubling of mortality was seen at the presence of peripheral vascular disease (PVD) or chronic obstructive pulmonary disease (COPD), each of found among 3 to 4% of the cohort.

Table 3. Mortality per 1,000 Person-years. Age-adjusted Rates, among 14,458 CHD Patients.

	Men		Women	
	Yes	No	Yes	No
Past MI	23	13	24	14
Current Angina	24	16	26	15
Diabetes	34	18	47	15
PVD	50	20	56	21
Stroke	77	20	24	22
COPD	49	20	45	22

The presence and severity of functional incapacity, representing primarily congestive heart failure, as well as the grading of anginal syndrome, are strong predictors of mortality in the screenees (Table 4).

Examining the association between screening lipid levels and mortality, we restricted the analysis to screenees who were not included in BIP and thus unlikely to be affected in a similar manner to patients half of whom have been receiving bezafibrate. Mortality rose with rising serum cholesterol and triglycerides in these patients, and declined with increasing HDL-C. Except for the latter, the relationship with CHD death were markedly attenuated when overall mortality was looked at. We have performed multivariate analysis of CHD and total mortality in patients with "desirable," "borderline high," as well as "elevated" cholesterol, dividing the latter into patients below or above 275 mg/dl. The adjusted risk is consistent with a gradually increasing risk of CHD death but an approximately equal risk of total mortality in all these boundaries.

When these associations were examined separately by sex, a small mortality increase of about 20% is seen among the men, while, paradoxically, the relative risk (RR) among the women with cholesterol above 200 mg/dl, admittedly far from significant, were in the "wrong" direction, specifically 0.75, 0.89, and 0.71 among those at the three cholesterol ranges above 200 as shown in table 5. This could certainly be the fruit of chance, although these trends closely resemble those observed in a 10.5 year follow up recently reported on a smaller group of patients in Framingham, Massachusetts [7]. Clearly, longer research on our screenees would be instrumental to confirm or refute the initial trends.

Table 4. Morality per 1000 Person-years. Age-adjusted Rates, among 14,458 CHD Patients.

	Men		Women	
	N	Odds ratio	N	Odds ratio
New York Heart Association Functional Classification				
Class I	17	1.0	18	1.0
II	27	1.6	24	1.4
III	43	2.2	54	3.0
Angina				
None		1.0		1.0
Grade I	20	1.2	16	1.0
II	25	1.5	31	2.1
III	49	3.0	57	4.3

Table 5. The 2.25-year Risk of Mortality in Patients by serum Cholesterol - Relative Hazard Adjusted by Multiple Variables*

Cholesterol	Relative Mortality Hazard (and 90% CI)	
(mg/dl)	All-cause	CHD
< 200	1.00	1.00
200-239	0.99 (0.82-1.18)	1.36 (1.03-1.80)
240-274	1.18 (0.97-1.49)	1.71 (1.28-2.29)
>275	1.12 (0.88-1.41)	1.69 (1.20-2.38)

* Multiple adjustment by Cox proportional hazards model for co-existing cardiac and circulatory morbidity, smoking, diabetes, and HDL cholesterol.

It is important to note that a parallel analysis by calculated LDL cholesterol rather than by total cholesterol yielded an even weaker association with mortality.

Discussion

Taken together, the results of a 2.25-year follow-up of the BIP screenees represent the largest reported mortality follow-up of CHD patients, men and women, with both clinical and lipid parameters assessed, in terms of person-years of follow-up. The limitations are clear: A follow up 2.25 years may be too short to provide complete valid information on a long-term association between post-CHD lipid levels and mortality; mortality may have occurred too close to the cholesterol measurement for the latter to be free from an effect of an already existing disease; and we have no information, at present, on nonfatal events in the screenee. Still, the findings appear to be thought provoking. We do not really have sizeable data on the effect of reducing slightly elevated or intermediate cholesterol in CHD patients. Clinical studies like BIP, HIT, which use fibrate derivatives, and three studies using pravastatin, are examining he effect of therapy in patients with an upper limit of serum cholesterol for inclusion. The latter three are CARE [8], examining 4,159 patients with cholesterol between 180 and 250 mg/dl, the LIPID trial of 9,014 MI patients aged 31-75 with cholesterol between 4 and 7 mmol/L, and the GISSI Intervention of 6,000 patients in Italy with cholesterol limits between 200 and 250 mg/dl all concentrate on the efficacy of correcting alleged dyslipidemia in the "normal to borderline cholesterol" range. Our observations make the expectation of their results all the more exciting.

References

1.   Miller GJ, Miller NE. Plasma-high-density-lipoprotein concentration and the development of ischaemic heart disease. Lancet 1975;i:16-19.
2.   Arntzenius AC, Kromhout D, Barth JD, et al. Diet, lipoprotein and the progression of coronary atherosclerosis. The Leiden Intervention Trial. N Engl J Med 1985;312:805-811.
3.   Frick ME, Elo O, Haapa K, et al. Helsinki Heart Study: Primary-prevention trial with gemfibrozil in middle-aged men with dyslipidemia: Safety of treatment, changes of risk factors and incidence of coronary heart disease. N Engl J Med 1987;317:1237-1245.
4.   Brown G, Albers JJ, Fisher LD, et al. Regression of coronary artery disease as a result of intensive lipid-lowering therapy in men with high levels of apolipoprotein B. N Engl J Med 1990;323:1289-1298.
5.   Bush TL, Riedel D. Screening for total cholesterol. Do the National Cholesterol Education Program's recommendations detect individuals at high risk of coronary heart disease. Circulation 1991;83:1283-1287.
6.   Goldbourt U, Behar S, Reicher-Reiss H, et al. Rationale and design of a secondary prevention trial of increasing serum high-density lipoprotein cholesterol and reducing triglycerides in patients with clinically manifest atherosclerotic heart disease (the Bezafibrate Infarction Prevention Trial). Am J Cardiol 1993;71:909-915.
7.   Wong ND, Wilson PWF, Kannel WB. Serum cholesterol as a prognostic factor after myocardial infarction: The Framingham Study. Ann Intern Med 1991;115:687-693.
8.   Sacks FM, Pfeffer MA, Moye L, et al for the CARE investigators. Rationale and design of a secondary prevention trial of lowering normal plasma cholesterol levels after acute myocardial infarction: The Cholesterol and Recurrent Events Trial (CARE). AM J Cardiol 1991;68:1436-1446.

TRIGLYCERIDES AND THE FIBRINOLYTIC SYSTEM

Elena Tremoli, Luigi Sironi, Marina Camera, Luisa Mannucci, Livia Prati, Cristina Banfi, Damiano Baldassarre, and Luciana Mussoni
Enrica Grossi Paoletti Center
Institute of Pharmacological Sciences
University of Milan
Via Balzaretti 9
20133 Milan
ITALY

Introduction

The fibrinolytic system is devoted to the removal of fibrin clots and it constitutes a physiological mechanism against the deposition of thrombi within the vascular tree [1]. Plasmin, the central enzyme of the fibrinolytic system is generated from its precursor, plasminogen, through the action of plasminogen activators, tissue type (t-PA) and urinary type (U-PA) plasminogen activators. The activity of plasminogen activators is regulated by several inhibitors, i.e. alfa-2-antiplasmin and plasminogen activator inhibitor type-1 (PAI-1) [2]. So far, impaired fibrinolytic activity has been reported to be mainly due to altered levels of the specific inhibitor of plasminogen activation, PAI-1. Deficiency of PAI-1 has been reported to be associated with bleeding disorder, due to uncontrolled t-PA activity on fibrin clots [3]. On the other hand, increased levels in blood of PAI-1 have shown to be associated with venous thrombosis and to predispose to arterial thrombosis [4]. Indeed, the elevated levels of PAI-1 reported in young patient survivors of myocardial infarction have been demonstrated to be an independent risk of recurrent infarction in the same individuals [5]. In addition, PAI-1 levels seem to be associated with the major features of Syndrome "X" and in particular with hyperinsulinemia, the biological marker of insulin resistance, thus providing a plausible mechanism for the atherothrombotic occlusions associated with the syndrome [6,7].

Moreover an association between elevated triglyceride levels and alterations of the coagulation or fibrinolytic system has been previously reported. Specifically, in patients with hypertriglyceridemia, reduction of plasma fibrinolytic capacity has been documented in several studies [8-11]. This aspect is of particular relevance in view of the role of plasma triglycerides as risk factor for cardiovascular disease [12]. Case-control studies have shown a positive correlation between triglyceride levels and incidence of cardiovascular disease and

A.M. Gotto et al. (eds), Multiple Risk Factors in Cardiovascular Disease, 379-384.
© 1995 *Kluwer Academic Publishers and Fondazione Giovanni Lorenzini.*

most prospective studies have confirmed this relationship [12]. The Framingham study indicates that men and women with triglyceride levels > 1.7 mM and high density lipoprotein (HDL) levels < 1.03 mM have a high rate of coronary heart disease [13]. On the other hand, the results of the PROCAM study indicate that hypertriglyceridemia is a powerful risk factor when excessive triglycerides coincide with high ratio (> 5.0) of plasma low density to high density lipoprotein cholesterol [14]. In this article the relationship between triglycerides and the fibrinolytic system, with particular attention to PAI-1 biosynthesis, will be discussed.

Studies in Patients with Hypertriglyceridemia

Studies performed in patients with cardiovascular disease have suggested that a direct relationship between plasma triglyceride levels and reduced fibrinolytic activity existed [15]. These studies, however, could not discriminate between the impact of plasma triglycerides and that of the ischemic disease on the different components of the fibrinolytic system. In an attempt to determine whether the hypertriglyceridemic state could directly influence the fibrinolytic activity as well as the levels of the individual components of the fibrinolytic system, we have performed a study in patients with hypertriglyceridemia as the only risk factor for cardiovascular disease [11].

The results of this study indicate that in hypertriglyceridemic patients total fibrinolytic and t-PA activities are within the normal range, whereas levels of t-PA antigen under basal condition (7.9 ± 0.7 and 11.8 ± 0.8 ng/ml for controls and patients respectively, $p < 0.01$) and following venous occlusion (18.7 ± 1.4 and 29.1 ± 2.1 respectively, $p < 0.01$) are significantly increased with respect to values found in plasma of a group of normotriglyceridemic subjects, matched with the patients for all the variables known to affect the fibrinolytic system, such as age, body mass index, and insulin levels. Interestingly, not only the levels of t-PA antigen were increased, but also the release of t-PA following venous occlusion was higher in plasma of hypertriglyceridemics than in controls (Figure 1).

In addition to increased basal t-PA antigen levels, basal PAI-1 antigen levels, the specific and rapid t-PA inhibitor, were also significantly higher in hypertriglyceridemics (Figure 1). PAI-1 antigen levels in patients were doubled and this increase paralleled that of PAI activity. In fact, PAI-1 antigen levels significantly correlated with PAI activity ($r=0.65$, Figure 2). The observation that both t-PA antigen and PAI-1 antigen levels are elevated offers a plausible explanation to the lack of alteration in total fibrinolytic activity found in our group of hypertriglyceridemic patients. On the other hand, it should be considered that PAI-1 antigen levels and, more recently, t-PA antigen have both been proposed as potential risk factors for vascular disease [16-18].

At present, we have no explanation for the enhanced levels of t-PA antigen observed in the group of hypertriglyceridemics. One might consider, however, that t-PA antigen is released from vascular endothelium in response to several stimuli, including cathecolamines. Thus, one might envision that the elevated levels of t-PA antigen found in hypertriglyceridemics reflect endothelial cell perturbation that might occur in this pathological condition. This hypothesis, however, does not fully explain the phenomenon, since in hypertriglyceridemic patients the increment in t-PA antigen, following stimulation of the vascular bed (i.e. following venous occlusion), is also enhanced, indicating that t-PA antigen biosynthesis and/or release is also increased in this pathological condition.

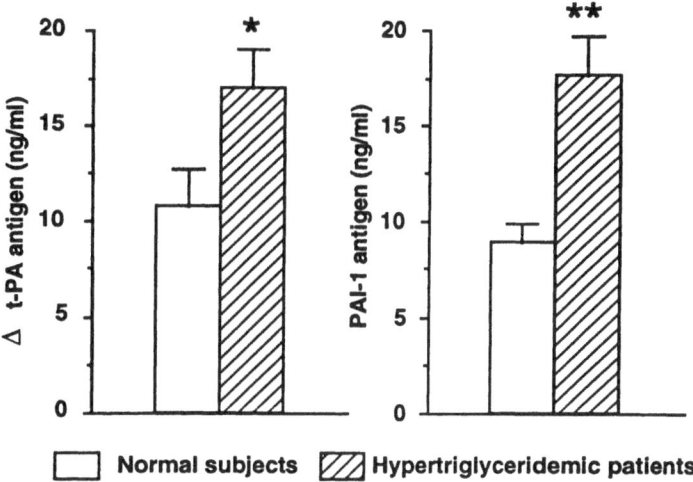

Figure 1. Increments in t-PA antigen (Δ-t-PA antigen) following venous occlusion and PAI-1 antigen levels in 27 normolipidemic subjects (open bars) and 30 hypertriglyceridemic patients (hatched bars). The data are the average ± SEM. ** $p < 0.01$ and * $p < 0.05$.

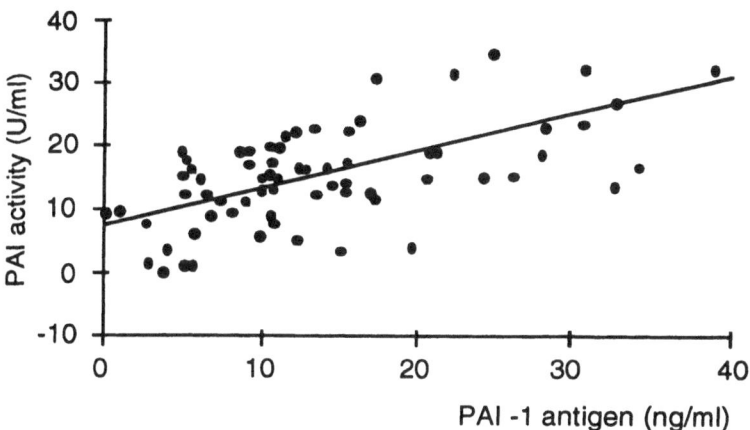

Figure 2. Scatter plot showing correlation between PAI activity and PAI-1 antigen levels in normo- and hypertriglyceridemic subjects.

When the relation between the fibrinolytic parameters and serum lipid profile was considered, a significant and direct correlation between PAI-1 antigen levels and plasma triglycerides was observed (r=0.40, p < 0.01). The observation of a linear relationship between these two variables, although not proving a causal relationship, suggested that triglycerides, and most likely, triglyceride-rich lipoproteins (very low density lipoproteins, VLDL) might influence PAI-1 biosynthesis by competent cells. Therefore in an attempt to elucidate this relationship, a series of studies were performed in cultured endothelial cells and in a hepatoma cell line that possesses most of the characteristics of human hepatocytes, i.e. HepG2 cells.

Studies in Endothelial Cells and in Hepg2 Cells

PAI-1 is a serine protease inhibitor synthesized by several cells types, including vascular cells, i.e. endothelial and smooth muscle cells, and liver cells and the synthesis of PAI-1 by competent cells is regulated by several substances [19]. To explain the link between PAI-1 and plasma triglyceride levels, *in vitro* studies in cultured human umbilical vein endothelial cells were performed [11,20]. The data indicate that VLDL, the major lipoprotein subfraction responsible for triglyceride transport, increase PAI-1 biosynthesis in endothelial cells. This effect is more pronounced when cells are incubated with VLDL isolated from plasma of hypertriglyceridemic patients [11,20]. The greater effect of VLDL from hypertriglyceridemic patients, compared with that of VLDL isolated from plasma of normolipidemic subjects, may be due to the presence in the patient's plasma of larger VLDL particle size containing newly transferred apolipoprotein E that has a high affinity for the apolipoprotein B/E receptor present on endothelial cells [20].

In vitro studies performed in HepG2 cells, have shown that the effect of VLDL on PAI-1 is not confined to endothelial cells, but rather represents a more general mechanism capable of regulating PAI-1 biosynthesis [11]. In fact VLDL are also capable of increasing PAI-1 release by HepG2 cells. Moreover the effect of VLDL isolated from hypertriglyceridemic donors is more pronounced on HepG2 cells than on endothelial cells (Figure 3).

The increased release of PAI-1 antigen by VLDL in HepG2 cells was accompanied by increase in PAI-1 mRNA expression [21]. These observations raise the possibility that this atherogenic lipoprotein subfraction is directly involved with an as yet unidentified mechanism in the regulation of PAI-1 biosynthesis not only in the vascular tree, but also at the hepatic level. No information, however, is available on the molecular mechanism(s) responsible for PAI-1 induction by VLDL in both cell types.

Conclusions

The available data indicate that the metabolic alterations that occur in hypertriglyceridemia result in an imbalance of the fibrinolytic system.

Interestingly, in the absence of clinical manifestations of cardiovascular disease, elevated triglyceride levels do not result in a reduction of total fibrinolytic activity due to

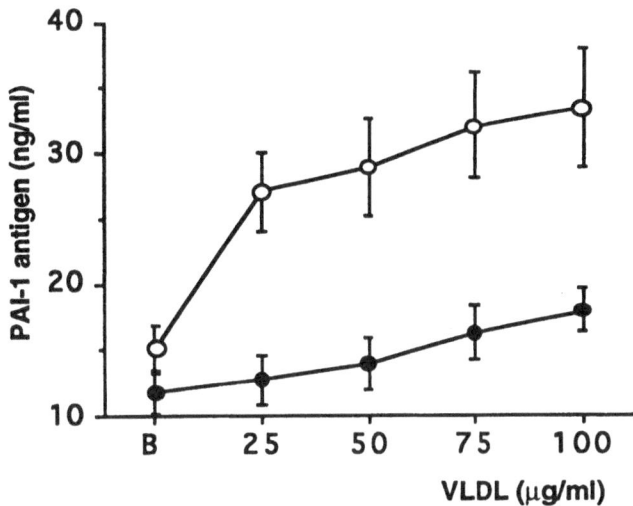

Figure 3. Plot showing effects of different concentrations of VLDL from hypertriglyceridemic patients on PAI-1 antigen release by endothelial cells (-•-) and HepG2 cells (-○-).

concomitant elevation in plasma of both t-PA and PAI-1. Thus one can speculate that reduction in fibrinolytic activity is not a primary phenomenon but is consequent to the prolonged enhancement in the synthesis of both t-PA and PAI-1. Indeed, as previously described, t-PA and PAI-1 are currently considered predictive of future vascular events. Interestingly, t-PA antigen levels have been proposed to be an independent marker of stroke, whereas for myocardial infarction the association between t-PA antigen and risk has been explained by the existence of other known risk factors. As for PAI-1 increment, the *in vitro* data obtained with VLDL and endothelial or HepG2 cells, indicate that the biosynthesis of this protein is directly regulated by this lipoprotein fraction. The mechanism responsible for this regulation remains to be elucidated.

References

1. Bachman F. In: Colman RW, Hirsh J, Marder VJ, Salzman EW, editors. Haemostasis and thrombosis: Basic principles and clinical practice. Philadelphia: JB Lippincott Company, 1994;1592-1622.
2. Bachman F, Sprengers ED, Kluft C. Plasminogen activator inhibitors. Blood 1987; 69:381-87.
3. Diéval J, Nguyen G, Gross S, Delobel J, Kruithof EKO. A lifelong bleeding disorder associated with a deficiency of plasminogen activator inhibitor type 1. Blood 1991;77:528-32.
4. Juhan-Vague I, Alessi MC. Plasminogen activator inhibitor 1 and athero-thrombosis. Thromb Haemost 1993;70:138-41.

5.   Hamsten A, Walldius G, Szamosi A, Blomback M, de Faire U, Dahlen G, Landou C, Wiman B. Plasminogen activator inhibitor in plasma: Risk factor for recurrent myocardial infarction. Lancet 1987;2:3-9.

6.   Laakso M. The possible pathophysiology of insulin resistance syndrome. Cardiovascular Risk Factors 1993;3:55-66.

7.   Juhan-Vague I, Alessi MC, Vague P. Increased plasma plasminogen activator inhibitor 1 levels. A possible link between insulin resistance and atherothrombosis. Diabetologia 1991;34:457-62.

8.   Andersen P, Arnesen H, Hjerman I. Hyperlipoproteinaemia and reduced fibrinolytic activity in healthy coronary high-risk men. Acta Med Scand 1981; 209:199-202.

9.   Mehta J, Metha P, Lawson D, Saldeen T. Plasma tissue plasminogen activator inhibitor levels in coronary artery disease. J Am Coll Cardiol 1987;9:263-268.

10.   Aznar J, Estelles A, Tormo G, Sapena P, Tormo V, Blanch S, Espana S. Plasminogen activator inhibitor activity and other fibrinolytic variables in patients with coronary artery disease. Br Heart J 1988;59:535-41.

11.   Mussoni L, Mannucci L, Sirtori M, Camera M, Maderna P, Sironi L, Tremoli E. Hypertriglyceridemia and regulation of fibrinolytic activity. Arterioscler Thromb 1991;12:19-27.

12.   Austin MA. Plasma triglyceride as a risk factor for coronary heart disease. The epidemiological evidence beyond. Am J Epidemiol 1989;129:249-259.

13.   Castelli WP. Epidemiology of triglycerides: A view from Framingham. Am J Cardiol 1992;70:3H-9H.

14.   Assman G, Shulte H. Role of triglycerides in coronary artery disease: Lessons from the prospective cardiovascular Munster study. Am J Cardiol 1992;70:10H-13H.

15.   Tremoli E. Triglycerides and fibrinolytic activity. Cardiovascular Risk Factors 1993;3:333-335.

16.   Ridker PM, Vaughan DE, Stampfer MK, Manson JE, Hennekens CH. Endogenous tissue-type plasminogen activator and risk of myocardial infarction. Lancet 1993;341:1165-1168.

17.   Dawson S, Henney A. The status of PAI-1 as a risk factor for arterial venous thrombotic disease: A review. Atherosclerosis 1992;95:105-17.

18.   Humphries S, Them A, Wiman B, Hamsten A, Nilsson J. Secretion of plasminogen activator inhibitor 1 from cultured human umbilical vein endothelial cells is induced by very low density lipoprotein. Arteriosclerosis 1990;10:1067-73.

19.   Loskutoff DJ. Regulation of PAI-1 gene expression. Fibrinolysis 1991;5:197-206.

20.   Stiko-Rahm AB, Wiman A, Hamsten A, Nilsson J. Secretion of plasminogen activator inhibitor 1 from cultured human umbilical vein endothelial cells is induced by very low density lipoprotein. Arteriosclerosis 1990;10:1067-1073.

21.   Mussoni L, Sironi L, Prati L, Baldassarre D, Camera M, Tremoli E. Plasminogen activator inhibitor type 1 mRNA expression is increased by triglyceride rich lipoproteins in human hepatoma cells. Thromb Haemost 1993;69:30.

APOLIPOPROTEIN E AND ALZHEIMER'S DISEASE

Guido Franceschini, Laura Calabresi, Cesare R. Sirtori, Giovanni B. Frisoni,
Cristina Geroldi, Angelo Bianchetti, Marco Trabucchi, Stefano Govoni.
Center E. Grossi Paoletti, Institute of Pharmacological Sciences
University of Milan and
Alzheimer's Disease Unit
Istituto S. Cuore-FBF and Geriatric Research Group
Brescia
ITALY

Alzheimer's disease (AD) accounts for half of all cases of senile dementia. Its prevalence increases steeply with age, from less than 1% at age 65 to 15% in the ninth decade [1]. Until last year, advances in understanding the genetics of the disease had been confined to rare familial AD, which accounts for less than 1% of all cases of AD. Recent work has shown a significant association between AD and apolipoprotein E (apoE) [2,3]. We report here on a similar association of apoE with other forms of dementia, and discuss possible mechanisms behind this association.

Apolipoprotein E

ApoE is a major protein component of human plasma lipoproteins, being a constituent of liver-synthesized very low density lipoproteins (VLDL), and of a subclass of high density lipoproteins (HDL) [4]. ApoE readily redistributes among plasma lipoproteins, by this way becoming a major component of chylomicron remnants, which transport dietary lipids to the liver. A major physiological role of apoE is to function as a ligand for lipoprotein receptors. At least two different receptors, the low density lipoprotein (LDL) receptor and the LDL-receptor related protein (LRP), can recognize apoE [4,5]. Lipoprotein binding to receptors initiates cellular uptake and degradation of the lipoproteins, the internalized cholesterol becoming a major regulatory factor of cell cholesterol homeostasis. Once enriched in cholesterol, cells can deplete themselves of excess cholesterol by secretion of apoE-containing lipoproteins [6], while lipid-free apoE in the extracellular space generates pre- HDL particles, which act as acceptors of cell cholesterol [7].

In addition to its primary function in the redistribution of lipids among tissues, apoE has a major role in neural physiology. The brain has the highest amount of apoE mRNA among extrahepatic tissues, apoE mRNA being distributed throughout all brain regions [8]. ApoE is synthesized and secreted mainly by astrocytes and oligodendrocytes of the central

A.M. Gotto et al. (eds), Multiple Risk Factors in Cardiovascular Disease, 385-391.

ApoE is synthesized and secreted mainly by astrocytes and oligodendrocytes of the central nervous system (CNS), and its synthesis is increased several fold following nerve injury [9]. The apoE present extracellularly between nerve fibers is either associated with lipids, forming cholesterol- and phospholipid-rich particles, or in a lipid-free form. The observation of a receptor-dependent uptake of apoE-containing lipoproteins by growth cones of neuronal cells [10] suggested a major role for apoE in redistributing lipids between different cells, and modulating cholesterol homeostasis, within the brain. A model was thus proposed, by which apoE helps in sequestrating lipids from degenerating axons; these are then reutilized for nerve regeneration [11]. This property does not seem to be unique to apoE, since nerve regeneration occurs at a normal rate in apoE-deficient mice [12]. Indeed, the synthesis of apoD is also increased following nerve injury, while apoA-I and apoA-IV can filtrate from plasma into the cerebrospinal fluid, thus substituting for apoE in its function within the nervous system [13].

Human apoE is a single polypeptide chain of 299 residues (Mr=34,200). In humans, the gene for apoE, which has been mapped on chromosome 19q13.2 [14], is polymorphic, with three common alleles designated ε2, ε3, and ε4. The relative frequencies of the apoE alleles are quite similar among Caucasian populations (ε2=0.08, ε3=0.77, and ε4= 0.15), while significant variations in allele frequencies were observed in Amerindians, Chinese, and Japanese populations [15]. The apoE alleles code for three major apoE isoforms, designated E2, E3, and E4, respectively. The ancestral form of the protein is apoE3, and this has cysteine at residue 112 and arginine at residue 158, whereas apoE4 and apoE2 have arginine and cysteine, respectively, at both sites [16]. This polymorphism results in six apoE phenotypes; three homozygous, i.e. E4/4, E3/3, and E2/2, and three heterozygous, E3/4, E2/3, and E2/4 (Figure 1).

The apoE2 isoform has lower affinity for the LDL receptor than has either apoE3 or apoE4 [4]. Although both ApoE3 and apoE4 bind with equal effectiveness to the LDL receptor, they associate preferentially with different classes of plasma lipoproteins: apoE4 with VLDL and apoE3 with HDL [17]. Indeed, apoE4-containing lipoproteins are cleared from the circulation at a faster rate than the ones with apoE3. The increased catabolism of apoE4-containing remnants would result in a down-regulation of LDL receptors in the liver, thus explaining the repeated observation of increased plasma total and LDL cholesterol levels in subjects carrying the ε4 allele [15]. If the same mechanisms operate also within the CNS, the ε 4/4 individuals should accumulate cholesterol-containing lipoproteins in the cerebrospinal fluid.

Similarly to other lipid-transport proteins, the apoE sequence contains several repeat units of 11 or 22 amino acids, presumed to exist in amphipathic α-helical conformation [18]. Lipid-free apoE readily self-associates in solution, likely because of hydrophobic interactions between amphipathic helices. Extensive characterization of apoE revealed that it contains two independently folded structural domains, each with different physical and functional properties [11]. The amino-terminal domain (residues 1-191) behaves like a globular soluble protein; it is responsible for the receptor-binding function of apoE and binds lipids only weakly. The three-dimensional structure of this domain has been characterized by x-ray crystallography and contains five α-helices, four of which are arranged in a four-helix bundle

4/4   3/3   2/2   3/4   2/3   2/4

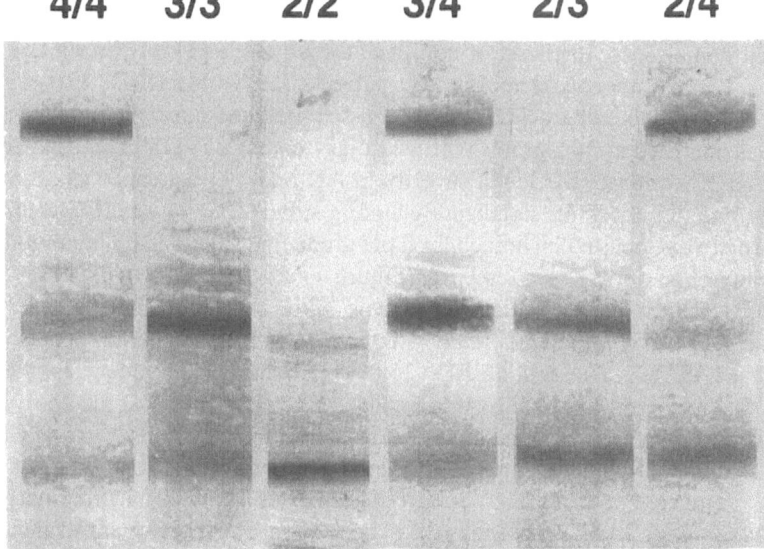

Figure 1. Phenotyping of apoE by isoelectric focusing and Western blotting. Plasma was delipidated and samples were applied to a polyacrylamide gel with an immobilized pH 4-6 gradient. After isoelectric focusing, proteins were transferred to a nitrocellulose membrane and immunodected by a sheep anti-apoE antibody.

[19]. The carboxyl-terminal domain (residues 216-299) is highly helical in structure, mediates the binding of apoE to lipids, but is not involved in apoE-receptor interactions. Although structurally and functionally distinct, the two domains interact with each other, conformational changes in one domain significantly altering the structural/functional properties of the other one.

ApoE and Alzheimer's Disease

Alzheimer's disease is an irreversible neurodegenerative disorder characterized neuropathologically by the presence of amyloid-containing senile plaques, neurofibrillary tangles, and loss of synapses and neurons [20]. Senile plaques are composed of aggregates of a 39-42 residue peptide, A4, which is derived from the amyloid precursor protein (APP) [21]. Numerous genetic factors have been identified, which underlie familial AD. Mutations in the APP have been found in a small percentage of families who have early-onset AD (EOAD) [22], while other cases of familial EOAD have been associated with an as yet unidentified gene on chromosome 14 [23]. Familial late-onset AD (LOAD) has been reported to be associated with a locus on chromosome 19 [24]. No specific genetic factors have been instead identified in sporadic AD.

The most recent breakthrough in AD research was the discovery of an increased frequency of the ε4 allele of apoE in familial LOAD [2], an earlier onset of the disease being associated with an increased number of copies of the ε4 allele [3]. Following this line, we determined the apoE phenotype in 157 AD patients (19 with EOAD, 33 with familial LOAD, and 104 with sporadic LOAD) and 70 age-sex matched controls. In addition, apoE phenotype was analyzed in 34 patients with vascular dementia (VD), diagnosed according to NINDS-AIREN criteria. Dementia severity in AD and VD patients was of moderate-severe degree, and did not differ significantly among subgroups. The apoE phenotype was assessed by isoelectric focusing on immobilized pH gradients, followed by immunodetection with a polyclonal anti-apoE sheep antibody (Figure 1).

ApoE3/3 was the most frequent phenotype among control subjects (75.7%), VD (50.0%), and AD (43.9%) patients. Only 3 controls were E4/4 homozygotes (4.3%), compared to 12 VD (31.6%), and 42 AD (26.8%) patients. The frequencies of the apoE alleles in the examined groups are shown in Table 1. The distribution of the apoE alleles in elderly controls was remarkably similar to that reported for control Italian and Caucasian populations. A four-fold higher frequency of the ε4 allele was found in the whole series of AD patients compared to controls. Subgroup analysis showed that the increased ε4 frequency is confined to LOAD patients, while those with EOAD have a prevalence of the ε4 allele not significantly different from that of controls. The E4/4 homozygotes and the E4/- heterozygotes had a 14-fold and 5.5.-fold higher risk of developing AD, respectively, than -/- individuals. A similarly elevated prevalence of the ε4 allele was also found in VD patients (Table 1). Among these, E4/E4 homozygotes had a 10-fold higher risk of VD, while in heterozygotes the relative risk did not differ significantly from -/- subjects (OR=2.5).

The present data confirm the previously reported association of the ε4 allele of apoE with sporadic and familial LOAD [1,2,25]. The relatively normal frequency of the ε4 allele in EOAD is also in accordance with previous findings, and suggests that, when a strong genetic factor is present, the ε4 allele loses its predisposing effect. Taken together, the epidemiological studies may well support the concept that the ε4 allele plays an important role in AD and it probably represents a major risk factor for the disease [26].

A risk factor must have a biologically plausible relation to disease in order to be etiologic. Antibodies against apoE decorate senile plaques [27], which are the hallmark of AD, and apoE co-localizes with amyloid deposits in individuals with AD [28]. This last finding does not seem specific for AD, since apoE is also found in the amyloid lesions of patients with other neurological diseases, such as Creutzfeldt-Jacob disease [29]. Moreover, apoE is only one of the several proteins that consistently localize with amyloid fibrils [21]. In vitro, apoE4 binds with more avidity than apoE3 to the A4 peptide, the site of interaction with A4 having been identified in the carboxyl-terminal domain of apoE [11]. Although it is curious that an amino acid change in the amino-terminal domain alters the binding of the carboxyl-terminal portion of apoE to A4, this finding is a further demonstration of the interaction of the two major apoE domains in determining the structural/functional properties of the whole apoE. It has also been suggested that the risk factor for AD is not apoE4, but the lack of a protective factor, i.e. apoE2 or apoE3, that increases the risk of developing AD [30]. Indeed, additional in vitro studies demonstrate that apoE3, but not

Table 1. ApoE Allele Frequencies in the Examined Subjects

Groups	alleles	ε2	ε3	ε4
Elderly controls	140	.07 ± .02	.84 ± .03	.09 ± .02
Alzheimer's Disease	314	.02 ± .01	.57 ± .03	.41 ± .03
EOAD	38	.00 ± .00	.84 ± .06	.16 ± .06
Familial LOAD	66	.00 ± .00	.48 ± .06	.52 ± .06
Sporadic LOAD	208	.03 ± .01	.54 ± .03	.42 ± .03
Vascular Dementia	68	.01 ± .01	.57 ± .06	.41 ± .06

Values represent frequencies ± SEM

apoE4, binds to Tau protein, thus preventing Tau hyperphosphorylation and the development of neurofibrillary tangles [11]. However, binding to Tau *in vivo* would require apoE, which is normally secreted through the Golgi system, to be present in the cytoplasmic compartment of the cell.

The observation of a similarly increased frequency of the ε4 allele of apoE in patients with VD, a neurodegenerative disorder with different etiopathogenetic mechanisms and clinical course, also argues against a specific association of the ε4 allele with AD. The impact of the apoE alleles on VD might be explained by the consistent association between the individual apoE genotype and plasma total and LDL cholesterol levels [15], individuals with the 2/2 genotype having the lowest, while individuals carrying the ε4 allele have the highest average level. This association is believed to explain the higher risk for coronary heart disease and stroke in E4/E4 subjects [15], and may also explain the high risk of VD found in the present study. However, an alternative and unifying explanation cannot be excluded [31]. Because of the major role of apoE in the control of repair processes following nerve regeneration [11], one can hypothesize that the individual apoE genotype might affect the efficiency of these processes, independently of the nature of injury, i.e., primary degenerative or vascular. Moreover, since apoE is the major cholesterol-carrying protein in the cerebrospinal fluid, and an adequate cholesterol content in cell membranes is required for several fundamental cell functions, it can be speculated that alterations of cell cholesterol homeostasis, possibly related to the apoE genotype, are involved in neurological diseases. Indeed, the cell membranes isolated from the cortical gray matter of AD patients contain 30% less cholesterol than those from age-sex matched controls [32]. This difference results in a significant reduction of the lipid bilayer width and fluidity, which, in turn, may strongly affect both endogenous (neurotransmitter, hormones, second messengers) and exogenous (drugs) regulation of brain cell function. The demonstration of a genetic link between apoE phenotype, cell cholesterol homeostasis, and neurodegeneration would also open new strategies for the treatment of AD and other neurodegenerative disorders, aimed at controlling brain cholesterol metabolism.

References

1. Skoog I, Nilsson L, Palmertz B, Andreasson LA, Svanborg A. A population based study of senile dementia in 85 year olds. N Engl J Med 1993;328:153-158.
2. Strittmatter WJ, Saunders AM, Schmechel D, et al. Apolipoprotein E: high-avidity binding to -amyloid and increased frequency of type 4 allele in late-onset familial Alzheimer disease. Proc Natl Acad Sci USA 1993;90:1977-1981.
3. Corder EH, Saunders AM, Strittmatter WJ, et al. Gene dose of apolipoprotein E type 4 allele and the risk of Alzheimer's disease in late onset families. Science 1993;261:921-923.
4. Mahley RW. Apolipoprotein E: Cholesterol transport protein with expanding role in cell biology. Science 1988;240:622-630.
5. Kowal RC, Herz J, Weisgraber KH, Mahley RW, Brown MS, Goldstein JL. Opposing effects of apolipoprotein E and C on lipoprotein binding to low density lipoprotein receptor-related protein. J Biol Chem 1990;265:10771-10779.
6. Huang Y, vonEckardstein A, Wu S, Maeda N, Assmann G. A plasma lipoprotein containing only apolipoprotein E and with mobility on electrophoresis releases cholesterol from cells. Proc Natl Acad Sci USA 1994;91:1834-1838.
7. Hara H, Yokoyama S. Role of apolipoproteins in cholesterol efflux from macrophages to lipid microemulsion: proposal of a putative model for the pre- high-density lipoprotein pathway. Biochemistry 1992;31:2040-2046.
8. Elshourbagy NA, Liao WS, Mahley RW, Taylor JM. Apolipoprotein E mRNA is abundant in the brain and adrenals, as well as in the liver, and is present in other peripheral tissues of rats and marmosets. Proc Natl Acad Sci USA 1985;82:203-207.
9. Snipes GJ, McGuire CB, Norden JJ, Freeman JA. Nerve injury stimulates the secretion of apolipoprotein E by nonneuronal cells. Proc Natl Acad Sci USA 1986;83:1130-1134.
10. Ignatius MJ, Shooter EM, Pitas RE, Mahley RW. Lipoprotein uptake by neuronal growth cones *in vitro*. Science 1987;236:959-962.
11. Weisgraber KH, Roses AD, Strittmatter WJ. The role of apolipoprotein E in the nervous system. Curr Opin Lipidol 1994;5:110-116.
12. Popko B, Goodrum JF, Bouldin TW, Zhang SH, Maeda N. Nerve regeneration occurs in the absence of apolipoprotein E in mice. J Neurochem 1993;60:1155-1158.
13. Boyles JK, Notterpek LM, Anderson LJ. Accumulation of apolipoproteins in the regenerating and remyelinating mammalian peripheral nerve. J Biol Chem 1990;265:17805-17815.
14. Olaisen B, Teisberg P, Gedde-Dahl T. The locus for apolipoprotein E (apoE) is linked to the complement component C3(C3) locus on chromosome 19 in man. Hum Genet 1982;62:233-236.
15. Davignon J, Gregg RE, Sing CF. Apolipoprotein E polymorphism and atherosclerosis.

Arteriosclerosis 1988;8:1-21.

16. Weisgraber KH, Rall SC, Mahley RW. Human E apoprotein heterogeneity: cysteine-arginine interchanges in the amino acid sequence of the apo-E isoforms. 1981;256:9077-9083.

17. Weisgraber KH. Apolipoprotein E distribution among human plasma lipoproteins: role of the cysteine-arginine interchange at residue 112. J Lipid Res 1990;31:1503-1511.

18. Segrest JP, Jones MK, De Loof H, Brouillette CG, Venkatachalapathi YV, Ananthramaiah GM. The amphipathic helix in the exchangeable apolipoproteins: a review of secondary structure and function. J Lipid Res 1992;33:141-166.

19. Wilson C, Wardell MR, Weisgraber KH, Mahley RW, Agard DA. Three-dimensional structure of the LDL receptor-binding domain of human apolipoprotein E. Science 1991;252:1817-1822.

20. Selkoe DJ. The molecular pathology of Alzheimer's disease. Neuron 1991;6:487-498.

21. Fraser PE, Lévesque L, McLachlan DR. Biochemistry of Alzheimer's disease amyloid plaques. Clin Biochem 1993;26:339-349.

22. Goate A, Chartier-Harlin M-C, Mullan M, et al. Segregation of a missense mutation in the amyloid precursor protein gene with familial Alzheimer's disease. Nature 1991;349:704-706.

23. Schellenberg GD, Bird TD, Wijsman EM, et al. Genetic linkage evidence for a familial Alzheimer's disease locus on chromosome 14. Science 1992;258:668-671.

24. Pericak-Vance MA, Bebout JL, Gaskell PC, et al. Linkage studies in familial Alzheimer disease: evidence for chromosome 19 linkage. Am J Hum Genet 1991;48:1034-1050.

25. Saunders AM, Strittmatter WJ, Schmechel D, et al. Association of apolipoprotein E allele 4 with late-onset familial and sporadic Alzheimer's disease. Neurology 1993;43:1467-1472.

26. Scott J. Apolipoprotein E and Alzheimer's disease. Lancet 1993;342:696.

27. Wisniewski T, Frangione B. Apolipoprotein E: a pathological chaperone protein in patients with cerebral and systemic amyloid. Neurosci Lett 1992;135:235-238.

28. Rebeck GW, Reiter JS, Strickland DK, Hyman BT. Apolipoprotein E in sporadic Alzheimer's disease: allelic variation and receptor interactions. Neuron 1993;11:575-580.

29. Nmba Y, Tomonaga M, Kawasaki H, Otomo E, Ikeda K. Apolipoprotein E immunoreactivity in cerebral amyloid deposits and neurofibrillary tangles in Alzheimer's disease and kuru plaque amyloid in Creutzfeldt-Jacob disease. Brain Res 1991;541:163-166.

30. Talbot C, Lendon C, Craddock N, Shears S, Morris JC, Goate A. Protection against Alzheimer' s disease with apoE 2. Lancet 1994;343:1432-33.

31. Frisoni GB, Bianchetti A, Govoni S, et al. Association of apolipoprotein E E4 with vascular dementia. JAMA 1994;271:1317.

32. Mason RP, Shoemaker WI, Shaienko L, Chambers TE, Herbette LG. Evidence for changes in the Alzheimer's disease brain cortical membrane structure mediated by cholesterol. Neurobiol Aging 1992;13:413-419.

APOLIPOPROTEIN AI: A NATURAL KIDNEY-PROTECTIVE AGENT?

James R. Paterniti, Jr., Bryan F. Burkey, Dennis France, Hongxing Wong*, Xiaowen Ma, Barbara Brand, Colleen Abuhani, Margaret R. Diffenderfer*, Julian B. Marsh*, and Edward A. Fisher*
Department of Atherosclerosis and Vascular Biology
Preclinical Research
Sandoz Research Institute
Sandoz Pharmaceuticals Corporation
East Hanover, NJ 07936
and
*Biochemistry Department
Medical College of Pennsylvania
Philadelphia, PA 19129
USA

Introduction

Hyperlipoproteinemia is a common feature of nephrotic syndrome and other glomerular diseases in both humans and experimental animals [1-3]. In both animals and humans, isolated hyperlipoproteinemia does not usually produce significant kidney damage. However, when hypertension, diabetes, or preexisting kidney damage has been established, hyperlipoproteinemia becomes an important determinant of disease progression, and this constellation of risk factors contributes to heart disease seen in patients with renal disease [4-6].

Renal disease and coronary artery disease share not only common risk factors, but many cellular and molecular events as well [for reviews see 2,7]. In humans, elevated high density lipoprotein (HDL) cholesterol and apolipoprotein (apo) AI levels are clearly associated with a decreased risk of coronary artery disease. In mice, the transgenic overexpression of human apo AI markedly decreased diet-induced aortic fatty streak lesions, that are thought to model early atherosclerotic disease [8].

We have undertaken a series of studies in human apo AI transgenic rats to examine the consequences of elevating apo AI and HDL cholesterol pools on early events in experimental nephrosis. In this report, we demonstrate that hepatic overexpression of human apo AI in rats suppresses the edema and hyperlipoproteinemia associated with experimental nephrosis, providing a model in which to examine other effects of apo AI on

393

A.M. Gotto et al. (eds), Multiple Risk Factors in Cardiovascular Disease, 393-401.
© 1995 *Kluwer Academic Publishers and Fondazione Giovanni Lorenzini.*

experimental renal disease.

Materials and Methods

INDUCTION OF EXPERIMENTAL NEPHROSIS

The effect of overexpression of human apo AI on lipid and lipoprotein metabolism was assessed in three groups of male Sprague Dawley rats (n = 10 per group), 7 to 11 weeks of age: (low-TrG) low-expressing human apo AI transgenic rats (16.0 ± 4.7 mg/dL human apo AI); (high-TrG) high-expressing human apo AI transgenic rats (284.2 ± 113.4 mg/dL human apo AI); and (non-TrG) non-transgenic littermates (see Table 1). A detailed description of these transgenic animals has been published [9]. Experimental nephrosis was induced in one-half of the rats by bolus intraperitoneal injections of puromycin aminonucleoside (PAN) at 65 mg/kg body weight in saline, on two consecutive days. All other animals were injected with equivalent volumes of saline. Within eight days, the response to PAN treatment was readily apparent as peritoneal edema, which could be graded over a range of slight to severe. Animals were sacrificed eight days after the initial injection of PAN or saline. Whole blood for serum isolation and lipoprotein analysis and liver for mRNA measurements were collected at the time of sacrifice. All animal studies were performed under a protocol approved by the Animal Care Committee of the Medical College of Pennsylvania and the Sandoz Animal Care and Use Committee.

QUANTITATION OF SERUM APO AI

Levels of human and rat apo AI were determined by separate competition ELISAs. Standard curves were made by serial dilution of human or rat serum containing known amounts of apo AI. The human apo AI assay was linear over the range of 1.5 - 24 μg apo AI per well. The rat apo AI assay was linear in the range of 0.9 - 15 μg of apo AI per well.

NONREDUCING SDS PAGE ANALYSIS OF SERUM PROTEINS

Rat serum or urine (3 μL) was mixed into Tris-SDS sample solubilization buffer to yield a 50 μL final volume. Samples were heat denatured at 80° C for 15 minutes, and loaded on an 11% SDS polyacrylamide gel. Proteins, resolved by electrophoresis at 75V for 6 hours, were visualized by staining with Coomassie Brilliant Blue.

ISOLATION AND ANALYSIS OF HEPATIC RNA

Total RNA was isolated from rat liver by a modified guanidine salt-based procedure previously described [10]. Rat and human apo AI mRNA levels were determined by Northern blot hybridization. The intensity of the hybridization signal was normalized to elongation factor 1 α, as described by Lu and Werner [11], and expressed as relative to this control.

Values are given as the mean +/- standard error of the mean. Statistical differences between treatment groups were sought by using Student's T test.

Results

EFFECT OF OVEREXPRESSION OF HUMAN APO AI ON PAN-INDUCED EDEMA

Eight days following the initial injection, hypoalbuminemia and albuminuria were seen in all three PAN-injected groups when proteins were resolved by nonreducing SDS PAGE. All rats receiving PAN displayed peritoneal edema while their saline-treated counterparts appeared normal. The edema in all high-TrG nephrotic rats was judged slight, whereas all nephrotic low-TrG and non-TrG animals showed severe edema.

RAT AND HUMAN APO AI PROTEIN AND mRNA LEVELS

As previously reported [12,13], total apo AI increased following the induction of nephrosis (Table 1). However, a more pronounced total apo AI elevation occurred in low-TrG and especially in high-TrG nephrotic rats, where apo AI replaced albumin as the major serum protein. The increase in total apo AI in the low-TrG and high-TrG nephrotic rats was primarily due to increased human apo AI levels. Rat apo AI actually decreased in the nephrotic high-TrG group.

We have shown previously that the genetic construct used to produce low-TrG and high-TrG rats drove the expression of human apo AI in the liver, but not in the intestine [9]. Hepatic rat (not shown) and human apo AI mRNA levels (Table 1) were measured by Northern blot hybridization in control and nephrotic rats. Similar to previous reports [14,15], the induction of experimental nephrosis increased the steady state levels of rat apo AI mRNA by 4- to 7-fold over the controls. By contrast, human apo AI mRNA levels were elevated 21-fold in low-TrG rats and 65-fold in high-TrG rats. These data demonstrate that rat and human apo AI mRNA and protein were differentially elevated by the induction of experimental nephrosis.

EFFECTS OF HUMAN APO AI ON PAN-INDUCED HYPERLIPOPROTEINEMIA

Consistent with the model [3], marked elevation of total cholesterol (+460%), phospholipid (+212%)(not shown), and triglyceride (+627%) occurred in non-TrG rats following the induction of experimental nephrosis. The degree of lipid elevation in nephrotic non-TrG rats and nephrotic low-TrG rats was virtually identical (Table 1).

In control high-TrG rats, expression of human apo AI raised circulating levels of cholesterol 51.2% and phospholipid 66.5% (not shown) compared with non-TrG rats, while triglycerides were unchanged (Table 1). The increased serum levels of cholesterol and phospholipid in high-TrG rats reflected expansion of the HDL pool (see below) and were consistent with our previous report [9]. By contrast, with non-TrG and low-TrG rats, the induction of experimental nephrosis in high-TrG animals produced a modest elevation

Table 1. Effect of human apo AI overexpression on levels of rat and human apo AI protein, human apo AI mRNA, cholesterol, and triglyceride in serum taken from rats eight days after PAN-(nephrotic) or saline-(control) injections. The change from the control in each group is expressed as the ratio; N/C (nephrotic/control). When two groups are compared by Student's T-test, (a) indicates $p < 0.001$, (b) indicates $p < 0.01$, and (c) indicates no significant difference.

	Serum Apolipoprotein AI Protein*, mRNA (units ±SEM), and Lipid Levels* (*mg/dL ± SEM)				
	Rat Apo AI Protein	Human Apo AI Protein	Human Apo AI mRNA	Cholesterol	Triglyceride
non-TrG					
control	75.2 ± 10.0	-	-	116.9 ± 5.0	78.3 ± 11.5
nephrotic	162.4 ± 26.6	-	-	654.9 ± 52.3	568.9 ± 49.1
N/C	2.16 (b)			5.6 (a)	7.27 (a)
low-TrG					
control	81.2 ± 10.4	16.0 ± 4.7	0.15 ± 0.06	110.6 ± 7.2	70.0 ± 11.4
nephrotic	127.4 ± 9.1	330.8 ± 51.7	3.16 ± 0.27	569.3 ± 71.0	505.7 ± 54.8
N/C	1.57 (b)	20.68 (b)	21.1	5.15 (a)	7.22 (a)
high-TrG					
control	71.8 ± 17.7	284.2 ± 113.4	1.19 ± 0.80	194.5 ± 35.6	70.1 ± 10.7
nephrotic	38.3 ± 5.9	1307.5 ± 186.0	77.03 ±	296.1 ± 41.4	223.7 ± 68.9
N/C	0.53 (c)	4.60 (b)	64.7	1.52 (c)	3.19 (c)

(+52%) of total serum cholesterol and a decrease in phospholipid levels. Total serum triglyceride increased 219% (control: 70.1 mg/dL versus nephrotic: 223.7 mg/dL). However, this elevation was less than one-half of the response of nephrotic non-TrG or low-TrG rats, and was not statistically significant ($p = 0.092$). Thus, overexpression of human apo AI in the high-TrG rats suppressed the hyperlipoproteinemia associated with experimental nephrosis.

To obtain lipoprotein profiles, serum samples were fractionated by FPLC gel permeation chomatography and lipoprotein peaks determined by elution volume and cholesterol content. Induction of experimental nephrosis increased all lipoprotein classes. Lipoprotein profiles of low-TrG control and nephrotic rats were virtually identical to the respective profiles of non-TrG rats (data not shown). Overexpression of human apo AI in high-TrG control rats expanded the HDL cholesterol pool (Figures 1A and 1B). While some increase in non-HDL cholesterol fractions occurred in high-TrG rats with experimental nephrosis, hyperbetalipoproteinemia was suppressed (compare Figures 1A and 1B). HDL cholesterol levels in high-TrG rats were unchanged (142.4 ± 33.4 mg/dL in controls versus 140.5 ± 21.2 mg/dL in nephrotics). However, HDL particles isolated from high-TrG nephrotic animals tended to elute ahead of control HDL on FPLC, indicating an increased particle size.

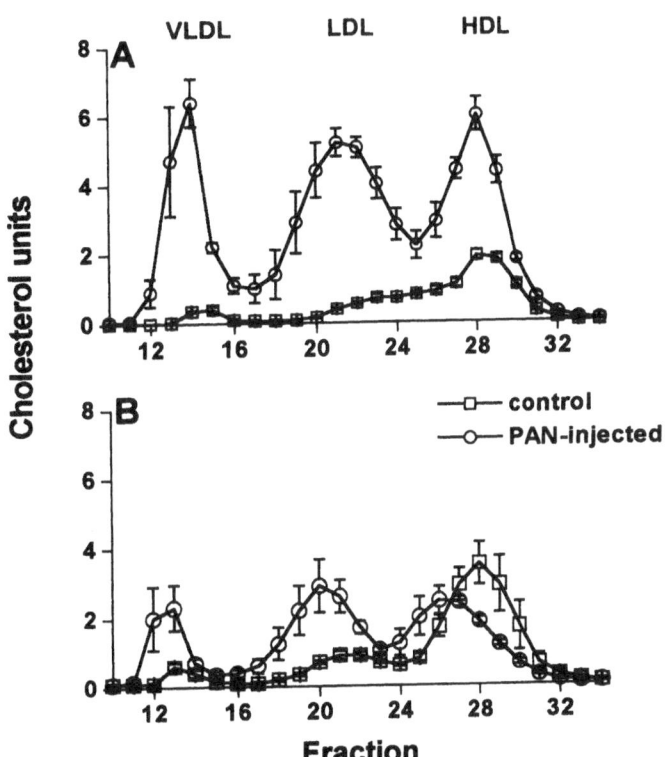

Figure 1. Analysis of lipoprotein profiles from low-TrG (A) and high-TrG (B) rat sera by gel filtration chromatography. Individual rat serum samples were fractionated by FPLC over a Superose 6 sizing column into 40 fractions. Total cholesterol from each fraction was assessed enzymatically, the absorbance at 490 nm was assigned whole number-values using a linear relation and the profiles plotted. Open squares (□) are saline-injected control rats and open circles (○) are PAN-injected nephrotic rats. Each profile is the mean of five individual profiles, with error bars representing the standard error of the mean. The elution position of human VLDL, LDL, and HDL is indicated at the top of profile A.

Discussion

EFFECTS OF OVEREXPRESSION OF HUMAN APO AI ON EDEMA IN EXPERIMENTAL NEPHROSIS

The mechanisms which drive fluid volume expansion in the nephrotic syndrome have been extensively studied [16]. Intravenous administration of albumin or other plasma expander macromolecules will decrease edema, at least temporarily [17]. Earlier work in humans with nephrotic syndrome has shown that plasma lipid levels will also decline when plasma expanders are given [18].

In the present study, overexpression of human apo AI did not prevent the induction of experimental nephrosis. Hypoalbuminemia and albuminuria (not shown) were qualitatively similar in non-TrG and both TrG lines. However, we demonstrate for the first time that genetic overproduction of a serum protein suppresses the edema and hyperlipoproteinemia associated with experimental nephrosis. The obvious decrease in visible ascites in high-TrG animals can be explained by the high serum levels of apo AI. In spite of urinary losses of both lipid-poor (free) apo AI and HDL [19], hepatic apo AI production was so overwhelming that serum apo AI levels reached 1346 mg/dL. We argue that the oncotic pressure was raised sufficiently so that little edema was evident in these rats.

EFFECTS OF EXPERIMENTAL NEPHROSIS ON APO AI GENE EXPRESSION AND ON SERUM APO AI LEVELS

While the fundamental mechanisms underlying the hepatic response to proteinuria are unknown at present, studies have shown increased steady-state levels of mRNA for several proteins [14]. The levels of apo AI mRNA are elevated to a greater extent than other apolipoproteins upon the induction of nephrosis [14].

In this study, prior to PAN treatment, all lines expressed essentially identical levels of rat hepatic apo AI mRNA (not shown). As reported previously, these levels rose four to seven fold upon the induction of nephrosis [14,15]. PAN treatment amplified human apo AI mRNA levels 21-fold in low-TrG and 65-fold in high-TrG animals (Table 1). Thus, both transgenic lines showed a striking differential response of rat and human apo AI mRNA levels to experimental nephrosis. Prior studies in the PAN nephrosis model [14], the Heymann nephitis model, and the Nagase analbuminemic rat [20] indicated that elevation of rat hepatic apo AI mRNA was associated with an increased transcriptional rate for the apo AI gene. An intriguing possibility is that rat and human apo AI genes develop different transcriptional responses to experimental nephrosis. This hypothesis is currently under study.

A variety of evidence supports the view that apo AI mRNA levels are critical determinants of apo AI production rates [21,22]. Comparing the high-TrG control group with low-TrG rats, baseline serum apo AI levels were four fold higher, while the corresponding mRNA levels increased eight fold. This difference probably reflects variable urinary loss of apo AI.

Overexpression of the human apo AI gene did not appreciably affect the response to nephrosis of hepatic mRNA for rat apo AI, though the high-TrG rats had lower average levels than low- or non-TrG rats (not shown). The baseline serum levels of rat apo AI protein were not decreased in the high-TrG rats as had been observed by Rubin et al. [8] in apo AI transgenic mice. However, when high-TrG rats were rendered nephrotic, there was a significant (47%) decrease in serum rat apo AI level (Table 1). Based on changes in HDL discussed below, it is likely that the excess human apo AI displaced rat apo AI from HDL into a nonlipoprotein fraction. In this form, rat apo AI would be more readily lost to the urine and would not be expected to accumulate in plasma.

EFFECTS OF OVEREXPRESSION OF HUMAN APO AI ON LIPOPROTEINS IN NEPHROTIC RATS

Nephrotic non-TrG and low-TrG rats showed the expected increases in all lipoprotein classes, including triglyceride-rich fractions. However, the effects of high levels of apo AI on nephrotic hyperlipoproteinemia were dramatic. Triglyceride and non-HDL cholesterol levels showed only a modest increase, and the associated lipoprotein peaks were blunted (Table 1 and Figure 1B). HDL cholesterol levels were unchanged (Figure 1B).

Several mechanisms might explain the amelioration of nephrotic hyperlipoproteinemia by high levels of apo AI. The overproduction of apo AI reduced edema in high-TrG rats, probably by restoring oncotic pressure. Appel et al. have shown a significant inverse relationship between plasma cholesterol and oncotic pressure in patients with nephrotic syndrome [23]. This relationship probably reflects a regulatory influence of oncotic pressure on hepatic lipoprotein production [20]. Interestingly, an osmosensing signal transduction pathway has recently been described in yeast which regulates the activity of protein phosphorylation cascades [24]. Such a pathway could exist in liver to monitor oncotic pressure and control the production of albumin and other proteins. Another possibility is that high rates of apo AI production in liver interfere with the secretion of apo B-containing lipoproteins. For example, as suggested by Verkade et al. [25], the sequestration of available phospholipid by apo AI would prevent the packaging of apo B. Alternatively, high levels of apo AI may offset the clearance defect which contributes to elevated levels of triglyceride-rich lipoproteins [3]. Future studies will focus on defining the effects of apo AI overexpression on lipoprotein production and clearance rates.

The present study has focused on early events in the nephrotic syndrome produced by PAN. At later times, though the glomerular lesions are repaired and proteinuria declines, progression to a glomerulonephritis with inflammatory and proliferative changes has been described [26]. Rubin et al. [8] have demonstrated that overexpression of human apo AI in mice suppressed the formation of aortic macrophage foam cell lesions. We have presented preliminary evidence that apo AI overexpression in rats decreased smooth muscle cell accumulation in the aorta following balloon injury [27]. In view of the strong analogies between atherosclerosis and kidney disease, further studies of the effects of apo AI overexpression on experimental nephrosis appear warranted.

Acknowledgements

The authors wish to thank Dr. David Weinstein for his helpful comments. This work was supported by grants (to JBM and EAF) from the Howard Heinz Endowment and the National Institutes of Health (HL 22633).

References

1.   Keane WF, Kasiske BL, O'Donnell MP. Hyperlipoproteinemia and the progression of renal disease. Am J Clin Nutr 1988;47:157-160.
2.   Wheeler DC, Zachariah V, Moorhead JF. Hyperlipoproteinemia in nephrotic syndrome. Am J Nephrol 1989;9(Suppl.I):78-84.
3.   Marsh JB. Lipoprotein metabolism in experimental nephrosis. J Lipid Res 1984;25: 1619-1623.
4.   Bierman EL. Atherogenesis in diabetes. Arterioscler Thromb 1992;12:647-656.
5.   Charney DI, Walton DF, Cheung AK. Atherosclerosis in chronic renal failure. Curr Opin Nephrol Hypertens 1993;2:876-882.
6.   Bernard DB. Extrarenal complications of the nephrotic syndrome. Kidney Int 1988; 33:1184-1202.
7.   Diamond JR, Karnovsky MJ. Focal and segmental glomerulosclerosis: Analogies to atherosclerosis. Kidney Int 1988;33:917-924.
8.   Rubin EM, Krauss RM, Spangler EA, Verstuyft JG, Clift SM. Inhibition of early atherogenesis in transgenic mice by human apolipoprotein A-I. Nature (Lond) 1991; 353:265-267.
9.   Swanson ME, Hughes TE, St Denny I, et al. High level expression of human apolipoprotein AI in transgenic rats raises total serum high density lipoprotein cholesterol and lowers rat apolipoprotein AI. Transgenic Research 1992;1:142-147.
10.   Zolfaghari R, Chen X, Fisher EA. Simple method for extracting RNA from cultured cells and tissue with guanidine salts. Clin Chem 1993;39:1408-1411.
11.   Lu X, Werner D. The complete cDNA sequence of mouse elongation factor 1 alpha mRNA. Nucleic Acid Research 1989;17:442-445.
12.   Calandra S, Gherardi E, Fainaru M, Guaitani A, Bartosek I. Secretion of lipoproteins, apoprotein A-I and apoprotein E by isolated and perfused liver of rat with experimental nephrotic syndrome. Biochim Biophys Acta 1981;665:331-338.
13.   Marsh JB, Sparks CE. Lipoproteins in experimental nephrosis: plasma levels and composition. Metabolism 1979;28:455-465.
14.   Marshall JF, Apostolopoulos JJ, Brack CM, Howlett GJ. Regulation of apolipoprotein gene expression and plasma high-density lipoprotein composition in experimental nephrosis. Biochim Biophys Acta 1990;1042:271-279.
15.   Tarugi P, Calandra S, Chan L. Changes in apolipoprotein A-I mRNA levels in the liver of rats with experimental nephrotic syndrome. Biochim Biophys Acta 1986;868: 51-61.
16.   Skorecki KL, Nadler SP, Badr KF, Brenner BM. Renal and systemic manifestations of glomerular disease. In: Brenner BM and Rector FC, Jr. editors. The Kidney (vol. 1, 4th ed.). Philadelphia:W. B. Saunders, 1991:891-928.
17.   Allen JC, Baxter JH, Goodman HC. Effects of dextran, polyvinylpyrrolidone and gamma globulin on the hyperlipidemia of experimental nephrosis. J Clin Invest 1961;40:499-508.
18.   Baxter JH, Goodman HC, Allen JC. Effects of infusions of serum albumin on serum

lipids and lipoproteins in nephrosis. J Clin Invest 1961;40:490-498.

19.   Glass CK, Pittman RC, Keller GA, Steinberg D. Tissue sites of degradation of apoprotein A-I in the rat. J Biol Chem 1983;259:7161-7167.

20.   Sun X, Jones H Jr, Joles JA, Van Tol A, Kaysen GA. Apolipoprotein gene expression in analbuminemic rats and in rats with Heymann nephritis. Am J Physiol 1992;262: F755-F761.

21.   Sorci-Thomas M, Prack MM, Dashti N, Johnson F, Rudel LL, Williamson DL. Apolipoprotein (apo) A-I production and mRNA abundance explain plasma apo A-I and high density lipoprotein differences between two nonhuman primate species with high and low susceptibilities to diet-induced hypercholesterolemia. J Biol Chem 1988;263:5183-5189.

22.   Hughes TE, Nottage BF, Mone MD, Paterniti JR Jr. Apolipoprotein A-I production is controlled at the mRNA level in transgenic mice and three cell lines. Arteriosclerosis 1990;10:774a

23.   Appel GB, Blum CB, Chien S, Kunis CL, Appel AS. The hyperlipoproteinemia of the nephrotic syndrome: relation to plasma albumim concentration, oncotic pressure, and viscosity. N Engl J Med 1985;312:1544-1548.

24.   Brewster JL, de Valoir T, Dwyer ND, Winter E, Gustin MC. An osmosensing signal transduction pathway in yeast. Science 1993;259:1760-1763.

25.   Verkade HJ, Fast DG, Rusinol AE, Scraba DG, Vance DE. Impaired biosynthesis of phosphatidylcholine causes a decrease in the number of very low density lipoprotein particles in the Golgi but not in the endoplasmic reticulum of rat liver. J Biol Chem 1993;268:24990-24996.

26.   Diamond JR, Ding G, Frye J, Diamond I-P. Glomerular macrophages and the mesangial proliferative response in the experimental nephrotic syndrome. Am J Pathol 1992;141:887-894.

27.   Burkey BF, Vlasic N, France D, et al. Elevated apoprotein A-I (Apo A-I) pools in human apo A-I transgenic rats decreases aortic smooth muscle cell proliferation following balloon angioplasty. Circulation 1992;86:I-472.

NONINVASIVE EVALUATION OF ARTERIAL REACTIVITY IN PATIENTS WITH PREMATURE ONSET CORONARY HEART DISEASE

Paolo Rubba, Cecilia Sapio, Paolo Pauciullo, Arcangelo Iannuzzi, Gabriella Iannuzzo, Domenico Iorio*, Nicola Spampinato*, Mario Mancini
Institute of Internal Medicine and Diseases of Metabolism Medical School
*Chair of Cardiovascular Surgery
Federico II University
Naples
ITALY

Introduction

Many research studies have been devoted in the last ten years to the evaluation of whether improved cardiovascular prognosis, after appropriate treatment with lipid-lowering drugs, could derive from regression of atherosclerotic lesions [1,2]. The main conclusion of these studies was that it is indeed possible to enhance regression of stenoses due to atherosclerotic plaques by administering a long-term lipid-lowering treatment that lasts at least 2-3 years. However, the extent of improvement in lumen diameter was found to be extremely limited (2-3% increase in lumen diameter). This is in contrast to the observed clinical benefits in terms of cardiovascular morbidity and has led to great interest in alternative mechanisms able to increase lumen diameter, in order to explain the clinical advantage [2].

In particular, two lines of research have been developed, aimed at the evaluation of new hypothetical mechanisms of the circulatory response to lipid-lowering treatment:

1)   lipid-lowering treatment might stabilize pre-existing lesions, making them less prone to thrombosis [3,4].

2)   reduction in circulating lipids might improve the functional properties of the arterial wall, leading to an improved regulation of blood flow in different arterial districts [5].

Coronary heart disease has been associated with increased vascular tone, mainly because of an impairment of endothelium-dependent relaxation. This endothelial dysfunction occurs before any definite atherosclerotic lesion is demonstrated. In animal models, the correction of hypercholesterolemia has been associated with hemodynamic improvement [5].

The present report will summarize personal contributions to the demonstration and development of the hypothesis of improved flow response to lipid-lowering treatment in patients with premature coronary heart disease.

403

A.M. Gotto et al. (eds), Multiple Risk Factors in Cardiovascular Disease, 403-407.

Patients and Methods

Twenty individuals were selected from a group of 40 male patients with premature coronary heart disease (onset of ischemic symptoms before age 50), to be compared with 20 age- and gender-matched healthy controls; both patient and control groups did not include heavy smokers (>10 cigarettes/day).

Muscle blood flow at the lower limb was determined by strain gauge plethysmography (Janssen Scientific Instruments, Periflow), at rest and during a reactive hyperemia test [6].

Twenty-one of the 40 patients with coronary heart disease had plasma cholesterol ≥ 200 mg/dl. Nine of them were randomly allocated to a six-month treatment with a moderate fat-controlled diet. The remaining twelve patients were allocated to combined treatment with fat-controlled diet and gemfibrozil (Genlip, Lusofarmaco, 600 mg bid). After six months of treatment, patients were reevaluated with regard to resting and postischemic flow.

Serum lipids were determined by enzymatic methods. HDL cholesterol was measured after precipitation.

Results

At the beginning of the study, mean serum cholesterol was 213 mg/dl in cases and 198 mg/dl in controls (difference is not statistically significant). Mean triglyceride and HDL cholesterol were 132 and 48 versus 100 and 56 mg/dl, in cases and controls respectively (difference is not statistically significant). The mean age was 50 years in both cases and controls.

Resting blood flow (median) at baseline was 3.80 ml/min/100 g tissue in patients with coronary heart disease versus 3.59 in controls (difference is not statistically significant). Median arterial flow measured during reactive hyperemia after a 5-minute arterial occlusion produced by a pneumatic cuff, was 20.4 ml/min/100 g tissue in patients versus 25.0 in controls (p=0.034, Kruskall-Wallis).

After a six-month lipid-lowering treatment (Table 1), serum cholesterol was approximately reduced by 15% after diet+gemfibrozil (p < 0.01) and by less than 5% (not significant) after diet alone. HDL cholesterol was not modified in any of the two groups. Resting arterial flow increased significantly only after diet+gemfibrozil (by about 70%, p < 0.05, paired t test). Postischemic peak flow was unmodified.

Discussion

In severe hypercholesterolemia, after repeat low density lipoprotein apheresis, pronounced reductions were demonstrated in serum cholesterol, with a significant increase in resting and postischemic blood flow above the calf muscle [6]. An acute cholesterol reduction by low-density lipoprotein apheresis was thus associated with potentially useful hemodynamic effects. They were likely to reflect a restoration of the endothelium-mediated vasodilation, which had been inhibited by high concentrations of low-density lipoprotein. This effect

Table 1. Intervention Study on Plasma Lipids.

	Intervention Study on Plasma Lipids Effects on Plasma Lipids and Vascular Parameters in Patients with Total Serum Cholesterol ≥ 200 mg/dl at Time 0			
	Diet N=9		Diet+Gemfibrozil N=12	
	T-0	T-6	T-0	T-6
Age (years)	49.5 ± 6.4		51.2 ± 5.4	
BMI (Kg/m^2)	28.8 ± 2.4	27.4 ± 2.9*	28.8 ± 2.9	27.7 ± 2.5***
SBP (mm/Hg)	127 ± 17	133 ± 14	137 ± 18	132 ± 19
Chol (mg/dl)	245 ± 54	236 ± 41	225 ± 23	189 ± 27**
HDL (mg/dl)	49.8 ± 13.0	43.1 ± 8.5	48.8 ± 8.4	47.0 ± 7.6
TG (mg/dl)	152 ± 76	144 ± 56	151 ± 98	87 ± 46**
RF (ml/min/dl)	4.85 ± 3.37	6.38 ± 3.81	3.32 ± 1.52	5.44 ± 2.66*
PF (ml/min/dl)	22.7 ± 8.5	21.8 ± 7.4	22.1 ± 6.3	21.9 ± 9.0

*p < .05; **p < 0.01; ***p < 0.001; mean ± SD.
Comparisons between baseline and 6-month values.
BMI= body mass index; PAS= systolic blood pressure; Chol= total cholesterol; HDL= HDL cholesterol; TG=total triglycerides; RF= lower limbs, blood flow at rest; PF= lower limbs, postischemic blood flow.

might be important in conditions of acute ischemia or impaired blood flow caused by thrombosis, microembolism, or arterial spasm. Improved adaptability to impaired perfusion might preserve cerebral and muscle tissues, and probably the myocardium as well, from irreversible necrotic changes [7].

Further studies are needed however to confirm these data in more patients with common, milder forms of hypercholesterolemia and to extend the observations to a more prolonged follow-up. This research has helped demonstrate, *in vivo* and in man, the validity of the hypothesis of improved blood flow regulation after lipid-lowering treatment. The evidence collected in the present study is not conclusive, but nevertheless encourages and further indicates that lipid-lowering treatment is useful to prevent a disease of major impact on public health, such as atherosclerotic cardiovascular disease.

There is much published evidence [8-16] along this line of investigation, obtained in both experimental and *in vitro* models. However, data *in vivo* in man are relatively few

[17-21], because of the difficulties in developing ethically acceptable protocols to test these hypotheses. In this regard, another useful new message emerging from the present research is that noninvasive methods for vascular diagnosis and monitoring might solve the problem of performing repeat observations on cardiovascular patients with little discomfort and limited expenses.

References

1.   Oliver MF. Clinical perspective of trials of regression of coronary atherosclerosis. Cardiovasc Risk Factors 1992;2:234-238.
2.   Loscalzo J. Regression of coronary atherosclerosis. New Engl J Med 1990;323: 1337-1339.
3.   Fuster V, Badimon L, Badimon JJ, Chesebro JH. The pathogenesis of coronary artery disease and the acute coronary syndromes (First of two parts). N Engl J Med 1992;326:242-250.
4.   Fuster V, Badimon L, Badimon JJ, Chesebro JH. The pathogenesis of coronary artery disease and the acute coronary syndromes (Second of two parts). N Engl J Med 1992;326:310-318.
5.   Rubba P, Mancini M. Hypercholesterolemia, blood rheology and hemodynamics. Curr Opin Lipidol 1990;1:341-345.
6.   Rubba P, Iannuzzi A, Postiglione A, et al. Hemodynamic changes in the peripheral circulation after repeat low density lipoprotein apheresis in familial hypercholesterol-emia. Circulation 1990;81:610-616.
7.   Rubba P, Pauciullo P, Mancini M. Lowering blood lipids to treat atherosclerosis: vascular tone, plaque, events and mortality. Cardiovascular Drug Ther 1993;7: 767-774.
8.   Andrews HE, Bruckdorfer KR, Dunn RC, Jacobs M. Low density lipoprotein inhibit endothelium dependent relaxation in rabbit aorta. Nature 1987;327:237-239.
9.   Wines PA, Schmitz JM, Pfister SL, et al. Augmented vasoconstrictor responses to serotonin precede development of atherosclerosis in aorta of WHHL rabbit. Arteriosclerosis 1989; 9:195-202.
10.   Shimokawa H, Kim P, Vanhoutte PM. Endothelium-dependent relaxation to aggregating platelets in isolated basilar arteries of control and hypercholesterolemic pigs. Circulation Res 1988;63:604-612.
11.   Tomita T, Ezaki M, Miwa M, Nakamura K, Inoue Y. Rapid and reversible inhibition by low density lipoprotein of the endothelium-dependent relaxation to hemostatic substances in porcine coronary arteries. Circulation Res 1990;66:18-27.
12.   Rabbani LE, Loscalzo J. The effects of hyperlipidemia and atherosclerosis on endothelial function and vascular reactivity. Curr Opin Lipidol 1991;2:259-265.
13.   Rossitch E, Alexander III E, Black PM, Cooke JP. L-Arginine normalizes endothelial function in cerebral vessels from hypercholesterolemic rabbits. J Clin Invest 1991;87:1295-1299.
14.   Kugiyama K, Kerns SA, Morriset JD, Roberts R, Henry PD. Impairment of

endothelium-dependent arterial relaxation by lysolecithin in modified low-density lipoproteins. Nature 1990;344:160-162.

15. Shuschke DA, Joshua IG, Miller FN. Comparison of early microcirculatory and aortic changes in hypercholesterolemic rats. Arteriosclerosis and Thrombosis 1991;11:154-160.

16. Harrison DG, Armstrong ML, Freiman PC, Heistad DD. Restoration of endothelium-dependent relaxation by dietary treatment of atherosclerosis. J Clin Invest 1987;80:1808-1811.

17. Rubba P, Postiglione A, Scarpato N, Iannuzzi A, Mancini M. Improved reactive hyperemia test after plasma-exchange. Atherosclerosis 1985; 56:237-242.

18. Creager MA, Cooke JP, Mendelsohn ME, et al. Impaired vasodilation of forearm resistance vessels in hypercholesterolemic humans. J Clin Invest 1990;86:228-234.

19. Henry PD, Bucay M. Effects of low-density lipoproteins and hypercholesterolemia on endothelium-dependent vasodilation. Curr Opin Lipidol 1991;2:306-310.

20. Chowienczyk PJ, Watts GF, Cockcroft JR, Ritter JM. Impaired endothelium-dependent vasodilation of forearm resistance vessels in hyper-cholesterolemia. Lancet 1992;340:1430-1432.

21. Celermajer DS, Sorensen KE, Gooch VM, et al. Non-invasive detection of endothelial dysfunction in children and adults at risk of atherosclerosis. Lancet 1992;340:1111-1115.

LONG-CHAIN ACYLCARNITINE AS MEMBRANE STABILIZER

Willem C. Hülsmann[1] and Alessandro Peschechera[2]
[1] Thoraxcenter
Erasmus University Rotterdam
THE NETHERLANDS
and
[2] Sigma-Tau
Pomezia
ITALY

Introduction

Long-chain acylcarnitine (LCAC) is a physiological membrane stabilizer in ischemic tissues. It is known to be formed in the carnitine palmitoyl transferase-1 (CPT-1) reaction in various cell types such as myocytes and vascular endothelial cells. CPT-1 becomes activated in stress, when insulin levels are low and stress hormone levels are high. This state not only stimulates lipolysis, which increases the availability of fatty acids, but also activates CPT-1 by phosphorylation of the enzyme. Increased production and excretion of LCAC by the addition of carnitine to cells that are not carnitine-deficient requires an explanation. Our explanation is based on the ability of (acyl)carnitine to bind to muscle membranes. The longer the acyl-group attached, the higher its affinity to bind. We have observed earlier that LCAC remains attached to plasmalemma of ischemic pig heart, even after repeated washing with medium devoid of carnitine. However, the presence of carnitine in the washing medium stimulates LCAC removal. Therefore it is possible that increasing the carnitine level in interstitium of muscle releases LCAC from muscle and makes it available to vascular endothelium in concentrations that might stabilize their membranes. This probably inhibits calcium overload, restricts edema, and promotes (re)flow. Improvement of flow by addition of carnitine to paced dog skeletal muscle has been observed by us employing microspheres and in Langendorff hearts by decrease of NADH surface fluorescence in ischemic areas, as will be further worked out below.

In summary, our explanation of improvement of tissue oxygenation and flow in imminent ischemia by carnitine supplementation to carnitine-sufficient organs is based upon plasmalemmal stabilization by low levels of LCAC.

A.M. Gotto et al. (eds), Multiple Risk Factors in Cardiovascular Disease, 409-412.
© 1995 Kluwer Academic Publishers and Fondazione Giovanni Lorenzini.

Effect of Long-Chain Acylcarnitine (LCAC) on Heart

The space between myocytes and capillary endothelium contains cell- and plasma-borne compounds. Enzymes present in this interstitium are, for example, lipoprotein lipase [1], ecto-5'-nucleotidase [2], and xanthine oxydase [3]. The activities of these enzymes may influence capillary flow. Adenosine, formed during the breakdown of adenine nucleotides in ischemia, affects flow and therefore edema [2]. It is also a precursor of (hypo) xanthine, which is the substrate for xanthine oxydase that generates oxygen free radicals (OFR) and therefore may interfere with vasoregulation. The breakdown of OFR in interstitium, by administration of superoxyde dismutase (SOD), during hypoperfusion of heart has been shown to improve perfusion efficiency [4,5]. This may be due to the ability of OFR to destroy the vasodilator endothelial-derived relaxing factor [6] and to lower adenosine levels [7] in interstitium.

Previous studies [4,8] led us to assume that vascular endothelium is relatively sensitive to products that accumulate during ischemia: lactic acid and OFR. However, recently this has become unlikely now we have found that cultured vascular endothelium is relatively resistent to lactic acidosis and OFR [9]. Therefore increased distances between capillary endothelium and myocytes resulting from contraction and gap increase, due to calcium overload of endothelial cells, have become a more likely explanation than cell damage [10]. This is supported by the observed rapid improvement of tissue oxygenation of ischemic areas of hypertrophic hearts by SOD administration [5]. Oxygen supply may also be improved by addition of long-chain fatty acids instead of SOD [5].

Recently, we found that not only L-carnitine but also aminocarnitine, was able to improve oxygenation of ischemic areas of hypertrophic rat Langendorff hearts. As L-carnitine is a substrate for LCAC synthesis and L-aminocarnitine an inhibitor of LCAC utilization [11], accumulation of LCAC and release from sarcolemma, may be a common factor [10]. Moreover, we found 10 years ago that LCAC may stabilize myocardial membranes during ischemia [12]. In Langendorff rat hearts 1 μM palmitoylcarnitine, present in the perfusion medium prior to global ischemia, prevented leakage of myoglobin and lactate dehydrogenase during reperfusion [12]. We also noted that it promoted restoration of contractile function in a number of cases, although apex displacement of the heart was less than before [12], indicating a lower level of intramyocytal calcium. However, when instead of 1 μM palmitoylcarnitine 5 μM had been used, the hearts suffered from calcium overload, judged by rapid arrest in systole prior to the no-flow period [12]. Therefore, administration of LCAC may be hazardous so that endogenous generation of LCAC and release by L-carnitine addition is preferred. Addition of its other substrate, fatty acid, is generally not required as endogenous lipolysis, particularly in stress when insulin levels are low, may provide fatty acids. When LCAC cannot be oxidized by addition of the carnitine palmitoyltransferase-2 inhibitor aminocarnitine, the heart is also not arrested even though LCAC accumulation and excretion from the heart may be abundant [11]. Hence we suppose that administration of either carnitine or aminocarnitine enhances release of LCAC from plasma membranes, to which (acyl)carnitine may be bound [13,14].

Influence of Insulin and Glucagon on Carnitine Effects

In paced musculus latissimus dorsi of dogs, L-carnitine infusion acutely improved the force of contraction [15]. As calcium fluxes may be increased by alkalinization of the cytosol of various cell preparations, we infused dogs with insulin (and glucose to avoid hypoglycemia) and observed that although this did not affect the force of contraction of the M.latissimus dorsi, the subsequent addition of L-carnitine had no effect on the paced muscle. In the absence of added insulin, D-carnitine instead of L-carnitine lowered the force of contraction of the M.latissimus dorsi, perhaps as D-carnitine is known to inhibit carnitine palmitoyl transferase-1 (CPT-1). The data gave us the impression that the vascular compartment rather than the muscle cells might have lost carnitine by ischemia. Further investigation with microspheres showed that during pacing the capillary flow in the M.latissimus dorsi had increased during L-carnitine infusion [16]. That insulin abolished the L-carnitine effect on M.latissimus dorsi, led us to consider the necessity of fatty acid supply for L-carnitine action. An additional effect of insulin is inhibition of LCAC formation by synthesis of malonyl-CoA, the physiological inhibitor of CPT-1 [17]. The synthesis of malonyl-CoA in cardiac myocytes may be accomplished by the presence of cytosolic acetyl-CoA carboxylase [18]. For vascular endothelial cells these data are not available. Yet, similar mechanisms may be expected to operate as we have observed, in bovine vascular endothelial cells in culture, secretion of LCAC after supplementation of the culture medium with oleate and L-carnitine. This process was found to be stimulated by epinephrine and inhibited by insulin (unpublished). That LCAC is formed in endothelial cells is in agrement with earlier observations of beta-oxidation in these cells [19]. Therefore, LCAC in interstitium of tissues may be derived from various cell types. In ischemic muscle the contribution comes mainly from the mitochondria-rich myocytes. It may be of interest to note that Inoue et al. [20] have recently observed that, although higher concentrations of palmitoylcarnitine cause calcium overload of endothelial cells, lower levels suppressed calcium transients induced by receptor agonists.

References

1.   Hülsmann WC, Dubelaar ML, DeWit LEA, Persoon NLM. Cardiac lipoprotein lipase: Effects of lipopolysaccharide and tumor necrosis factor. Mol Cell Biochem 1988;79:137-145.
2.   Rubio R, Berne RM, Dobson G Jr. Sites of adenosine production in cardiac and skeletal muscle. Am J Physiol 1975;225:938-953.
3.   Samra ZQ, Oguro T, Fontaine R, Ashraf M. Immunocytochemical localization of xanthine oxidase in rat myocardium. J Submicroscop Cytol Pathol 1991;23:379-390.
4.   Hülsmann WC, Dubelaar ML. Early damage of vascular endothelium during cardiac ischemia. Cardiovasc Res 1987;21:674-677.
5.   Hülsmann WC, Ashruf JF, Bruining H, Ince C. Imminent ischemia in normal and hypertrophic rat Langendorff hearts; effect of fatty acids and superoxide dismutase

monitored by NADH surface fluorescence. Biochim Biophys Acta 1992;1181:273-278.

6.   Gryglewski RJ, Palmer RJ, Moncada S. Superoxide anion involved in the breakdown of endothelial-derived relaxing factor. Nature 1986;320:454-456.

7.   Kitakaze M, Hori M, Katashima S, et al. Superoxide dismutase enhances both adenosine release and coronary hyperemic flow through protection of 5'-nucleotidase against its degradation during reperfusion following ischemia in dogs. Biorheology 1993;30:359-370.

8.   Hülsmann WC, Dubelaar ML. Carnitine requirement of vascular endothelial and smooth muscle cells in imminent ischemia. Mol Cell Biochem 1992;116:125-129.

9.   Peschechera A, Ferrari LE, Arrigoni-Martelli E, Hülsmann WC. Uptake and release of carnitine by vascular endothelium in culture; effects of protons and oxygen free radicals. Mol Cell Biochem, in press.

10.   Hülsmann WC, Peschechera A, Arrigoni-Martelli E. Carnitine and cardiac interstitium. Cardioscience 1994;5:67-72.

11.   Hülsmann WC, Schneydenberg CTWM, Verkley AJ. Accumulation and excretion of long-chain acylcarnitine by rat hearts; studies with aminocarnitine. Biochim Biophys Acta 1991;1097:263-269.

12.   Hülsmann WC, Dubelaar ML, Lamers JMJ, Maccari F. Protection by acylcarnitines and phenylmethylsulfonylfluoride of rat hearts subjected to ischemia and reperfusion. Biochim Biophys Acta 1985;847:62-66.

13.   Paulson DJ, Traxler J, Schmidt M, Nooman J, Shug AL. Protection of the ischemic myocardium by L-propionylcarnitine: Effects on the recovery of cardiac output after ischemia and reperfusion, carnitine transport and fatty acid oxidation. Cardiovasc Res 1986;20:536-541.

14.   Lamers JMJ, DeJonge-Stinis JT, Verdouw PD, Hülsmann WC. On the possible role of long-chain fatty acylcarnitine accumulation in producing functional and calcium permeability changes in membranes during myocardial ischemia. Cardiovasc Res 1987;21:313-322.

15.   Dubelaar ML, Lucas CMBH, Hülsmann WC. Acute effect of L-carnitine upon cardiac muscle force tests in the dog. Am J Physiol 1991;260:E189-E193.

16.   Dubelaar ML, Lucas CMBH, Hülsmann WC. The effect of L-carnitine on force development of the latissimus dorsi muscle in dogs. J Cardiac Surg 1991;6(Suppl. 1):270-275.

17.   McGarry JD, Foster DW. Regulation of hepatic fatty acid oxidation and ketone body formation. Ann Rev Biochem 1980;49:395-420.

18.   Scholte HR, Luyt-Houwen IEM, Dubelaar ML, Hülsmann WC. The source of malonyl-CoA in rat heart; the calcium paradox releases acetyl-CoA carboxylase and not propionyl-CoA carboxylase. FEBS Lett 1986;198:47-50.

19.   Hülsmann WC, Dubelaar ML. Aspects of fatty acid metabolism in vascular endothelial cells. Biochimie 1988;70:681-686.

20.   Inoue N, Hirata K, Akita H, Yokoyama M. Palmitoyl-L-carnitine modifies the function of vascular endothelium. Cardiovasc Res 1994;28:129-134.

PROTECTIVE EFFECTS OF MODERATE CONSUMPTION OF ALCOHOL ON THE INCIDENCE OF CORONARY HEART DISEASE

Michael H. Criqui
Department of Family and Preventive Medicine
University of California, San Diego
9500 Gilman Drive
La Jolla, California 92093-0607
USA

In order to open this session, I'd like to share with you some thoughts from a recent research project we competed, as well as some insights about the possible mechanism of moderate alcohol consumption's effect on CHD incidence.

An Ecological Study of Alcohol and CHD Mortality

Along with a medical student trained initially as a nutritionist, Brenda Ringel, we looked at coronary and total mortality in 21 industrialized countries with an annual per capita Gross Domestic Product of $9500 or greater [1]. We separately examined the years 1965, 1970, 1980, and 1988. As expected, animal fat consumption was positively and vegetable consumption and fruit inversely associated with CHD mortality. Among alcoholic beverages, only wine showed a strong inverse association with CHD mortality, and this relationship was stronger and more consistent in multivariate analyses than any other food or beverage variable. However, wine ethanol showed a stronger inverse correlation than total wine volume, suggesting ethanol was more important than nonethanol constituents present in wine.

Wine, however, was unrelated to total mortality; only fruit showed a beneficial effect. This result reflects the close association between the average wine consumption levels in various countries and extent of alcohol abuse. Moderate (defined as up to 2 drinks per day) drinkers do have increased longevity but countries with large numbers of moderate drinkers, also have many heavier drinkers, who have sharply reduced longevity. Therefore, the use of alcohol for cardioprotective purposes cannot be encouraged.

413

A.M. Gotto et al. (eds), Multiple Risk Factors in Cardiovascular Disease, 413-415.
© 1995 *Kluwer Academic Publishers and Fondazione Giovanni Lorenzini.*

Does Alcohol Affect CHD Risk Via HDL Cholesterol?

There has been considerable speculation as to the biological effect or effects responsible for the reduction of CHD in moderate drinkers. In 1983, we presented preliminary data from the prospective Lipid Research Clinics (LRC) Follow-up Study that about half of the protective effect of moderate alcohol consumption could be attributed to higher HDL cholesterol in drinkers [2]. This conclusion was based on demonstration that the inverse regression coefficient for alcohol from the Cox survival model for CHD death was attenuated by approximately 50% when HDL cholesterol was simultaneously entered into the model. We published the final LRC data on this question in 1987 [3], and we replicated this finding almost exactly in the prospective Honolulu Heart Study [4]. A report from the prospective Multiple Risk Factor Intervention Trial (MRFIT) data, utilizing virtually identical analyses, also found an HDL "pathway" of approximately 50% [5]. Finally, a retrospective case-control study also found a pathway of approximately 50% for HDL cholesterol, and in a subset found that adding apolipoprotein A-I and A-II to the model further attenuated the alcohol effect [6].

Now that an HDL pathway for alcohol's effect on CHD is assuming the status of scientific fact, we need to take a step back and ask a question. Does the statistical demonstration of a 50% reduction in the strength of the protective effect of moderate alcohol consumption for CHD when HDL cholesterol is added to the statistical model prove that alcohol has a protective effect via increased HDL? The answer is not necessarily. Although an HDL pathway is certainly consistent with this finding and perhaps even likely, it is also possible that an unmeasured variable(s) could change in stepwise fashion with alcohol consumption in parallel with HDL, and this unmeasured variable could be responsible for the protective effect. For example, alcohol has been shown to affect several factors involved in thrombosis [3].

I trust these introductory comments have set the stage for what I hope will be a spirited roundtable discussion.

References

1.   Criqui MH, Ringel BL. Invited plenary lecture, "Does Diet/Alcohol Explain the Difference?" in Symposium: Regional Variation in Coronary Heart Disease Rates - The French Paradox, presented at the 66th Scientific Sessions of the American Heart Association, Atlanta, GA, November 9, 1993.

2.   Criqui MH. Alcohol and Cardiovascular Mortality. In: Kaplan RM, Criqui MH, editors. Behavioral Epidemiology and Disease Prevention. New York: Plenum, 1985.

3.   Criqui MH, Cowan LD, Tyroler HA, et al. Lipoproteins as mediators for the effects of alcohol consumption and cigarette smoking on cardiovascular mortality: Results from the Lipid Research Clinics Follow-up Study. Am J Epidemiol 1987;126:629-37.

4.   Langer RD, Criqui MH, Reed DM. Lipoproteins and blood pressure as biological

pathways for effect of moderate alcohol consumption on coronary heart disease. Circulation 1992;85:910-5.

5.   Suh I, Shaten BJ, Cutler JA, Kuller LH. Alcohol use and mortality from coronary heart disease: The role of high-density lipoprotein cholesterol: The Multiple Risk Factor Intervention Trial Research Group. Ann Intern Med 1992;116:881-7.

6.   Gaziano JM, Buring JE, Breslow JL, et al. Moderate alcohol intake, increased levels of high-density lipoprotein and its subfractions, and decreased risk of myocardial infarction. N Engl J Med 1993:329:1829-34.

ALCOHOL CONSUMPTION: WEIGHING THE CARDIOVASCULAR BENEFIT WITH THE OVERALL HEALTH RISK

Eric B. Rimm
Departments of Epidemiology and Nutrition
Harvard School of Public Health
Boston, Massachusetts 02115
USA

Introduction

To understand the overall health consequences of alcohol consumption, it is crucial to consider the cardiovascular benefit as well as the adverse risk of cirrhosis, breast cancer, colon cancer, accidents, violence, and other chronic and acute conditions. Much attention has been given to both sides of the spectrum. On the benefit side, in several reviews [1,2] a consistent inverse association between alcohol and coronary heart disease has been thoroughly explored. The inverse association for cardiovascular disease is found quite consistently within populations throughout the world. Because cardiovascular disease is the primary cause of death for men and women in the United States [3] and in many Westernized countries, the beneficial effects of alcohol consumed at the rate of one to two drinks per day on rates of cardiovascular disease are of substantial public health importance. Conversely, the known adverse associations between alcohol and cirrhosis, liver cancer, and cancers of the upper airway and digestive tract, and the recent evidence which suggests that alcohol may play an important role in breast cancer [4-6] and some forms of colon cancer [7] also fuel the public health debate.

One way to weigh the benefits and harm of alcohol on disease is to examine the epidemiological evidence relating alcohol to total mortality [8]. This oversimplifies the true effects of alcohol consumption, since the benefits from reducing nonfatal coronary disease cannot be accounted for nor can the ill-effects of alcoholism, accidents, or domestic abuse. Furthermore, since some populations may be at higher risk of alcohol-related cancers or at lower risk of cardiovascular disease due to age, gender, or lifestyle variables such as diet or exercise, a single statement about the health effects of alcohol may not apply to all populations. In this review, I will discuss several of these issues. I cannot provide a thorough review of all the literature on alcohol and chronic disease, although several have been published elsewhere [1,2,5,7,9,10]. Some of this review is taken from a recent summary of alcohol as an essential component in the Mediterranean diet [Rimm and Ellison,

417

A.M. Gotto et al. (eds), Multiple Risk Factors in Cardiovascular Disease, 417-425.
© 1995 *Kluwer Academic Publishers and Fondazione Giovanni Lorenzini.*

in press].

Cardiovascular Disease

The inverse association between moderate alcohol consumption and cardiovascular disease has been consistently reported in over 30 observational studies among populations ranging from the United States to Yugoslavia and from New Zealand to Finland [2]. Most available data suggests a U- or J-shaped association between daily quantity of alcohol consumed and incidence of coronary disease. For instance, Klatsky et al. [11] reported that participants who consumed 1-2 drinks/day were at 30% lower risk of cardiovascular mortality than abstainers. However, among consumers of 6 or more drinks per day, the rates of coronary disease were similar to those of abstainers. In our studies among 44,059 male health professionals and 85,881 female nurses [12,13], we reported a similar inverse association at 1 to 2 drinks per day for risk of both fatal and nonfatal coronary disease. Rather than a U-shaped association, in our large cohorts we reported a linear inverse association. We did not see a higher risk of coronary disease among men and women consuming in excess of 4 drinks per day probably due to the short follow-up period, the small numbers of heavy drinkers, and the nature of the participants in these professional cohorts.

In the past, some concern was raised about including individuals in the nondrinkers group who may have recently stopped drinking due to illnesses such as hypertension or diabetes, since these people would be at higher risk of coronary disease [14,15]. To eliminate this problem Klatsky et al. used lifetime nondrinkers as a reference group [11,16] and still found 1-2 drinks per day to reduce risk of coronary mortality. In a subanalyses from our study [12] we excluded men who reported at baseline any cardiovascular disease, cancer (except nonmelanoma skin cancer), hypertension, gout, diabetes, high cholesterol, high triglycerides, tachycardia, heart rhythm disturbances, or other heart disease. We still found a strong inverse association between alcohol and fatal and nonfatal coronary disease.

Because of the beneficial effect of alcohol on lipids, it is not surprising that this or other hypothesized biases do not play a major role in explaining the inverse association between alcohol and coronary disease in most populations. Several mechanisms which may explain the cardioprotective effects of alcohol have been clearly elucidated. Alcohol raises levels of HDL-2 and HDL-3 cholesterol [17] which are consistently inversely associated with coronary heart disease [18]. Among the epidemiologic studies where data are available on both alcohol intake and HDL-cholesterol [17,19,20], results for statistical modelling suggest that the association between alcohol and HDL-cholesterol explains 30-50% of the overall reduction in coronary heart disease attributable to alcohol. Other hemostatic mechanisms associated with reduced thrombosis [21-24] may explain much of the rest of the cardioprotective effects of alcohol.

In general, the association between alcohol and ischemic stroke parallels that of alcohol and coronary heart disease discussed above. Among the prospective studies that have differentiated type of stroke, men and women who consume 1 to 3 drinks per day are at the same or lower risk of ischemic stroke compared with abstainers or with those who drink substantially more [9,10,25]. For the subclasses of hemorrhagic stroke, where the pathophysiology of the disease relates to anti-aggregatory mechanisms, alcohol is positively associated even at moderate levels of consumption. Since in most western countries hemorrhagic stroke accounts for about 15% of cerebrovascular deaths [3, 26], the association between alcohol and total stroke in most studies is generally flat or U-shaped, with the nadir occurring among individuals who consume 1-3 drinks per day.

Cancer

Cancers of the upper airway and of the digestive tract, including the oropharynx, esophagus, liver, and colon, are the major sites which have been linked to alcohol consumption. Alcohol consumption at or above 3 drinks per day is associated with higher mortality rates of stomach, esophageal, pharyngeal, and oral cancer [8]. The rates of these rare cancers increase substantially at levels of heavier alcohol consumption, and for the upper airway occur almost exclusively among heavy drinkers who are also cigarette smokers.

COLON CANCER

In a recent review of alcohol consumption and risk of colorectal cancer, Kune and Vitetta [7] summarize 52 major studies published in the last 35 years. Most case-control (which have used population controls) and cohort studies have reported an approximate two-fold increase in risk of colon and/or rectal cancer among participants drinking two or more drinks per day. Since diet most certainly plays an important role in the etiology of colon cancer [27-31], making conclusions about alcohol consumption or beverage type without accounting for macro- or micronutrient intake may yield misleading results. For instance, a number of previous studies which have collected information on beverage type concluded that the strongest risk of colon cancer is associated with beer rather than spirits or wine [7]. However, since beer drinkers have different diet and lifestyle characteristics [32] than consumers of wine or spirits, it is essential to carefully control for these factors before concluding that beer rather than alcohol *per se* is associated with elevated colon cancer risk. In our study of alcohol, diet and risk of adenomatous colon polyps, precursors of colon cancer, Giovannucci et al. [31] found that a high folate diet strongly attenuated the association between alcohol and colon polyps. Since vegetables and fruits are the main sources of folate, individuals who consume 2 drinks per day may not be at higher risk of colon cancer if they consume recommended amounts of fruits and vegetables.

BREAST CANCER

There have been over 40 epidemiologic studies of the association between alcohol and breast cancer. In a recent review, Rosenberg et al. [5], interpreted the evidence cautiously, but concluded that if chance were a viable explanation for the consistently reported null or positive associations, then more studies with inverse associations should be expected. The results of a meta-analysis suggest an approximate 25% increase in risk among women drinking two drinks per day compared with abstainers [6]. In case-control comparisons that used community-based controls most studies have found an increase in breast cancer risk only for reported alcohol consumption above 4 drinks per day [33]. Although only conducted among US women, results from most [5], but not all [34], prospective cohort studies have suggested a positive association between alcohol and breast cancer even at levels less than three drinks per day. For example, among 89,538 women in the Nurses' Health Study followed for four years, Willett et al. [4] reported a relative risk of 1.6 (95% CI 1.3, 2.0) among women consuming 15 or more grams of alcohol per day compared to abstainers.

Breast cancer is one of the more controversial diseases where it is important to weigh the cardiovascular benefit with the adverse risk. Clearly, premenopausal women have much lower rates of cardiovascular disease than men of similar age, and therefore may not gain as much benefit from alcohol. It is only 10 to 15 years after menopause that rates of cardiovascular disease are similar between genders. Since breast cancer rates in women start to rise in their midthirties, if alcohol is an important determinant of risk of pre and postmenopausal breast cancer [4,35], then much of the adverse effects of alcohol may be realized before the long term benefit can be gained. Other factors, such as postmenopausal estrogen use [35], obesity [36], and reproductive factors [4] that may modify the effect of alcohol on breast cancer need to be studied further.

To understand better the role of alcohol and its effect on breast cancer, further research is needed in several areas: measuring the effects of alcohol among subpopulations of women with specific dietary patterns, determining the importance of alcohol consumed in adolescence (since early- life drinking patterns may effect hormonal and developmental growth), and a deeper understanding of the mechanism(s) which may explain alcohol's effect on breast cancer.

Morbidity

Morbidity related to alcohol or alcohol abuse is the most commonly discussed argument against a policy of alcohol acceptance for cardiovascular benefits. It is estimated that up to half of the yearly 50,000 motor vehicle deaths and countless nonfatal accidents in the United States are alcohol-related [37]. Alcohol is also an important contributor to falls, fires, and other accident rates [38]. Men and women who consume alcohol are also more likely to be involved in domestic abuse. Unlike cardiovascular disease, much of adverse alcohol-related events are acute and related to binge drinking or heavy episodic drinking rather sustained use. Rice et al. [39] estimated the direct and indirect costs of alcohol abuse in 1988 in the United States to be $85.8 billion. This estimate does not take into account the financial impact of the beneficial role that alcohol may have on the lipid profile and coronary heart disease or that alcohol may reduce the risk of diabetes [40,41] or gallstones [42].

Much of the adverse effects of alcohol on morbidity are restricted to individuals who abuse alcohol. Since alcohol abuse or heavy alcohol consumption does not afford any long-term cardioprotective benefits [8,16], individuals who drink 1 to 2 drinks per day should not be advised to increase their consumption to further reduce their risk of cardiovascular mortality. Unfortunately, there are no good screening methods to identify individuals who may develop alcohol problems. Since up to 10% of individuals who drink in the United States may be considered alcoholics [38], clearly there is a tendency for abuse among populations who start by drinking moderately. Brewer et al. [43] found that drivers killed in motor vehicle accidents where alcohol was involved were 11 times more likely to have a previous arrest for driving while impaired than drivers killed in a non-alcohol-related accident. Stricter laws and lower tolerance for alcohol on the roadways may be an important tool for reducing alcohol-related automobile fatalities as well as identifying individuals who abuse alcohol.

Total Mortality and Life Expectancy

As outlined above, alcohol reduces the risk of overall cardiovascular disease and may somewhat increase the risk of cancer at several sites. In countries where cardiovascular disease is the leading cause of death in both men and women, one to two alcoholic drinks per day are associated with lower risk of total mortality [8,11,44-47] and increase life expectancy [48]. In the largest study to date, Boffetta and Garfinkel followed 276,802 men for 12 years in the American Cancer Society prospective study [8]. In that study, men consuming up to 5 drinks/day had significantly lower risk of coronary heart disease death compared with abstainers, whereas total cancer deaths were significantly increased at consumption levels of 3 or more drinks per day. For overall mortality, men drinking from less than 1 drink per day up to 2 drinks per day were at lowest risk of death.

In a review of nine follow-up cohort studies giving total mortality data in reports between 1986 and 1992 [49], almost all showed that at least one category of alcohol consumption was associated with total mortality rates lower than that of abstainers. While some studies included "ex-drinkers" in the zero alcohol category, others, such as the Japanese Physician's Study [47], the Busselton Study in Australia [44], and the studies from Kaiser Permanente in California [11], used lifetime abstainers as the referent group. Those studies also found that mild or moderate drinkers had lower total mortality rates than lifetime abstainers. Coate, using data from the National Health and Nutrition Examination survey in 1971-74 and the follow-up survey in 1982-88, found that white men consuming up to 2 drinks per day at the initial survey increased their time until death from any cause by about 3 percent [48].

Data on the relationship between alcohol consumption and total mortality among women are much more limited than they are among men. In the few studies that have included women, the alcohol-mortality relationship is similar to that of men [16]. However, since women do not metabolize alcohol as efficiently as men and are, on average, smaller, levels of consumption related to maximum reduction in total mortality would be expected to be somewhat lower. Also as stated above, depending on the population or on other lifestyle characteristics, the increased risk of breast cancer may make the nadir of the overall U-shaped association between alcohol and total mortality at a lower level of consumption.

Summary

For most adults, consumption of alcohol is an enjoyable and controllable part of their lifestyle. The substantially amount of epidemiological data suggests that for these people, drinking one to two drinks per day yields lower rates of morbidity and mortality than individuals who drink more or less than this level. For individuals who are currently nondrinkers, alcohol should not be recommended since a significant percentage of individuals may develop problems of alcohol abuse. At high levels of consumption, rates of many chronic diseases are increased as are death rates due to acute alcohol-related events (i.e. accidents, domestic abuse, suicide, etc). In addition, former alcohol abusers or those with certain diseases or conditions should be advised to limit alcohol consumption. Although still not fully elucidated, the risk versus the benefit for alcohol consumption among women may be dependent on the strength of other risk factors an individual woman may have for breast cancer or cardiovascular disease. The available evidence suggests that one drink per day or less may be optimal. Overall, moderate alcohol consumption, as defined above, is consistently found to lower cardiovascular disease, marginally increase the risk of some forms of cancer, yielding an overall protective effect for total mortality.

References

1.   Maclure M. A demonstration of deductive meta-analysis: Ethanol intake and risk of myocardial infarction. Epidemiol Rev 1994; in press.

2.   Moore RD, Pearson TA. Moderate alcohol consumption and coronary artery disease: A review. Medicine 1986;65:242-67.

3.   National Center for Health Statistics. Births, marriages, divorces, and deaths for February 1994. Monthly vital statistics report; vol 43 no. 2. Hyattsville, Maryland: Public Health Service. 1994.

4.   Willett WC, Stampfer MJ, Colditz GA, Rosner BA, Hennekens CH, Speizer FE. Moderate alcohol consumption and the risk of breast cancer. N Engl J Med 1987;316:1174-80.

5.   Rosenberg L, Metzger LS, Palmer JT. Alcohol consumption and risk of breast cancer: A review of the epidemiologic evidence. Epidemiologic Reviews 1993;15:133-44.

6.   Longnecker MP. Alcoholic beverage consumption in relation to risk of breast cancer: Meta-analysis and review. Cancer Causes and Control 1994;5:73-82.

7.   Kune GA, Vitetta L. Alcohol consumption and the etiology of colorectal cancer: A review of the scientific evidence from 1957 to 1991. Nutr Cancer 1992;18:97-111.

8.   Boffetta P, Garfinkel L. Alcohol drinking and mortality among men enrolled in a American Cancer Society prospective study. Epidemiology 1990;1:342-8.

9.   Rimm EB, Stampfer MJ. Prospective studies of moderate alcohol consumption and the risk of coronary disease in stroke in women and men. In: Ventra J, van der Hiej DG, editors. Alcohol and cardiovascular disease: Proceedings of an international

symposium, Scheveningen, Netherlands, 2 October 1991. Pudoc, Wageningen, 1992;1-18.

10.   van Gijn J, Stampfer MJ, Wolfe C, Algra A. The association between alcohol and stroke. In: Verschuren PM, editor. Health issues related to alcohol consumption. Washington: ILSI Press. 1993;43-79.

11.   Klatsky AL, Armstrong MA, Friedman GD. Risk of cardiovascular mortality in alcohol drinkers, ex-drinkers, and nondrinkers. Am J Cardiol 1990;66:1237-42.

12.   Rimm EB, Giovannucci EL, Willett WC, et al. A prospective study of alcohol consumption and the risk of coronary disease in men. Lancet 1991;338:464-68.

13.   Stampfer MJ, Colditz GA, Willett WC, Speizer FE, Hennekens CH. A prospective study of moderate alcohol consumption and the risk of coronary disease and stroke in women. N Engl J Med 1988;319:267-73.

14.   Shaper AG, Wannamethee G, Walker M. Alcohol and mortality in British men: Explaining the U-shaped curve. Lancet 1988;2:1267-1273.

15.   Shaper AG, Wannamethee G, Walker M. Alcohol and coronary heart disease: A perspective from the British Regional Heart Study. Int J Epidemiol 1994;23:482-494.

16.   Klatsky AL, Armstrong MA, Friedman GD. Alcohol and mortality. Ann Int Med 1992;117:646-54.

17.   Gaziano JM, Buring JE, Breslow JL, et al. Moderate alcohol intake, increased levels of high-density lipoprotein and its subfractions and decreased risk of myocardial infarction. N Engl J Med 1993;329:1829-1834.

18.   Stampfer MJ, Sacks FM, Salvini S, Willett WC, Hennekens CH. A prospective study of cholesterol, apolipoproteins, and the risk of myocardial infarction. N Engl J Med 1991;325:373-81.

19.   Suh I, Shaten J, Cutler JA, Kuller L. Alcohol use and mortality from coronary heart disease: The role of high-density lipoprotein cholesterol. Ann Int Med 1992;116:881-887.

20.   Langer RD, Criqui MH, Reed DM. Lipoproteins and blood pressure as biological pathways for effect of moderate alcohol consumption on coronary heart disease. Circulation 1992;85:910-915.

21.   Meade TW, Vickers MV, Thompson SG, et al. Epidemiologic characteristics of platelet aggregability. Br Med J 1985;290:428-432.

22.   Seigneur M, Bonnet J, Dorian B, et al. Effect of the consumption of alcohol, white wine, and red wine on platelet function and serum lipids. J Applied Cardiol 1990;5:215-222.

23.   Sumi H, Hamada H, Tsushima H, Mihara H. Urokinase-like plasminogen activator increased in plasma after alcohol drinking. Alcohol & Alcoholism 1988;23:33-43.

24.   Renaud SC, Beswick AD, Fehily AM, Sharp DS, Elwood PC. Alcohol and platelet aggregation: The Caerphilly prospective heart disease study. Am J Clin Nutr 1992;55:1012-1017.

25.   Camargo CA Jr., Williams PT, Vranizan KM, Albers JJ, Wood PD. The effect of moderate alcohol intake on serum apolipoproteins A-I and A-II: A controlled study.

JAMA 1985;253: 2854-7.

26. Wolf PA, Cobb JL, D'Agostino RB. Epidemiology of stroke. In: Barnett HJM, Mohr JP, Stein BM, Yatsu FM, editors. Stroke, pathophysiology, diagnosis, and management. New York: Churchill Livingston, 1992;3-27.

27. Block G, Patterson B, Subar A. Fruit, vegetables, and cancer prevention: A review of the epidemiologic evidence. Nutr Cancer 1992;18:1-29.

28. Willett WC, Stampfer MJ, Colditz GA, Rosner BA, Speizer FE. Relation of meat, fat, and fiber intake to the risk of colon cancer in a prospective study among women. N Engl J Med 1990;323:1664-72.

29. Giovannucci E, Rimm EB, Stampfer MJ, Colditz GA, Ascherio A, Willett WC. Intake of fat, meat, and fiber in relation to risk of colon cancer in men. Cancer Res. 1994;54:2390-2397.

30. Giovannucci E, Stampfer MJ, Colditz GA, Rimm EB, Speizer FE, Willett WC. Relation of diet to the risk of colorectal adenoma in men. JNCI 1992;84:91-98.

31. Giovannucci E, Stampfer MJ, Colditz GA, et al. Folate, methionine and alcohol intake and risk of colorectal adenoma. JNCI 1993;85:875-884.

32. Klatsky AL, Armstrong MA, Kipp H. Correlates of alcoholic beverage preference: Traits of persons who choose wine, liquor or beer. Br J Addict 1990;85:1279-1289.

33. Roth HD, Levy PS, Shi L, Post E. Alcoholic beverages and breast cancer: Some observations on published case-control studies. J Clin Epidemiol 1994;47:207-216.

34. Schatzkin A, Carter CL, Green SB, et al. Is alcohol consumption related to breast cancer? Results from the Framingham Heart Study. Journal of the National Cancer Institute 1989;81:31-35.

35. Gapstur SM, Potter JD, Sellers TA, Folsom AR. Increased risk of breast cancer with alcohol consumption in postmenopausal women. Am J Epidemiol 1992;136:1221-1231.

36. Schatzkin A, Jones DY, Hoover RN, et al. Alcohol consumption and breast cancer in the epidemiologic follow-up study of the first National Health and Nutrition Examination Survey. N Engl J Med 1987;316:1169-73.

37. McGinnis JM, Foege WH. Actual causes of death in the United States. J Am Med Assoc 1993;270:2207-2212.

38. Angell M, Kassirer JP. Alcohol and other drugs - toward a more rational and consistent policy (editorial). N Engl J Med 1994;331:537-539.

39. Rice DP, Kelman S, Miller LS. The economic cost of alcohol abuse. Alcohol Health & Research World 1991;15:307-315.

40. Stampfer MJ, Colditz GA, Willett WC, et al. A prospective study of moderate alcohol drinking and risk of diabetes in women. Am J Epidemiol 1988;128:549-58.

41. Rimm EB, Chan J, Stampfer MJ, et al. A prospective study of alcohol and smoking and risk of non-insulin-dependent diabetes among US men (abstract). Am J Epidemiol 1994;139:S15.

42. Maclure KM, Hayes KC, Colditz GA, Stampfer MJ, Speizer FE, Willett WC. Weight, diet and risk of symptomatic gallstones in middle-aged women. N Engl J Med 1989;321:563-9.

43. Brewer RD, Morris PD, Cole TB, Watkins S, Patetta MA, Popkin C. The risk of dying in alcohol-related automobile crashes among habitual drunk drivers. N Engl J Med 1994;331:513-517.

44. Cullen K. The Busselton Population Studies. Conference Proceedings. The Medicinal Virtues of Alcohol in Moderation. Sydney, Australia, October 30-November 1, 1991:110-119.

45. de Labry LO, Glynn RJ, Levenson MR, Hermos JA, LoCastro JS, Vokonas PS. Alcohol consumption and mortality in American male population: Recovering the U-shaped curve - Findings from the Normative Aging Study. J Studies on Alcohol 1992;53:25-32.

46. Scherr PA, LaCroix AZ, Wallace RB, et al. Light to moderate alcohol consumption and mortality in the elderly. J Am Geriatr 1992;40:651-657.

47. Kono S, Ikeda M, Tokudome S, Nishizumi M, Kuratsune M. Alcohol and mortality: a cohort study of male Japanese physicians. Int. J. Epidemiol 1986;15:527-532.

48. Coate D. Moderate drinking and coronary heart disease mortality: evidence from NHANES I and the NHANES I follow-up. Am J Public Health 1993;83:888-890.

49. Ellison RC. Does moderate alcohol consumption prolong life? New York: American Council on Science and Health. 1993;.

ALCOHOL AND ATHEROSCLEROSIS

Alberico L. Catapano
Institute of Pharmacological Sciences
Centro per lo Studio, la Prevenzione e
la Terapia delle Vasculopatie Aterosclerotiche
University of Milan
Milan
ITALY

Introduction

Epidemiologic data generally show an inverse correlation between coronary heart disease risk and moderate alcohol intake (variously defined but generally corresponding to 2 to 4 drinks per day). The potentially drastic effects of excessive alcohol intake on health, however, preclude any recommendation that patients increase their alcohol consumption. Equally, there may be no basis for proscribing moderate alcohol intake.

The mechanism by which moderate alcohol intake "protects" remains unclear. Perhaps the best available hypothesis relates to the increased concentration of high-density lipoprotein (HDL) cholesterol associated with moderate alcohol intake; however, recently some interesting observations have appeared indicating that moderate alcohol consumption could favorably interfere with the coagulation system as well as with the pheripheral resistance to insulin.

Pathogenesis of Atherosclerosis

RISK FACTORS

Hypercholesterolemia, hypertension, and cigarette smoking are major risk factors that predispose one to premature atherosclerosis. Additional risk factors include obesity, diabetes mellitus, and low high-density lipoprotein (HDL) levels. Cigarette smokers and hypertensive persons have the most extensive anatomic disease. Although we still do not understand in full the mechanism linking these risk factors to the disease process, rapid progress has been made in recent years in understanding how lipoproteins relate to atherosclerosis.

A.M. Gotto et al. (eds), Multiple Risk Factors in Cardiovascular Disease, 427-436.
© 1995 *Kluwer Academic Publishers and Fondazione Giovanni Lorenzini.*

ATHEROGENIC LIPOPROTEINS

Two classes of lipoproteins have been demonstrated to be proatherogenic: low-density lipoprotein (LDL) and ß-very-low-density lipoprotein (ß-VLDL). Elevated LDL is probably the most common basis for hypercholesterolemia in the general population, but only a small percentage of these cases represent familial hypercholesterolemia.

Epidemiologic data on the negative correlation between coronary heart disease and HDL levels are persuasive. A low HDL level predicts risk for coronary heart disease as well as or better than a high LDL level. Using a combination of the two significantly improves one's predictions. The most widely accepted explanation for this inverse correlation is that HDL play a role in reverse cholesterol transport, the transport of cholesterol away from tissue (presumably including the arteries) and back to the liver for excretion in the bile.

EVENTS OCCURRING IN THE ARTERIAL WALL

The earliest lesion of atherosclerosis is the fatty streak, which begins beneath an intact layer of endothelial cells. The fatty streak consists essentially of lipid-loaded cells, the so-called "foam cells." These arise primarily from circulating monocytes. In a sense then, understanding the genesis of the fatty streak reduces to understanding how monocyte-macrophages acquire lipids.

Monocyte-macrophages cannot take up native LDL fast enough to become foam cells [1]. Yet patients in whom the only lipoprotein abnormality is elevated LDL show fatty-streak lesions typical of those seen in patients with other forms of hypercholesterolemia-typical foam cell lesions. Chemical modification of LDL generates a form of LDL that is taken up rapidly enough to generate foam cells from monocyte-macrophages. The uptake occurs by a specific saturable receptor, the acetyl LDL receptor. There is no evidence, however, that acetylated LDL (oxidized LDL) can be generated *in vivo*. On the other hand, a biologic modification of LDL might account for its ability to generate foam cells [2].

In addition to its role in foam-cell formation, oxidized LDL is potentially more atherogenic than native LDL in other ways. First, oxidized LDL has chemotatic activity toward monocytes, in part because of its lysolecithin content, and this could contribute to the recruiment of circulating monocytes to a developing fatty-streak lesion. Secondly, oxidized LDL inhibits the mobility of tissue macrophages and might thus prevent their exit back to the plasma compartment. Thirdly, this modified form of LDL is higly cytotoxic, at least in the absence of protective serum proteins. Evidence that oxidative modification of LDL can occur *in vivo* is accumulating and has been extensively reviewed [3-4].

Effects of Alcohol on Lipoprotein Metabolism

EFFECTS OF ALCOHOL ON LDL-CHOLESTEROL METABOLISM

Population studies relating alcohol consumption to LDL-cholesterol levels have generally found an inverse correlation, but the strength of this relationship is quite variable [5]. There is little trend in LDL levels over the range of moderate alcohol consumption (1 to 3 bottles of beer, glasses of wine, or shots of liquor per day). At high levels of alcohol consumption, LDL levels generally appear to decrease [6], and alcohol may constitute a significant proportion of caloric intake (up to 40-60% of calories in some persons with alcoholism), often at the expense of fat and cholesterol. A second theory concerns the possible role of alcohol-related acetaldehyde in LDL oxidation. Although this may speed LDL clearance by macrophage receptor, it may also increase the atherogenecity of LDL [3-4]. Studies aiming at explaining the protective effect of alcohol against coronary heart disease have not identified LDL metabolism as the probable mechanism through which alcohol acts [7]. On the other hand, the lowering of LDL with high levels of alcohol consumption may relate to an impairment of liver function.

EFFECTS OF ALCOHOL ON TRIGLYCERIDE-RICH LIPOPROTEIN METABOLISM

Alcohol consumption exerts a paradoxical effect on the metabolism of triglyceride-rich lipoproteins, mainly chylomicrons and VLDL cholesterol. Population studies often fail to show any correlation between alcohol consumption and fasting levels of either VLDL or plasma triglycerides [5]. Over the range of moderate use, there appears to be little correlation between plasma triglycerides and alcohol consumption. However, heavy alcohol use is the second most prevalent secondary cause of hypertriglyceridemia.

The magnitude of the rise in triglycerides after alcohol ingestion is related to the fasting triglyceride level, suggesting a role for underlying, abnormalities of triglyceride metabolism. A substantial proportion of patients with alcohol-induced pancreatitis have elevated fasting serum triglyceride levels during abstinence [8,9]. After consuming a fatty meal, these patients shows markedly higher and more delayed postprandial levels of triglycerides than normal controls [10]. These studies point to an interaction of dietary fat, alcohol, and metabolic or genetic predisposition in causing severe hypertriglyceridemia and may affect three major pathways of lipid metabolism: the exogenous triglyceride pathway, the free fatty acid pathway, and the endogenous triglyceride-rich lipoprotein pathway [11,12,13].

EFFECTS OF ALCOHOL ON HDL METABOLISM

HDL shows a consistent, direct relationship to alcohol intake [5-14] across the range of moderate alcohol consumption. Teetotalers have significantly lower levels of HDL cholesterol than persons consuming three drinks per day. These findings could be explained by differences in diet, obesity, and exercise among groups. However, recent data have confirmed this finding and indicate an independent effect of alcohol on plasma HDL [15]. High-density lipoprotein is thought to play an important role in preventing atherosclerosis by removing free cholesterol from the arterial wall. Alcohol may enhance this reverse-cholesterol-transport pathway in two ways. First, by enhancing lipoprotein lipase and hepatic triglyceride lipase activity, alcohol may speed the removal of triglycerides from HDL_2 to form new HDL_3 particles [16]. Second, by inducing liver microsomal oxidases, alcohol may increase synthesis of apo A-I and apo A-II, with subsequent increased secretion of HDL particles. Evidence from clinical trials supports this mechanism [17]. Thirdly, alcohol consumption also lowers cholesteryl ester transfer activity (CETP). This protein mediates the exchange of esterified cholesterol from HDL to VLDL and LDL. Decreasing its activity results in increased HDL cholesterol.

One argument raised against alcohol reducing atherosclerotic risk via effects on HDL metabolism is the hypothesis that alcohol raises only HDL_3 cholesterol, whereas HDL_2 is the fraction inversely correlated with risk. This finding though is not consistent in all studies. However, data linking only the HDL_2 subfraction with coronary heart disease risk were derived from relatively few studies [18,19]. More recent studies suggest that HDL_2 and HDL_3 are both inversely related to coronary heart disease risk [20,21]. Additional studies suggest that apo A-I levels, and not HDL subfractions, best predict atherosclerosis [22].

Does the effect of alcohol on HDL cholesterol account for all its cardioprotective effects? Criqui and coworkers [7] found that the relative risk for cardiovascular disease was 0.8 for alcohol consumers when smoking and alcohol were included in a multivariate model. When HDL cholesterol level was added to the model, the adjusted relative risk associated with alcohol consumption increased to 0.91 and lost its statistical significance, prompting the authors to conclude that at least half the effect of alcohol on risk was mediated by HDL cholesterol. This finding was recently confirmed by epidemiological data [15].

MORBIDITY AND MORTALITY DATA

The end point of most studies is clinical coronary heart disease, myocardial infarction, angina pectoris, or death from coronary heart disease.

EPIDEMIOLOGIC STUDIES OF ALCOHOL USE AND HEART DISEASE

Three types of epidemiologic studies have explored the relation between alcohol intake and coronary heart disease: case-control studies, longitudinal or prospective studies, and evaluations of alcohol consumption and coronary angiographic measurement of atherosclerosis and coronary stenosis. Strong evidence associates at least moderate alcohol intake with a lower risk for myocardial infarction and perhaps with a lower risk for death from coronary heart disease [23,24,25]. Kannel [24], Criqui [25], and Moore and Pearson [23] have reviewed case-control studies comparing histories of alcohol consumption of patients with myocardial infarction with those of controls. These studies generally show a lower risk for myocardial infarction among persons consuming one to seven drinks per day, with the relative risk approximately 0.5. This lower risk remains consistent after adjusting for many confounding factors, especially smoking, blood pressure, and serum cholesterol levels.

Prospective studies also show a lower risk for myocardial infarction or death from coronary heart disease among alcohol consumers, including both young and old men and women. The highest risk for coronary heart disease is usualy noted for drinkers compared with nondrinkers. In the Framingham study [24,26,27], the 24-year coronary heart disease mortality for men varied from 28.3 in heavy smokers consuming no alcohol to 5.7 in nonsmokers consuming 200 to 500 g of alcohol per week. The Nurses Health Study of women aged 34 to 59 years also evaluated the relation between alcohol consumption and the risk for coronary heart disease and stroke [28]. After about 4 years of follow-up, an inverse relation was found between alcohol intake and nonfatal myocardial infarction or fatal heart disease. Higher differences in risk were found primarily between drinkers and nondrinkers of alcohol. The inverse relation between alcohol intake and coronary heart disease risk remained consistent after adjusting for the other confounding risk factors.

The association between alcohol use and coronary heart disease risk, especially death, may differ from that for myocardial infarction. Dyer and colleagues [29] reported a much higher risk for sudden death among problem than nonproblem drinkers. Persons who had stopped drinking had higher rates of sudden death and coronary heart disease mortality than did those who continued to drink; the presumption was that problem drinkers stopped because of health problems. Similary, in the Puerto Rico Heart Study [30], the sudden death rate from coronary heart disease was much higher and the nonsudden death rate much lower in drinkers than in nondrinkers. However, alcohol consumers had lower rates of angina pectoris and myocardial infarction. In a study of women who died suddenly before age 60, the prevalence of alcoholism was 27% among sudden-death cases, only 2% among controls, and 3% among myocardial infarction survivors [31].

Several Scandinavian studies [32,33] have evaluated the relation between heavy alcohol consumption and both myocardial infarction and sudden death from coronary heart disease. Wilhelmsen and coworkers [33] studied all deaths from 1968 to 1974 among men aged 35 to 44 in Goteborg, Sweden. Among persons who died from ischemic heart disease, 26% had a history of alcohol problems, compared with only 10% of controls, and 37% had been detained for drunkenness, compared with 15% of controls. In a Finnish study of 4,532 men aged 40 to 64, the 314 deaths during 5 years of follow-up included 140 from coronary heart disease, 62% of them sudden [34]. Among men free from coronary heart disease at entry into the study, the incidence of sudden death from this cause was significantly lower in abstainers than in alcohol users. Among men with a history of coronary heart disease, the rate from this cause was significantly higher among men who consumed more than 200 g of alcohol per month. Because the autopsy rate was about 40%, some sudden deaths from coronary heart disease may have been misclassified.

In the Multifactor Primary Prevention Trial in Goteborg [35], heavy alcohol consumers were more likely to be smokers and to do heavy physical work. During 11.8 years of follow-up, no relation was found between alcohol consumption and myocardial infarction among smokers. However, deaths from coronary heart disease were highest among smokers with a history of alcoholism, a relative risk of 4.2% (95% CI, 3.0% to 7%). Both sudden and nonsudden deaths were higher among alcohol drinkers. Multivariate analysis showed that smoking and alcohol intake were independently associated with coronary heart disease deaths.

Few studies have evaluated the relation of alcohol intake to mortality from different causes within the same cohort. Preliminary data after 10.5 years of follow-up in the Multiple

Risk Factor Intervention Trial (MRFIT) [36] showed an inverse relationship between the number of alcoholic drinks per week and death from coronary heart disease. This trial specifically excluded heavy drinkers. No relation was found between alcohol consumption and total or cancer mortality. In a multiple logistic regression analysis, alcohol consumption was significantly inversely related only to coronary heart disease mortality.

Marmot [37] also analyzed alcohol consumption and cardiovascular and total mortality and observed a U-shaped relationship, with the highest total mortality among nondrinkers and consumers of less than 34 g (approximately 1.5 oz) of alcohol per day. Shaper and colleagues [38] also evaluated this U-shaped relationship by following 7,735 British men aged 40 to 59 for 7.5 years. Among the 504 deaths, the higest total and cardiovascular mortality was found among abstainers or occasional drinkers and among those consuming more than 42 drinks per week. The association between alcohol and cardiovascular disease mortality was primarily limited to men with cardiovascular conditions on entry into the study. These results suggest that men with cardiovascular conditions are more likely to stop drinking. On the other hand, Klatsky and coworkers [39] evaluated risk for coronary heart disease among former drinkers and lifelong nondrinkers in the Kaiser Permanente Health Plan study. Both groups had a higher risk for hospitalization and death from coronary heart disease than did drinkers.

Camacho and colleagues [40] found no link between alcohol consumption and total or coronary heart disease mortality in the follow-up of 6,928 paticipants in the Human Population Laboratory in Alameda County, California. Ex-drinkers had lower total and coronary heart disease mortality than lifetime nondrinkers. In a recent work conducted on 14,253 people aged 20 or more, living in Copenhagen [41], a U-shaped curve for the risk of mortality as a function of alcohol consumption was found. Nondrinkers were at higher risk (30%) as compared to moderate drinkers. Other studies have compared lifelong abstainers with ex-drinkers [42]. Ex-drinkers were more likely to be men, to smoke heavily, to be less sociable, and to have more negative life problems. Abstainers were more likely to be religious and puritanic, to live in rural areas, to have lower income and less education, and to come from families with histories of drinking problems. Ex-drinkers include two subgroups: those who stopped because of health problems and those who stopped because of a desire for a healthier lifestyle. Unfortunately, no current studies satisfactorily deal with the possible confounding factors of health status, social behavior, and being a nondrinker or ex-drinker. However, long-term follow-up in some studies, such as 24 years for the Framingham Study [27] or 10.5 years for the MRFIT [3], and results of the Kaiser Permanente study [39] suggest that inclusion of sick ex-drinkers in the nondrinker category may not completely explain the lower risk among moderate drinkers than among nondrinkers.

The mechanism accounting for the possibly lower risk for heart attack among the alcohol consumer may relate to the extent of atherosclerosis and the risk for thrombosis or occlusion. In angiographic studies, drinkers had lower coronary oclusion scores than nondrinkers [43]. Studies by Fried and coworkers [44] suggest that drinkers have larger coronary arteries than abstainers. Heavy alcohol use has also benn related to decreased platelet aggregation. In the Northwich Park Study, Meade and colleagues [45] reported lower fibrinogen levels and higher fibrinolytic activity in both male and female drinkers than in nondrinkers. Preliminary data from the Health Women Study shown an inverse relation between alcohol intake and fibrinogen levels. Drinkers also had lower platelet aggregation than nondrinkers. Thus, higher HDL-cholesterol levels, lower platelet aggregation, and possible effects of alcohol on other clotting factors including tPA [46] could explain the reduced risk for coronary heart disease among drinkers.

On the other hand, many studies note that alcohol consumption is related to high blood pressure levels [47]. High blood pressure in alcohol users is also associated with increased risk for stroke, especially hemorhage [48]. Alcohol may also increase left ventricular hypertrophy [49].

Conclusions

Given present evidence, a recommendation to increase alcohol consumption at large would probably be unjustifiable. However, a large body of evidence associates moderate alcohol intake with decreased overall risk for mortality. The unique risk of alcohol consumption during pregnancy and the failure of most studies to consider risk associated with binge drinking, even among moderate drinkers, should also be considered in evaluating individual drinking behavior. Finally, mechanisms by which alcohol effects lipoprotein metabolism have important implications and require further studies.

Acknowledgements

This work was supported in part by MPI (Publication n. 953546). The author thanks Miss Maddalena Marazzini for typing the manuscript.

References

1. Brown MS, Goldstein JL. Lipoprotein metabolism in the macrophage: Implication for cholesterol deposition in atherosclerosis. Annu Rev Biochem 1983;52:223-262.
2. Henriksen T, Mahoney EM, Steinberg D. Interactions of plasma lipoproteins with endothelial cells. Ann NY Acad Sci 1982;401:102-116.
3. Steinberg D, Parthasarathy S, Carew TE, Khoo JC, Witztum JL. Beyond cholesterol: Modifications of low density lipoprotein that increase its atherogenicity. N Engl J Med 1989;320:915-924.
4. Roma P, Bernini F, Fogliatto R, et al. Defective catabolism of oxidized LDL by J774 murine macrophages. J Lipid Res 1992;33:819-829.
5. Castelli WP, Gordon T, Hjortland MC, et al. Alcohol and blood lipids. The Cooperative Lipoprotein Phenotyping Study. Lancet 1977;2:153-155.
6. Hulley SB, Gordon S. Alcohol and high density lipoprotein cholesterol. Causal inference from diverse study designs. Circulation 1981;64(Suppl.III):57-63.
7. Criqui MH, Cowan LD, Tyroler HA, et al. Lipoproteins as mediators for the effects of alcohol consumption and cigarette smoking on cardiovascular mortality: Results

from the Lipid Research Clinic Follow-Up Study. Am J Epidemiol 1987;126:629-637.

8. Cameron JL, Capuzzi DM, Zuidema GD, Margolis S. Acute pancreatitis with hyperlipemia: The incidence of lipid abnormalities in acute pancreatitis. Ann Surg 1973:177:483-489.

9. Buch A, Buch J, Carlsen A, Schmidt A. Hyperlipidemia and pancreatitis. World J Surg 1980;4:307-314.

10. Cameron JL, Capuzzi DM, Zuidema GD, Margolis S. Acute pancreatitis with hyperlipidemia: Evidence for a persistent defect in lipid metabolism. Am J Med 1974;56:482-487.

11. Baraona E, Lieber CS. Effect of ethanol on lipid metabolism. J Lipid Res 1979;20: 289-315.

12. Sabesin SM. Lipid and lipoprotein abnormalities in alcoholic liver disease. Circulation 1981;64(Suppl.III):72-84.

13. Borowsky SA, Perlow W, Baraona E, Lieber CS. Relationship of alcoholic hypertriglyceridemia to stage to liver disease and dietary lipid. Dig Dis Sci 1980;25: 22-27.

14. Christian JC, Carmelli D, Castelli WP, et al. High density lipoprotein cholesterol. A 16-year longitudinal study in aging male twins. Arteriosclerosis 1990;10:1020-1025.

15. Gaziano JM, Buring JE, Breslow JL, et al. Moderate alcohol intake, increased levels of high density lipoprotein and its subfractions and decreased risk of myocardial infaction. New Engl J Med 1993;329:1829-1834.

16. Taskinen M-R, Vilimaki M, Nikkila EA, Kuusi T, Ehnholm C, Ylikahri R. High density lipoprotein subfractions and post heparin plasma lipases in alcoholic men before and after ethanol withdrawal. Metabolism 1982;31:1168-1174.

17. Amarasuriya RN, Gupta AK, Civen M, Horng Y-C, Maeda T, Kashyap ML. Ethanol stimulates apolipoprotein A-I secretion by human hepatocytes: Implications for a mechanism for atherosclerosis protection. Metabolism 1992;41:827-832.

18. Miller NE, Hammet F, Saltissi S, et al. Relation of angiographically defined coronary artery disease to plasma lipoprotein subfractions and apolipoproteins. Br Med J 1981;282:1741-1744.

19. Ballentyne FC, Clark RS, Simpson HS, Ballentyne D. High density and low density lipoprotein subfractions in survivors of myocardial infarction and in control subjects. Metabolism 1982;31:433-437.

20. Salonen JT, Seppanen K, Rauramaa R. Serum high density lipoprotein cholesterol subfractions and the risk of acute myocardial infarction: A population study in Eastern Finland (Abstract). Circulation 1989;80(Suppl.II):281.

21. Stampfer MJ, Sacks FM, Hennekens CH. A prospective study of lipids and apolipoproteins and risk of myocardial infaction (Abstract). Circulation 1989;80 (Suppl.II):281.

22. Dai WS, LaPorte RE, Hom DL, et al. Alcohol consumption and high density lipoprotein cholesterol concentration among alcoholics. Am J Epidemiol 1985;122: 620-627.

23. Moore RD, Pearson TA. Moderate alcohol consumption and coronary artery disease. A review. Medicine (Baltimore) 1986;65:242-267.
24. Kannel WB. Alcohol and cardiovascular disease. Proc Nutr Soc 1988;47:99-110.
25. Criqui MH. The role of alcohol in the epidemiology of cardiovascular diseases. Acta Med Scand 1987;717(Suppl.)73-85.
26. Worf PA, Kannel WB, Verter J. Current status of risk factors for stroke. Neurol Clin 1983;1:317-343.
27. Friedman LA, Kimball AW. Coronary heart disease mortality and alcohol consumption in Framingham. Am J Epidemiol 1986;124:481-489.
28. Stampfer MJ, Colditz GA, Willett WC, Speizer FE, Hennekens CH. A prospective study of moderate alcohol consumption and the risk of coronary disease and stroke in women. N Engl J Med 1988;319:267-273.
29. Dyer AR, Stamler J, Paul O, et al. Alcohol consumption, cardiovascular risk factors, and mortality in two Chicago epidemiologic studies. Circulation 1977;56:1067-1074.
30. Kittner SJ, Garcia-Palmieri MR, Costas R Jr, Cruz-Vidal M, Abbott RD, Havlik RJ. Alcohol and coronary heart disease in Puerto Rico. Am J Epidemiol 1983;117:538-350.
31. Beard CM, Griffin MR, Offord KP, Edwards WD. Risk factors for sudden unexpected cardiac death in young women in Rochester. Minnesota, 1960 through 1974. Mayo Clinic Proc 1986;61:186-191.
32. Rosengren A, Wilhelmsen L. Alcoholic registration and cardiovascular morbidity and mortality: A prospective study in middle-aged Swedish men. Acta Med Scand 1987;717(Suppl.):87-92.
33. Wilhelmsen L, Elmfeldt D, Wedel H. Cause of death in relation to social and alcoholic problems among Swedish men aged 35-44 years. Acta Med Scand 1983;213:263-268.
34. Suhonen O, Aromaa A, Reunanen A, Knekt P. Alcohol consumption and sudden coronary death in middle-aged Finnish men. Acta Med Scand 1987;221:335-341.
35. Rosengren A, Wilhelmsen L, Pennert K, Berglund G, Elmfeldt D. Alcoholic intemperance coronary heart disease and mortality in middle-aged Swedish men. Acta Med Scand 1987;222:201-213.
36. The MRFIT Research Group. Risk factors and mortality in the Multiple Risk Factor Intervention Trial after 10.5 years of follow-up (Abstract). J Am Coll Cardiol 1989;13:11A.
37. Marmot MG. Alcohol and coronary heart disease. Intl J Epidemiol 1984;13:160-167.
38. Shaper AG, Phillips AN, Pocock SJ. Walker M. Alcohol and ischaemic heart disease in middle-aged British men. BMJ 1987;294:733-737.
39. Klatsky AL, Armstrong MA, Friedman GD. Alcohol and cardiovascular deaths (Abstract). Circulation 1989;80(Suppl.II):614.
40. Camacho TC, Kaplan GA, Cohen RD. Alcohol consumption and mortality in Alameda Country. J Chron Dis 1978;40:229-236.

41. Grønbæk M, Deis A, Sørensen TIA, Becker U, Borch-Johnsen K, Müller C, Schnohr P, Jensen G. Influence of sex, age, body mass index, and smoking on alcoholic intake and mortality. BMJ 1994;308:302-306.
42. Ferrence RG, Truscott S, Whitehead PC. Drinking and the prevention of coronary heart disease: findings, issues and public health policy. J Stud Alcohol 1986;47:394-408.
43. Barboriack JJ, Anderson AJ, Hoffmann RG. Smoking, alcohol and coronary occlusion. Atheroclerosis 1982;43:277-282.
44. Fried LP, Moore RD, Pearson TA. Long-term effects of cigarette smoking and moderate alcohol consumption on coronary artery diameter. Mechanisms of coronary artery disease independent of atherosclerosis or thrombosis? Am J Med 1980;80:37-44.
45. Meade TW, Imerson J, Stirling Y. Effects of changes in smoking and other characteristics of clotting factors and the risk of ischaemic heart disease. Lancet 1987;1:986-988.
46. Ridker PM, Vaughan DE, Stampfer MJ, Glynn RJ, Hennekens CH. Association of moderate alcohol consumption and plasma concentration of endogenous tissue-type plasminigen activator. JAMA 1994;272:929-933.
47. Flegal KM, Cauley JA. Alcohol consumption and cardiovascular risk factors. In: Galanter M, editor. Recent developments in alcoholism. Vol 3. New York: Plenum Press; 1985:165-180.
48. Camargo CA. Moderate alcohol consumption and stroke: The epidemiologic evidence. Stroke 1989;20:1611-1626.
49. Manolio TA, Levy D, Garrison RJ, Castelli W, Kannel WB. Relationship of alcohol ingestion to left ventriculum mass: The Framingham study (Abstract). Circulation 1989;80(Suppl.II):678.

INDEX

Medical Science Symposia Series

1. A.M. Gotto, C. Lenfant, R. Paoletti (eds.) and M. Soma (ass.ed.): *Multiple Risk Factors in Cardiovascular Disease.* 1992 ISBN 0-7923-1938-9
2. A.L. Catapano, A.M. Gotto, Jr., L.C. Smith and R. Paoletti (eds.): *Drugs Affecting Lipid Metabolism.* 1993 ISBN 0-7923-2232-0
3. T. Godfraind, S. Govoni, R. Paoletti and P.M. Vanhoutte (eds.): *Calcium Antagonists. Pharmacology and Clinical Research.* 1993
   ISBN 0-7923-2259-2
4. D. Galmarini, L.R. Fassati, R. Paoletti and S. Sherlock (eds.): *Drugs and the Liver: High Risk Patients and Transplantation.* 1993 ISBN 0-7923-2307-6
5. P.M. Vanhoutte, P.R. Saxena, R. Paoletti, N. Brunello (eds.) and A.S. Jackson (ass.ed.): *Serotonin. From Cell Biology to Pharmacology and Therapeutics.* 1993 ISBN 0-7923-2518-4
6. A.G. Dalgleish, A. Albertini and R. Paoletti (eds.): *The Impact of Biotechnology on Autoimmunity.* 1994 ISBN 0-7923-2724-1
7. P.G. Crosignani, R. Paoletti, P.M. Sarrel, N.K. Wenger (eds.), M. Meschia and M. Soma (ass.eds.): *Women's Health in Menopause.* Behaviour, Cancer, Cardiovascular Disease, Hormone Replacement Therapy. 1994
   ISBN 0-7923-3068-4
8. A.M. Gotto Jr., C. Lenfant, A.L. Catapano and R. Paoletti (eds.): *Multiple Risk Factors in Cardiovascular Disease.* 1995 ISBN 0-7923-3503-1

KLUWER ACADEMIC PUBLISHERS – DORDRECHT / BOSTON / LONDON